Innovations in Global Maternal Health:

Improving Prenatal and Postnatal Care Practices

Information Resources Management Association
USA

A volume in the Trending Topics
Book Series (TTBS) Book Series

IGI Global
DISSEMINATOR OF KNOWLEDGE

Published in the United States of America by
IGI Global
Medical Information Science Reference (an imprint of IGI Global)
701 E. Chocolate Avenue
Hershey PA, USA 17033
Tel: 717-533-8845
Fax: 717-533-8661
E-mail: cust@igi-global.com
Web site: http://www.igi-global.com

Library of Congress Cataloging-in-Publication Data

Names: Information Resources Management Association, editor, issuing body.
Title: Innovations in global maternal health : improving prenatal and postnatal care practices / Information Resources Management Association, editor.
Description: Hershey, PA : Medical Information Science Reference, [2020] | Includes bibliographical references and index. | Summary: "This book addresses the main issues facing women during pregnancy, childbirth, and the postpartum period. It also explores new techniques, tools, and solutions that can be used in a global capacity to support women regardless of their wealth or location"--Provided by publisher.
Identifiers: LCCN 2019039492 (print) | LCCN 2019039493 (ebook) | ISBN 9781799823513 (hardcover) | ISBN 9781799823520 (ebook)
Subjects: MESH: Maternal Welfare | Prenatal Care--methods | Postnatal Care--methods | Information Technology | Global Health
Classification: LCC RG940 (print) | LCC RG940 (ebook) | NLM WA 310.1 | DDC 362.19682--dc23
LC record available at https://lccn.loc.gov/2019039492
LC ebook record available at https://lccn.loc.gov/2019039493

British Cataloguing in Publication Data
A Cataloguing in Publication record for this book is available from the British Library.

Trending Topics Book Series (TTBS)

Mehdi Khosrow-Pour, D.B.A.
Information Resources Management Association, USA

ISSN:pending
EISSN:pending

MISSION

Every day all over the world, researchers are making groundbreaking discoveries that address current challenges and solve complex problems across a variety of fields. Due to advancements in technology, changes in demographics, adjustments to societal norms, the development of political and economic structures, and more, new theories, methods, strategies, techniques, and applications are constantly being established in response to both existing and evolving issues.

Based on the success of IGI Global's latest Trending Topics Campaign, which provides news snippets and trending research breakthroughs relevant to IGI Global content, IGI Global has launched this new book series, titled the **Trending Topics Book Series**, which offers small anthologies of reprinted IGI Global book chapters and journal articles hand-selected by IGI Global's Executive Editorial Board on topics currently trending and stirring up discussion and/or controversy.

Spanning across topics such as the multigenerational workforce, legislation for sustainability, emotional branding, privacy on mobile devices, robotics in healthcare, and bio-based product development, this book series aims to provide researchers, academicians, professionals, and students with the most up-to-date studies in order to advance knowledge across all industries.

COVERAGE

- Millennials
- Robotics in Healthcare
- Aging Workforce
- Eco-Cities
- Women in STEM Fields
- Privacy on Mobile Devices
- Inclusive Learning
- Library Budget Challenges
- Plan S and Open Access Movements
- Environmental Legislation and Sustainability

IGI Global is currently accepting manuscripts for publication within this series. To submit a proposal for a volume in this series, please contact our Acquisition Editors at Acquisitions@igi-global.com or visit: http://www.igi-global.com/publish/.

The Trending Topics Book Series (TTBS) Book Series (ISSN pending) is published by IGI Global, 701 E. Chocolate Avenue, Hershey, PA 17033-1240, USA, www.igi-global.com. This series is composed of titles available for purchase individually; each title is edited to be contextually exclusive from any other title within the series. For pricing and ordering information please visit http://www.igi-global.com/book-series/trending-topics-book-series/228608. Postmaster: Send all address changes to above address.

Titles in this Series

For a list of additional titles in this series, please visit:
https://www.igi-global.com/book-series/trending-topics-book-series/228608

Five Generations and Only One Workforce How Successful Businesses Are Managing a Multigenerational Workforce
Information Resources Management Association (USA)
Business Science Reference • © 2020 • 364pp • H/C (ISBN: 9781799804376) • US $215.00 (our price)

Developing Eco-Cities Through Policy, Planning, and Innovation Can It Really Work?
Information Resources Management Association (USA)
Engineering Science Reference • © 2020 • 374pp • H/C (ISBN: 9781799804413) • US $195.00 (our price)

IGI Global
DISSEMINATOR OF KNOWLEDGE

701 East Chocolate Avenue, Hershey, PA 17033, USA
Tel: 717-533-8845 x100 • Fax: 717-533-8661
E-Mail: cust@igi-global.com • www.igi-global.com

Table of Contents

Section 3
Postpartum Care

Preface

Whether they are in developed or developing nations, all women are susceptible of dying from complications in childbirth. According to the World Health Organization (WHO), approximately 830 women die each day from preventable causes related to pregnancy, with 99% of these deaths occurring in developing countries (World Health Organization, 2018). Despite better accessibility to care, developed countries are not exempt from maternal deaths, with the CDC reporting that about 700 women still die from pregnancy complications each year in the United States (Centers for Disease Control and Prevention, 2019). Many maternal deaths occur due to severe bleeding, infections, pre-eclampsia and eclampsia, and complications during delivery. While some of these complications are unavoidable, many develop during pregnancy and can be prevented or, when caught in time, treated. These difficulties are often a result of inaccessibility to care, inadequate health services, poor prenatal screening, uninformed mothers, etc. that in many cases is a direct consequence of the mother's geographical location (rural) and economic status (poor).

Various entities around the world have continuously called for a global effort to reduce the maternal mortality ratio by improving maternal health. These improvements range from a call for better healthcare systems in rural and poor areas to a greater understanding and improved identification and monitoring methods of risk factors that can lead to pregnancy-related deaths. Ensuring that all women have access to professional and skilled healthcare in the prenatal and postnatal phases as well as during childbirth can significantly improve the woman and baby's health. Additionally, it is important to note that simply promoting healthy habits during pregnancy and providing information on identifying risk factors to women can lead to healthier pregnancies.

In response to the need for advanced research that can offer innovative solutions to deal with these growing concerns and also as part of IGI Global's Trending Topics Book Series, which aligns with IGI Global's Trending Topics Campaign that showcases the latest research breakthroughs that are stirring up discussion and/ or controversy across a variety of fields, this publication, *Innovations in Global Maternal Health: Improving Prenatal and Postnatal Care Practices*, is comprised of reprinted IGI Global book chapters and journal articles that have been hand-selected by IGI Global's executive editorial board with the intent to adequately address the main issues facing women during pregnancy, childbirth, and the postpartum period.

The following chapters offer new techniques, tools, and solutions that can be used in a global capacity to support women regardless of their wealth or location. Such technological tools include better rural health monitoring, social media and internet forums that connect new and soon-to-be mothers, and apps that provide access to maternal health services and interventions for those suffering from postpartum depression. Additionally, maternal care models are examined in order to solve issues related to inadequate physician care practices. High risk pregnancies and maternal morbidity are also considered and the latest research on environmental risk factors that can cause unwanted side effects are discussed.

Through this book, readers will come to understand some of the latest practices currently in use that can combat maternal mortality and lead to healthier women and newborns. World health organizations, obstetricians, midwives, lactation consultants, doctors, nurses, hospital staff, directors, counselors, and therapists can benefit from the chapters within this publication that examine such items as breastfeeding, postpartum depression, clinical health systems, emergency care models, and risk factors. Academicians, researchers, and students will also find this title beneficial for developing solutions to inaccessible and unaffordable health services and for the identification, monitoring, and reduction of complications during pregnancy and immediately following childbirth.

This publication is organized into three sections that provide comprehensive coverage of important topics. The sections are:

1. Care Models and Technological Tools
2. Complications and Risks
3. Postpartum Care

The following paragraphs provide a summary of what to expect from this invaluable reference source:

Section 1, "Care Models and Technological Tools," opens this extensive reference source by highlighting the latest maternal care models and technologies that can be utilized by doctors and hospitals, or by the woman herself, that support her through her pregnancy and childbirth. The first chapter in this section, "A Clinical Recommendation System to Maternity Care," by Prof. Eliana Pereira from University of Minho, Portugal; Prof. Filipe Portela of University of Minho, Portugal & Porto Polytechnic, Portugal; and Prof. António Abelha of University of Minho, Portugal presents an overview of the clinical recommendation system for obstetric triage, the model developed, and the main results that were achieved. The second chapter,

"An Emerging Model of Pregnancy Care: The Introduction of New Technologies in Maternal Wellbeing," authored by Profs. Claudia Carissoli and Daniela Villani from Università Cattolica del Sacro Cuore, Italy and Prof. Giuseppe Riva from Università Cattolica del Sacro Cuore, Italy & I.R.C.C.S. Istituto Auxologico Italiano, Italy, examines new technologies—smartphones and tablets in particular—that play an increasingly important role in health intervention for pregnant women thanks to their spread, lower costs, and peculiar characteristics. The next chapter in this section, "The MAMICare Project: Monitoring Maternal and Child Health in Rural Areas," by Profs. Juan C. Lavariega, Gustavo A. Córdova, Lorena G. Gómez, and Alfonso Avila from Tecnológico de Monterrey, Mexico explores an information technology solution based on mobile devices and health sensors such as electrocardiogram, stethoscope, pulse-oximeter, and blood-glucose meter to automatically collect relevant health data for monitoring pregnancy. In the next chapter, "Cyber-Moms Facing Motherhood: Holding Functions and Regressive Movements in Parenting Websites," Prof. Valentina Boursier of the University of Naples Federico II, Italy; Prof. Valentina Manna from Association for Social Promotion Roots in Action, Italy; and Profs. Francesca Gioia, Federica Coppola, and Noemi Venosa from University of Naples Federico II, Italy present a study on web forum contributions to parenting skills and transitions to motherhood by exploring the manifest and latent contents of their interactions and the emotional connections between users own maternal experiences and the e-group dynamics. The following chapter, "Teaching Childbirth Support Techniques Using the Prepared Partner and Digital Birth: The Design and Development of Games for Dads-to-Be," by Prof. Alexandra Holloway from University of California – Santa Cruz, USA seeks to address the problem of limited access to childbirth preparation methods by introducing video games as a positive learning tool for birth partners to ensure that the mother is well-supported in her birth. In the final chapter, "MotherCare App for Expectant Mothers in Interior Parts of Pakistan," Prof. Muhammad Abdul Tawab Khalil of City University of Science and Information Technology, Pakistan and Profs. Saifullah Jan, Wajid Ali, and Adnan Khan from IQRA National University, Pakistan present the MothersCare app, a user-friendly app that offers a wide spectrum of maternal healthcare services and is designed to help expecting mothers in third world countries or rural areas who have difficulty seeking help during gestation.

Section 2, "Complications and Risks," examines environmental risk factors for pregnant women and the complications that they can cause during pregnancy and studies and solutions for preventing maternal morbidity and mortality. The first chapter in this section, "The Decision-Making Processes of Pregnant Women at High Risk," by Prof. Marta Ferraz from Entidade Reguladora da Saúde, Portugal; Prof. Ana Margarida Pisco Almeida from Universidade de Aveiro, Portugal; and Prof. Alexandra Matias from Universidade do Porto, Portugal presents the results of a study whose main purpose was understanding how the decision-making process of pregnant women with an associated maternal pathology is influenced by the search for information provided by institutional and/or commercial websites, other pregnant women through social networks, and opinions expressed by health professionals. The next chapter in this section, "County Socioeconomic Deprivation and Preterm Birth Risk Between White and Black Mothers in Georgia, USA," authored by Prof. Wei Tu from the Department of Geology and Geography, Georgia Southern University, Statesboro, USA, examines the association between county-level deprivation and PtB risk of three stratified racial groups: White, Black, and the others. In the next chapter, "A Predictive Analytic Model for Maternal Morbidity," Prof. Edgardo Palza from École de technologie supérieure, Canada; Profs. Jorge Sanchez and Guillermo Mamani from the Universidad Peruana Unión, Peru; Prof. Percy Pacora from the Hospital Nacional Docente Madre Niño "San Bartolomé", Peru; Prof. Alain Abran from École de Technologie Supérieure, Canada; and Prof. Jane Moon from the University of Melbourne, Australia present a predictive analytic model for preventing neonatal morbidity through the analysis of patterns of risky behavior regarding morbidity in newborns. The model aims to identify the factors that are causes of morbidity in newborns, based on data mining techniques, and developed using the CRISP-DM methodology. In the following chapter, "Scaling the Maternal and Newborn Survival Initiative (MANSI): Rural India," Profs. Deepa Fernandes Prabhu and Richard C. Larson from Massachusetts Institute of Technology, Cambridge, USA focus on a system analysis approach to the best practices for scaling and replicating of maternal and newborn survival initiative (MANSI), a field-tested pilot program for addressing high IMRs and MMRs. The authors conclude with a discussion of the prospects for and difficulties of replicating MANSI in other resource-constrained areas, not only in India but in other developing countries as well. The next chapter in this section, "Sustainable Development Goal 3 and Maternal Health in Nigeria: Any Hope of Meeting the Target by 2030?" by Prof. Idongesit Eshiet of the University of Lagos, Nigeria addresses the feasibility of Nigeria achieving Target 3.1 of Sustainable Development Goal 3, which aims at reducing maternal deaths to less than 70 per 100,000 live births by 2030. The chapter assesses the maternal health landscape of Nigeria and the measures taken by the government to address maternal health. The following chapter, "Health Effects of Pesticides on Pregnant Women and Children," authored by Profs. Mudasir Youssouf and Arun Kalia from Central University of Punjab, India; Prof. Zahid Nabi from Central University of Jammu, India; and Prof. Zubair A. Malik from Government HSS, India, discusses solutions for reducing the impact of pesticides on pregnant women through efforts that include risk assessment tools, encouragement of organic diets, educating parents working in agricultural fields from hazards of pesticides particularly in pregnancy and breastfeeding, implementation of integrated pest management (IPM) programs, and encouraging policies supporting IPM. The final chapter in this section, "Environmental Phthalate Exposure in Relation to Reproductive Outcomes and Other Health Endpoints in Humans," by Prof. Sameena of P. M. B. Gujarati Science College, India; Prof. Riyes Un Aziz from the Government Holkar College, India; and Prof. Aubid Bashir of Barkatullah University, India reviews the environmental impact of phthalate exposure in relation to reproductive behavior and its harmful effects during fetal development.

Section 3, "Postpartum Care," discusses tools and methods for promoting health during the postpartum period with a special focus on postpartum depression and breastfeeding support and awareness. The first chapter in this section, "An Analysis of Factors Affecting Postnatal Depression Intervention Adherence," by Profs. Omobolanle Omisade, Alice Good, Tineke Fitch, and Jim Briggs from the University of Portsmouth, Portsmouth, UK aims to establish the factors that determine adherence to postnatal depression intervention and support. It also intends to establish attitudes that women have towards postnatal depression intervention and support. In the second chapter, "Communicating 'What's Not Said': Mobile Apps for Psychological Wellbeing," the authors, Profs. Marguerite Barry, Kevin Doherty, and Gavin Doherty of Trinity College Dublin, Dublin, Ireland, offer insights into ethical approaches to design for projects that explore the potential for using mobile apps for reporting psychological wellbeing, especially for postpartum mothers. The discussion focuses on the practical and cultural issues that arise and explores how technologies can mediate self-knowledge and information in ways that might otherwise remain unsaid, but is crucial for successful outcomes both clinically and in design. The following chapter, "User Experiences and Perceptions of Internet Interventions for Depression," by Prof. Filip Drozd of the National Network for Infant Mental Health, Norway; Prof. Caroline Emilie Andersen from University of Oslo, Norway; Profs. Silje Marie Haga and Kari Slinning of the National Network for Infant Mental Health, Norway; and Prof. Cato Alexander Bjørkli from University of Oslo, Norway reviews qualitative research on user experiences with internet interventions for depression and presents original results from in-depth interviews from a preventive unguided intervention for postpartum depression. The next chapter in this section, "Complexity of Breastfeeding on Child/Maternal Health and Counseling Intervention," authored by Prof. Ogunlade Joseph Olurotimi from the College of Education Ikere Ekiti, Ekiti State, Nigeria, reviews the complexities of breastfeeding and its effects on the health of the mother and child and argues for a serious, dedicated, pragmatic, and coordinated counseling approach to foster a positive attitude towards breastfeeding to improve maternal and child health. In the final chapter, "Breastfeeding, Authority, and Genre: Women's Ethos in Wikipedia and Blogs," by Prof. Alison A. Lukowski from Christian Brothers University, USA and Prof. Erika M. Sparby from Northern Illinois University, USA, the authors are concerned with women's mis- or underrepresentation in knowledge cration and examine how Wikipedia's generic regulations determine that women's often experiential ethos is unwelcome on the site. Thus, women are often unable to construct knowledge on the "Breastfeeding" entry; their epistemological methods are ignored or banned by other contributors.

Although the primary organization of the contents in this work is based on its three sections, offering a progression of coverage of the important concepts, methodologies, technologies, applications, social issues, and emerging trends, the reader can also identify specific contents by utilizing the extensive indexing system listed at the end.

REFERENCES

Centers for Disease Control and Prevention. (2019, February 26). *Pregnancy-related deaths*. Retrieved from https://www.cdc.gov/reproductivehealth/maternalinfanthealth/pregnancy-relatedmortality.htm

World Health Organization. (2018, February 16). *Maternal mortality*. Retrieved from https://www.who.int/news-room/fact-sheets/detail/maternal-mortality

Section 1

Care Models and Technological Tools

Chapter 1
A Clinical Recommendation System to Maternity Care

Eliana Pereira
University of Minho, Portugal

Filipe Portela
University of Minho, Portugal & Porto Polytechnic, Portugal

António Abelha
University of Minho, Portugal

ABSTRACT

Nowadays in healthcare, the Clinical Decision Support Systems are used in order to help health professionals to take an evidence-based decision. An example is the Clinical Recommendation Systems. In this sense, a pre-triage system was developed and implemented in Centro Hospitalar do Porto in order to group the patients on two levels (urgent or outpatient). However, although this system is calibrated and specific to the urgency of obstetrics and gynaecology, it does not meet all clinical requirements by the general department of the Portuguese HealthCare (Direção Geral de Saúde). The main requirement is the need of having priority triage system characterized by five levels. Thus some studies have been conducted with the aim of presenting a methodology able to evolve the pre-triage system on a Clinical Recommendation System with five levels. After some tests (using data mining and simulation techniques), it has been validated the possibility of transformation the pre-triage system in a Clinical Recommendation System in the obstetric context. At the end the main indicators achieved with this system are presented in the Business Intelligence Platform already deployed. This paper presents an overview of the Clinical Recommendation System for obstetric triage, the model developed and the main results achieved.

DOI: 10.4018/978-1-7998-2351-3.ch001

INTRODUCTION

Currently, in health institutions, there is an increasing amount of information. The need of making decisions the most correct as possible, emerges the Decision Support Systems (DSS) as a way of supporting the decisions of healthcare professionals based on evidences. In this context are inserted the Clinical Recommendation Systems, whose objective is the use of various computational techniques to achieve a particular purpose (Mackway-Jones K., 1997) (Filipe Portela César Quintas, José Machado, José Neves, & Santos, 2013) and recommending a clinical action.

Furthermore, the triage systems used in hospital emergency units may be considered a Clinical Recommendation System. In the case of *Centro Hospitalar do Porto (CHP)*, the triage system aims to select the type of patients in terms of clinical urgency, prioritizing the treatment response speed, the type of assistance and response resources to the level of urgency. So patients with a higher level of urgency and with increased risk of worsening of the disease, are attended as soon as possible. The most commonly used triage systems are those with five levels of severity, such as the Emergency Severity Index (ESI), the Manchester Triage System (MTS) and the Canadian Triage Acuity Scale (CTAS). The main limitation of this type of scales is the lack of flexibility, since usually they are used only in general emergency units and they are not specific for other units (Murray, Bullard, & Grafstein, 2004) (Portela et al., 2013). Due to this lack of flexibility for specific specialties, particularly for the obstetrics specialty, a pre-triage system was developed in 2010 in order to categorize the patients on two levels: Urgent (URG) and Consultation (ARGO) (Portela et al., 2013). It should be mentioned that this system only performs a routing triage. This system can forward the patient to the urgency (URG) - if the clinical features justify it, or for consultation - in the less urgent cases.

On the other hand, it is currently recommended by the general department of the Portuguese HealthCare (*Direção Geral de Saúde (DGS)*), more specifically by the *Comissão Nacional da Saúde Materna, da Criança e do Adolescente (CNSMCA)*, the use of the priority triage system with five priority levels in the obstetric emergency units (Infantil, 2013).

Having in consideration these two factors a set of studies was developed (Pereira, Brandão, Salazar, et al., 2014) (Abelha, Pereira, Brandão, Portela, Santos, & Machado, 2014) involving Data Mining and Simulation techniques in order to evaluate if it would be possible transforming the existing pre-triage system in a Clinical Recommendation Triage System for Obstetric (CRTSO). The Business Intelligence Platform (Brandão et al., 2014; Pereira et al., 2014) will contains several indicators about triage process (% usage room, type of patient, waiting time (expected, real, average, by level, among others). Additionally the own CRTSO also can be considered a Business Intelligence system due the way of how it was developed and their main goals as is improving the decision making process by providing useful information in real-time (S. O. Filipe Portela, Manuel Filipe Santos, António Abelha, José Machado, 2015; F. Portela et al., 2011). Using CRTSO as a BI platform is also possible create indicators related with the waiting triage time and patient priorities. This information will be available in the emergency room in situated devices, being it updated in real-time.

In this article the proposed CRTSO is exposed, as well as all the methodology used in its construction.

Apart from the introduction this article consists of five section. The second section presents the Background and Related Work. In the third section is presented the research methodology used and the methods used for the development of CRTSO. In the fourth section is presented the CRTSO developed as well as some adjustments that are necessary to perform the same be functional. In the fifth section are discussed some crucial points and presented the main conclusions. Finally, the sixth section are presented the future research directions.

BACKGROUND AND RELATED WORK

In this section is presented the project background and the theoretical aspects of the main triage systems existing in the world.

Case Study Contextualization and the Pre-Triage System

This project designed as CRTSO was developed in partnership with the *Centro Hospitalar do Porto* (CHP), more specifically with the *Centro Materno Infantil do Norte* (CMIN), old *Maternidade Júlio Dinis* (MJD). CMIN was inaugurated in 2014 and covers the needs associated with the care of paediatrics, neonatology, gynaecology and obstetrics (GO). The CMIN is responsible for the inpatient unit, intensive and intermediate care, diagnostic areas, day hospital, births block and has a GO emergency department (Portela et al., 2013).

Due to the inefficiency of the Manchester Triage System (MTS) to triage specific cases, most concretely GO, a specific pre-triage system (Cabral et al., 2011; Filipe Portela, Alexandra Cabral, et al., 2013; Filipe Portela et al., 2010) for obstetrics emergency department was implemented in 2010. This system is characterized by a set of discriminators for the obstetrics urgency allowing a patients triage in two levels: Urgent Consultation (ARGO) and Urgent (URG) (Abelha, Pereira, Brandão, Portela, Santos, Silva, et al., 2014). In addition, this system is also characterized by six specific flowcharts (Pregnant ("Yes"), Postpartum Women ("No", "Yes"); Not Women ("No," No"); Pregnant Maybe ("Maybe); Voluntary Interruption of Pregnancy

(VIP) ("To IGO"); Cardiotocography (CTG) ("To CTG")). This measure allowed a significant reduction (7%) of women at the obstetric emergency department as can be seen in *Improving Quality of Services in Maternity Care Triage System* (Abelha, Pereira, Brandão, Portela, Santos, Silva, et al., 2014). This pre-triage system is supported by the Agency for Integration, Diffusion and Archive Clinic and Medical Information (AIDA), the interoperability platform of CHP (Peixoto, Santos, Abelha, & Machado, 2012). This interoperability platform (Marins et al., 2014) is based on the use of intelligent agents (Cardoso, Marins, Portela, Santos, et al., 2014) to enable communication among different systems. This multi-agent system (Cardoso, Marins, Portela, Abelha, & Machado, 2014) allows the standardization of clinical systems and overcomes medical and administrative complexity inherent to different sources of information (Pereira, Brandão, Portela, et al., 2014).

Triage Systems

As mentioned there are several triage systems currently implemented in healthcare institutions. However, the main limitation of this type of triage systems is the lack of flexibility, i.e., they are not able to respond to the requirements of specific emergency departments (Smithson et al., 2013). One such instance, are the patients that fall in the gynaecology and obstetrics specialties. They are characterized by specific symptoms and signs that are not evaluated by the general triage systems available today.

A literature review was carried out about the triage systems most used in the GO Units. In this case highlights the Manchester Triage System (MTS) and Obstetric Triage Accuracy Scale (OTAS). Manchester Triage System (MTS) is a general priorities triage system implemented in the majority of Portuguese and European institutions and Obstetric Triage Accuracy Scale (OTAS) is an obstetric priorities triage system.

Manchester Triage System

The Manchester Triage System (MTS) was introduced in the United Kingdom (UK) in 1996 and quickly became widespread in Europe. In mid of 2000 it was implemented in the United States of America (Portela et al., 2013). This system, as most of the triages systems, aims to identify in a practical and systematic way the severity criteria indicating the clinical priority of a patient should be treated as well as the respective maximum waiting time that each patient should be subject. MTS includes a set of fifty two flowcharts, containing a specific set of discriminators associating the patients to a given urgency class, as can be seen in table 1.

Table 1. MTS Nomenclature (adapted from (Grupo Português de Triagem, 2002))

Number	Name	Colour	Target Time
1	Emergent	Red	0
2	Very Urgent	Orange	15
3	Urgent	Yellow	30
4	Less Urgent	Green	60
5	Non- Urgent	Blue	120

According to the *Comissão Nacional de Saúde Materna da Criança e do Abolescente* (CNSMCA) evaluating the advantages and disadvantages of MTS in relation to obstetrics proved to be a difficult task. However, it can be identified that the flowchart 34 ("Pregnancy") is inappropriate for obstetric triage. Furthermore, some advantages was identified like the fact that the MTS be valid and universally accepted. The patients are triage into five levels of clinical priorities, and the focus is in the speed and in the objectivity. MTS also enables the monitoring of the implementation and development of quality and efficiency indicators (triage time, waiting time, managed care, list of priorities with the high and hospitalizations, etc.). It should be noted the fact of this system is being adopted in Portugal and it is currently linked to the Medical Support System (SAM) (Infantil, 2013).

Obstetrical Triage Acuity Scale

The Obstetrical Triage Acuity Scale (OTAS) has been shaped by the Canadian Triage and Acuity Scale (CTAS). It was introduced in 1999 and has undergone revisions in years 2006 and 2008 (Murray et al., 2004). The CTAS has a high degree of reliability and validity, however, this only includes a limited number of parameters obstetric which, in turn, does not reflect the diversity of women that go to obstetric triage units. Thus, in order to allow the creation of a tool encompassing a wide variety of patients in the obstetric units it was developed the OTAS. The parameters evaluated are shown in Table 2.

Thus, OTAS revised five specific parameters of pregnant women: Working Labour and Fluid, Haemorrhage, Hypertension, Fetal Assessment, other (Smithson et al., 2013). In this follow-up it was formed an expert group of physicians and nurses and it was analysed the classification system in order to safeguard the accuracy and integrity of the obstetric discriminators defined.

OTAS is the first comprehensive obstetric tool with an accurate classification, establishing reliability and validity in terms of obstetric triage. It is a renowned scale and already has a wide application in various obstetric triage units and general

Table 2. OTAS Nomenclature (adapted from (Smithson et al., 2013))

Number	Name	Colour	Target Time	Reassessment
OTAS 1	Recursive	Red	0	Immediate
OTAS 2	Emergent	Orange	15	All 10 min
OTAS 3	Urgent	Yellow	30	All 15 min
OTAS 4	Less Urgent	Green	60	All 15 min
OTAS 5	Non-Urgent	Blue	120	All 60 min

emergencies. OTAS provides care to a significant number of women in the obstetrics specialty (Smithson et al., 2013).

In general, this system has the advantage of considering separately the maternal and fetal reviews and separating the pregnancy labour from the pathology. This system is also well-structured for obstetrics in the definition of signs, symptoms and timing of care.

However, this system is not implemented in Portugal and it is not allowed a practice assessment, so it is unknown the OTAS compatibility with the existing systems in the Portugal GO Emergency Department (Infantil, 2013).

MATERIALS, METHODS, AND METHODOLOGIES

Being this project based in scientific studies, a research methodology was followed and a set of materials and methods were used in order to achieve the best model.

Research Methodology

The project presented throughout this chapter was developed using the research methodology *Design Research* (DR). The DR purpose is to guide and validate the construction of artefacts. This presupposes the action of a particular study based in a real problem. In this case, there is a problem requiring a solution being necessary design a solution (artefact) to the problem and assess it. In this sense, the researcher is not a mere observer but an individual who acts in the research context. He seeking to understand a given reality by using their creative potential to create solutions to real problems or needs (Wang & Hannafin, 2005). So this methodology is divided into five sequential steps: Awareness of Problem, Suggestion, Development, Evaluation and Conclusion. In this sense and following this methodologies CRTSO was developed.

Development Methodology of the Clinical Recommendation Triage System for Obstetric

To develop the CRTSO, several steps to assess (technically and scientifically) the feasibility of the proposal were carried out and they are presented in section entitled by *Triage Systems*.

The procedures performed are shown below.

Literature Review: Initially a survey was conducted about the existing triage systems in the Portuguese and World hospitals. In this context it was concluded that MTS are the most used in the Portuguese reality, and therefore, more suitable for analysis (Infantil, 2013). Specifically, the OTAS System constitutes a world reference for obstetric triage (Smithson et al., 2013).

Development of a CRTSO Proposal: In practical terms it was evaluated the evolution possibility of the pre-triage system into a CRTSO. First in the article entitled as *Improving Quality of Services in Maternity Care Triage System* (Abelha, Pereira, Brandão, Portela, Santos, Silva, et al., 2014) was presented the pre-triage system, their specific flowcharts and discriminators. Subsequently the process of evolution to a CRTSO it was evaluated by Data Mining (DM) techniques. In the article entitled as *Pre-Triage Decision Support Improvement in Maternity Care by means of Data Mining* (Pereira, Brandão, Salazar, et al., 2014) it was proven that the pre-triage system is calibrated for the patients triage on two levels (URG and ARGO), however it was found that the pre-triage system needs for some improvements. That said, it was developed a simulation algorithm intending to simulate a triage system with five priority levels. This algorithm was developed having as base the pre-triage system. In general as shown in the article entitled *Simulating A Multi-Level Priority Tri- age System For Maternity Emergency* (Abelha, Pereira, Brandão, Portela, Santos, & Machado, 2014) it was concluded that the transformation of the pre-triage system in to a CRTSO is viable. After the application of the algorithm developed to the data provided by the existing pre-triage system it was found that there are patients who fall into all levels of the priorities designed. This conclusion can also be withdrawn by observing the graph presented in the Figure 1.

Figure 1 presents the results obtained by the pre-triage System and the simulated system. By analysing figure 1 is possible observing that much of the URG pregnant is in level 3 and ARGO pregnant is in level 5. This analysis gives some confidence in concluding the viability assessment study of turning the pre-triage system into a CRTSO.

After these preliminaries studies, the proposal was developed using:

- OTAS system, because it already is a specific system of obstetric triage (Smithson et al., 2013).

Figure 1. Results of pre-triage system and the simulated system grouped by number of patients, for maximum waiting time and time average waiting (adapted from (Abelha, Pereira, Brandão, Portela, Santos, & Machado, 2014))

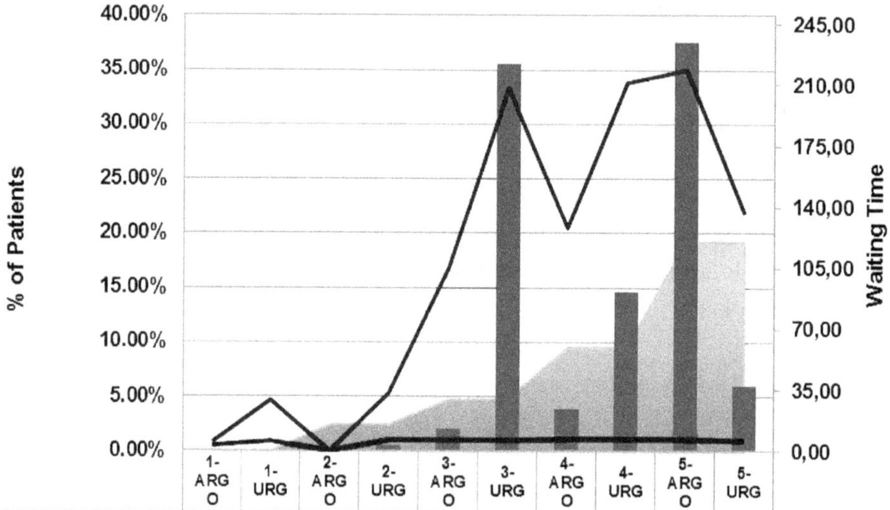

	1-ARGO	1-URG	2-ARGO	2-URG	3-ARGO	3-URG	4-ARGO	4-URG	5-ARGO	5-URG
Waiting Time (Target)	0,00	0,00	15,00	15,00	30,00	30,00	60,00	60,00	120,00	120,00
Patients in Triage	0.01%	0.10%	0.00%	0.47%	2.00%	35.51%	3.88%	14.57%	37.52%	5.94%
Waiting Time (MAX)	5,00	29,00	0,00	33,00	105,00	208,00	128,00	211,00	219,00	136,00
Waiting time (AVG)	3,00	5,50	0,00	6,37	5,98	6,37	6,50	6,90	7,09	6,06

- MTS system, because it is a standard Triage System for general emergency departments.
- Empirical knowledge of health specialists in obstetric area that currently work, or have already exercised triage activities.

Model Evaluation: In the evaluation process and after being designed the proposal of clinical CRTSO, three joint meetings were performed with all the professionals involved, with the following order of work:

- At the first meeting the system proposal was presented to all members.
- At the second meeting and after everybody involved in the work be framed on the subject, there was made an analysis of all flowcharts in order to proceed to their medical and scientific evaluation;
- At the third meeting, an agreement on the proposal made was achieved.

This process was time consuming but rewarding, since after the interaction made between the information system professionals and the healthcare professionals it was possible to obtain a final model sensitive and adapted to a specific reality: gynaecology service.

CLINICAL RECOMMENDATION SYSTEM FOR OBSTETRIC TRIAGE

This section presents the transformation model of pre-triage system into a CRTSO. Initially it is shown the nomenclature chosen for the CRTSO. Then the CRTSO developed is presented. Finally in the last topic of this section the overall adjustments to the proposal be functional are presented.

Nomenclature

The analysis of the nomenclature and definitions currently in use by the existing triage systems revealed the existence of some similarities but also some differences between the pre-triage systems. Two of the systems in analysis were the MTS and OTAS. The terms used were presented in Tables 1 and 2 respectively. With the analysis of these two systems was possible to quickly reach an agreement on a new nomenclature. In this regard, to each one of the new triage categories was assigned a level, a name, a colour, a target time (maximum wait time for the admission) and a re-evaluation time, as presented in Table 3.

This initial nomenclature will be re-calibrated in the future after testing the model by using real data. The main changes can be essentially in the target time and in the reassessment time.

Table 3. Clinical recommendation triage system for obstetrics nomenclature

Level	Name	Colour	Target Time	Reassessment
1	Emergent	Red	0	Immediate
2	Very Urgent	Orange	15	All 10 min
3	Urgent	Yellow	30	All 15 min
4	Less Urgent	Green	60	All 15 min
5	Non- Urgent	Blue	120	All 60 min

Model

Three different models have been developed taking into account the types of users: Pregnant ("Yes"), Postpartum, ("No", "Yes"), Not Postpartum Women ("No", "No") and Maybe Pregnant ("Maybe"), as described in the article entitled *Improving Quality of Services in Maternity Care Triage System* (Abelha, Pereira, Brandão, Portela, Santos, Silva, et al., 2014).

Due to similarities between issues/discriminators the six flowcharts were grouped in three different flowcharts, and the flowcharts "To VIP" and "To CTG" were extinguished of the triage system as is explained below.

As part of this work and due to confidentiality duties, only it is presented the model for the flowchart Pregnant ("Yes"). Although this fact the other two models also have been developed.

In Table 4, is represented the model developed for the flowchart of patients identified as Pregnant ("Yes").

In this system some relevant parameters are evaluated in order to distinguish the priority of pregnant woman ("Yes") taking into account the clinical characteristics at the triage time: labour, haemorrhage, hypertension, fetal assessment, the Glasgow Coma Scale (GCS), pain scale, fever and others variables as can be seen in Table 4.

In order to changing the pre-triage system to a CRTSO with five priority levels, the existing pre-triage system requires some changes:

Change in nomenclature of the existing discriminators:

- Uterine contractions > Rhythmic and Painful Contractions;
- Nausea / Vomiting > Uncontrollable Vomiting;
- Change the Colour of the skin > Jaundice;
- In general, the categorization of the other parameters evaluated in Table 4 was trivial between the pre-triage system and OTAS.

Add new discriminators:

- Discharge;
- Itching;
- Other conditions (contact with varicella and rubella);
- To IGO or Not Evolutionary Pregnancy: Women for IGO should be included in the type of pregnant patients. If this is not associated with a medical condition should be inserted in less urgent level (level 5);
- Dyspnoea;
- Imminent birth;

Table 4. Model of the Clinical Recommendation Triage System for Obstetrics, Flowchart Pregnant patients ("Yes")

Triage GO (Pregnant)	1 (Emergent)	2 (Very Urgent)	3 (Urgent)	4 (Less Urgent)	5 (Non- Urgent)
Target Time	**Immediate care**	**<=15 min**	**<= 30 min**	**<= 60 min**	**<=120 min**
Re-assessment	**Continuous Nursing Care**	**Every 15 min**	**Every 15 min**	**Every 30 min**	**Every 60 min**
Labor/Fluid	Imminent birth	Loss of amniotic fluid. Rhythmic and painful uterine contractions and week of pregnancy <35?	Loss of amniotic fluid and Rhythmic and painful uterine contractions		
Vaginal bleeding	Hemorrhage (Severe)?	Hemorrhage (Moderate)?	Hemorrhage (Scarce)?		
Blood Pressure	(Systolic> 160 and diastolic> 110) and / or (headache, visual changes or epigastric pain / right upper quadrant Pain)?		Systolic> 140 and diastolic> 90) and (headache or visual changes or epigastric pain / right upper quadrant)?	Ref. Tension Rise? Systolic> 140 and diastolic> 90?	
Fetal Assessment			Absence of fetal movements?	Decreased of fetal movements?	
Glasgow Coma Scale	Glasgow (3)?	Glasgow (4-5)?	Glasgow (6-8)?	Glasgow (9-12)?	Glasgow (13-15)?
Pain scale (local, intensity, duration)	Pain (10) and (abdominal pain or low back pain or pain in the lower abdomen)?	Pain (7-9 and (abdominal pain or low back pain or pain in the lower abdomen)?	Pain (4-6) and (abdominal pain or low back pain or pain in the lower abdomen)?	Pain (1-3) and (abdominal pain or low back pain or pain in the lower abdomen)?	Pain (0)?
Fever		>= 41, 0 °C	38,5 – 40,9 °C	37,5 °C – 38,4 °C	<37,4 °C?
Umbilical cord prolapse	Umbilical cord prolapse?				
Other	• Dyspnoea • Seizures?	• Lipothymy • Trauma in pregnant	• Uncontrollable vomiting? • Epigastric pain / right upper quadrant and weeks of gestation> 20? • Higher pain 1 week? • Jaundice and gestational weeks> 20? • General condition (Bad)?	• Epigastric pain / right upper quadrant and weeks of gestation <20? • Jaundice and weeks gestation <20 • Urinary symptoms? • General condition (Average)?	• General condition (Good) • To IGO or not Evolutionary Pregnancy • Combur? • Other situations (contact with chickenpox and rubella)?

Changing the type of variable:

- The parameters "Weeks of Pregnancy", "Blood Pressure" and "Fever" should become numeric (permit the choice of a value or enter a numerical value only).

General Adaptations

After the models development, a set of overall adjustments were designed to the three proposed models (one for each flowchart).

The first adjustment is in the fact of the flow discriminators described in the previous subsection (model) are not performed sequentially in the pre-triage system. Thus, it is suggested that during the implementation of this model should be imposed a condition, preventing the priority reduction by the system, or a recast where first it is asked the main discriminator and so forth, as can be seen in Figure 2.

Figure 2. Proposal for general clinical recommendation system for obstetric triage

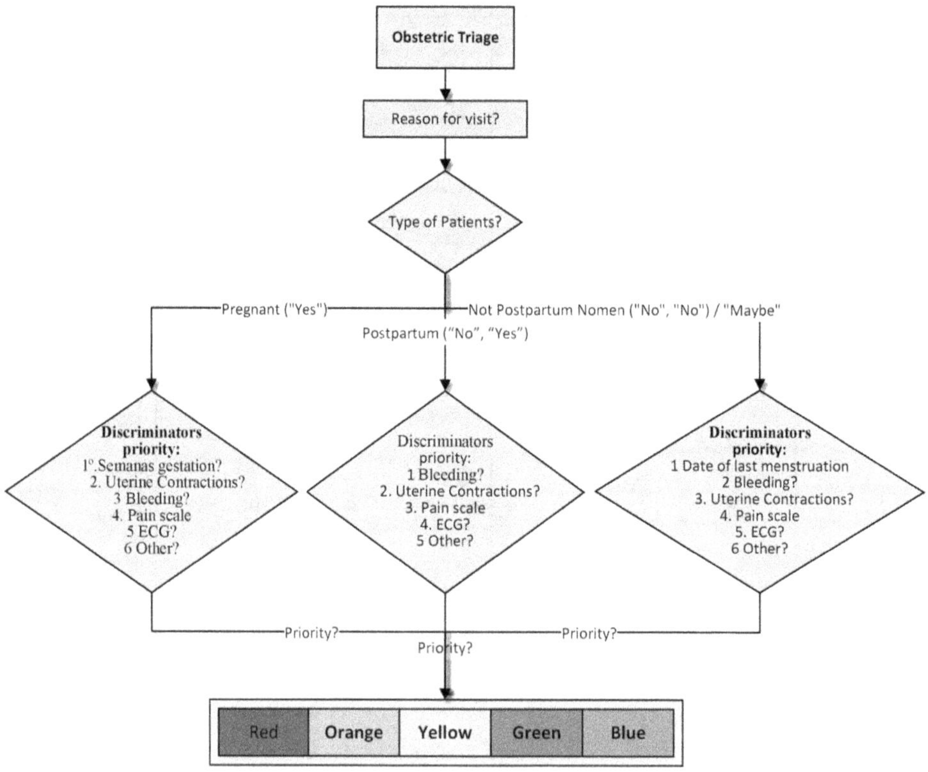

In Figure 2 is defined a set of priority questions, that must be doing to the patients when they are admitted to the emergency department. First should be asked to patient the reason for the visit the emergency department. In the case of bean emergent situation the patient is attended immediately, i.e., he is not submitted to the triage process.

Then the clinical professional should try to see what type of patient she is. She can be a Pregnant Woman ("Yes"), Postpartum Women ("Yes", "No") or not Pregnant Women ("No", "No") / Pregnant Maybe ("Maybe"). That said, should be carried out a set of priority questions, according to the chosen flowchart. Finally should be recommended the priority level.

The second adjustment is to the patients identified as Urgent Consultation (ARGO) in the pre-triage system. They should be distinguished with the Blue priority (level 5) and sent for urgent consultations as happen actually with pre-triage system. On the other hand, patients assigned to category Urgent (URG) in the pre-triage system must be distributed among the remaining four levels of priorities proposed (Red (level 1), Orange (level 2), Yellow (level 3) and Green (level 4)) being then referred to the obstetric emergency room according to their clinical condition (priority).

With this condition it can be can recommended a referral of the patients in more detail and more effectively, especially for urgent patients. They are now divided by different levels of clinical care.

Finally the classes of patients "To CTG" and "To IGO" were removed from the CMIN obstetric emergency. The patients "To CTG" are not considered urgent once the exams and pregnancy monitoring process are not an urgent situation. Relatively to the patients "To IGO", they are not also considered urgent cases, unless exceptions where the patients present situations inspiring urgent care (e.g. vaginal bleeding). In these situations the women should be placed on pregnant woman ("Yes") flowchart.

DISCUSSION AND CONCLUSION

The possible implementation of a CRTSO will provide significant benefits for CMIN while health institution as well as to the patients who use this health institution. It allows a patient categorization in five levels according to the level of clinical needs, prioritizing their care according their condition.

For the development of this proposal it was required an extensive work of literature review, planning, development and evaluation of the proposed CRTSO. Throughout this section it is made an analysis between the work developed and guidelines suggested by the CNSMCA regarding to the obstetric triage.

They were evaluated four points:

1. **Scientific gathering information on the various existing systems:** for this process it was conducted a scientific review on the existing triage systems in worldwide. In sub section *Triage System* were described the theoretical aspects of MTS and OTAS Systems and in the article entitled *by Improving Quality of Services in Maternity Care Triage System* (Abelha, Pereira, Brandão, Portela, Santos, Silva, et al., 2014) is described the pre-triage system implemented in CMIN.
2. **Knowledge criteria of the Portuguese reality through contact with triage systems in use**: on this topic, according to the study done by CNSMCA where a survey was conducted at 38 institutions Portuguese about the obstetric triage, it was identified that 34 of these institutions has the obstetric urgency and the general urgency separated. Of these, only 12 performed the obstetric triage. Usually it turns out the existence of these systems in hospitals where the flow of patients in obstetric emergency is high. It was also detected that there is a wide variety software with adaptations made as is the ALERT software with MTS, or very simplistic triage systems that only differentiate between urgent and non-urgent patients (Portela et al., 2013) (Infantil, 2013) (Abelha, Pereira, Brandão, Portela, Santos, Silva, et al., 2014).
3. **Defining criteria for the CRTSO developed:**
    a. *The most scientific and consensually internationally valid:* in this context the two systems valid at international level are: the OTAS and MTS. The first was developed for triage in obstetric emergency. The second is recognized at international level and it is in the Portuguese healthcare institutions. Then there is also the pre-triage system, which although it is not a global system, their efficiency has been demonstrated in the articles *Improving Quality of Services in Maternity Care Triage System* (Abelha, Pereira, Brandão, Portela, Santos, Silva, et al., 2014), *Pre-Triage Decision Support Improvement in Maternity Care by means of Data Mining* (Pereira, Brandão, Salazar, et al., 2014) and *Simulating Multi-Level Priority Triage System For Emergency Maternity* (Abelha, Pereira, Brandão, Portela, Santos, & Machado, 2014). It is characterized by a set of discriminators adapted to the CMIN and the reality of an obstetric emergency.
    b. *Must be compatible with the software applications of the Ministry of Health, i.e. interconnection to existing software level hospitals*: Given that the starting point is that the pre-triage system should be supported by AIDA which interlinks with other National Health systems (Medical Support System (SAM) Nursing Practice Support System (SAPE), etc.). In the future the CRTSO proposed will take up these features too.
    c. *Easy to learn and intuitive as possible:* The pre-triage system was already implemented in the MJD, since 2010 and it was subsequently transferred

to the CMIN. Being the CRTSO an adaptation of the pre-triage system, the healthcare professionals at CMIN are much familiarized with the system.

d. *Adapted or the ability to adapt to obstetric specialty, i.e., flowchart and discriminated specific for obstetrics:* The pre-triage system is characterized by having specific discriminators to obstetrics therefore the developed model also has this valence. In addition to the specific discriminators already used in pre-triage system this CRTSO has new discriminators. The existing discriminators, such as those added to the model went through a process of natural discussion to assess their viability.

4. **Defining the criteria for who does obstetric:** Usually this pre-triage process should be performed by health professionals: Nurse Specialist in maternal and child health or Physician specialist in obstetric. Once the triage process currently is carried out by experts in Obstetric, this feature also will be present in the new CRTSO.

It is important to note that although this CRTSO have been designed based on the MTS, OTAS and pre-triage system of CMIN, should not be classified as a priority triage system but as a Clinical Recommendation System (CRS). CRTSO only allows a recommend forwarding and a service order taking into account a range of clinical aspects of patients, however the final decision is always taken by the health professional responsible for this process.

It is therefore concluded that the proposed transformation of the pre-triage system into a CRTSO is a pioneer project with great potentialities. The main goal is not replace the MST but create an alternative to most specific departments as is GO emergency units.

FUTURE RESEARCH DIRECTIONS

In view of the project success, as future work is suggested one set of sequential steps:

1. Presenting of the this CRTSO in the CMIN to discuss its possible implementation and testing;
2. Contact the Portuguese Group of Triage (Grupo Português de Triagem, 2014), responsible institution for the implementation of triage systems in Portugal, in order to approve the CRTSO developed;
3. If approved by those two institutions should proceed to the implementation of the flowcharts associated to the respective discriminators and conditions specified for the transformation considered in the article. If the project is not

approved, should be made the necessary changes in order to approve the project, after the changes should be executed again the point 1 of this sequence.

4. Preparation of documents and specific protocols supporting the use of the system implemented, for example, a manual to support the healthcare professional in the triage process.
5. Performing periodic evaluations in order to make timeout adjustments to optimize the speed of attending patients in critical condition. One of the methodology to be followed it was focused in article entitled by *Pre-Triage Decision Support Improvement in Maternity Care by means of Data Mining* (Pereira, Brandão, Salazar, et al., 2014). This article used DM techniques to obtain prediction models. At same time it was developed a Business Intelligence platform to manage pre-triage indicators. This platform also can incorporate indicators from the CRTSO developed. This Business Intelligence platform can be consulted in the articles entitled by *Business Intelligence to Maternity Care* (Pereira, Brandão, Portela, et al., 2014) and it allows obtaining Key Indicator Performance (KPI) about the performance of the pre-triage system.
6. Developing data mining models (Filipe Portela, Filipe Pinto, & Santos, 2012; Santos & Portela, 2011) to improve the CRTSO models
7. Assessing the CRTSO using as example earlier studies (Filipe Portela, Jorge Aguiar, Manuel Filipe Santos, Álvaro Silva, & Fernado Rua, 2013)

The proposal CRTSO presented in this article aims the implementation in CMIN as a testing phase. However the objective is that in the future may be used by other health institutions that contemplate the obstetric emergency department.

ACKNOWLEDGMENT

This work is funded by National Funds through the FCT - Fundação para a Ciência e a Tecnologia (Portuguese Foundation for Science and Technology) within projects PEst-OE/EEI/UI0752/2014 and PEst-OE/EEI/UI0319/2014. The work of Filipe Portela was supported by a postdoctoral grant associated to FCT project INTCare II - PTDC/EEI-SII/1302/2012.

REFERENCES

Abelha, A., Pereira, E., Brandão, A., Portela, C. F., Santos, M. F., & Machado, J. (2014). Simulating a multi-level priority triage system for Maternity Emergency. *Proceedings of ESM - 28th European Simulation and Modelling Conference*, Porto, Portugal. EUROSIS.

Abelha, A., Pereira, E., Brandão, A., Portela, F., Santos, M. F., Silva, Á., & Braga, J. (2014). Improving Quality of Services in Maternity Care Triage System. *International Journal of E-Health and Medical Communications, 6(2), 10-26.*

Brandão, A., Pereira, E., Portela, F., Santos, M., Abelha, A., & Machado, J. (2014). Real-time Business Intelligence platform to maternity care. *Proceedings of IECBES 2014 - IEEE Conference on Biomedical Engineering and Sciences*, Sarawak, Malaysia (pp. 379-384). IEEE.

Cabral, A., Pina, C., Machado, H., Abelha, A., Salazar, M., Quintas, C., & .... (2011). Data Acquisition Process for an Intelligent Decision Support in Gynecology and Obstetrics Emergency Triage. In M. M. Cruz-Cunha, J. Varajão, P. Powell, & R. Martinho (Eds.), *Enterprise Information Systems* (Vol. 221, pp. 223–232). CCIS.

Cardoso, L., Marins, F., Portela, F., Abelha, A., & Machado, J. (2014). Healthcare interoperability through intelligent agent technology. *Procedia Technology, 16*, 1334–1341.

Cardoso, L., Marins, F., Portela, F., Santos, M., Abelha, A., & Machado, J. (2014). The Next Generation of Interoperability Agents in Healthcare. *International Journal of Environmental Research and Public Health, 11*(5), 5349–5371. doi:10.3390/ijerph110505349 PMID:24840351

Comissão Nacional de Saúde Materna da Criança e do Abolescente. (2013). *Triagem Obstétrica- modelo de Triagem*. Lisboa: Direção Geral de Saúde.

Grupo Português de Triagem. (2002). *Triagem no serviço de Urgência – Manual do Formador* (2nd ed.). Lisboa: BMJ Publishing Group.

Grupo Português de Triagem. (2014). Grupo Português de Triagem. Retrieved from http://www.grupoportuguestriagem.pt/jm/

Mackway-Jones, K., M. J. & W. J. (1997). Emergency triage: Manchester triage group. *BMJ (Clinical Research Ed.).*

Marins, F., Cardoso, L., Portela, F., Santos, M. F., Abelha, A., & Machado, J. (2014). Improving High Availability and Reliability of Health Interoperability Systems. In *New Perspectives in Information Systems and Technologies* (Vol. 2, pp. 207–216). Springer. doi:10.1007/978-3-319-05948-8_20

Murray, M., Bullard, M., & Grafstein, E. (2004). Revisions to the Canadian Emergency Department Triage and Acuity Scale implementation guidelines. *Cjem, 6*(6), 421–7. Retrieved from http://www.ncbi.nlm.nih.gov/pubmed/17378961

Peixoto, H., Santos, M., Abelha, A., & Machado, J. (2012). Intelligence in Interoperability with AIDA. In L. Chen, A. Felfernig, J. Liu, & Z. Raś (Eds.), *Foundations of Intelligent Systems SE - 31* (Vol. 7661, pp. 264–273). Springer Berlin Heidelberg; doi:10.1007/978-3-642-34624-8_31

Pereira, E., Brandão, A., Portela, C. F., Santos, M. F., Machado, J., & Abelha, A. (2014). Business Intelligence in Maternity Care. *Proceedings of the 18th International Database Engineering & Applications Symposium* (pp. 352–355). New York, NY, USA: ACM. 10.1145/2628194.2628248

Pereira, E., Brandão, A., Salazar, M., Portela, C. F., Santos, M. F., & Machado, J. … Jorge, B. (2014). Pre-Triage Decision Support Improvement in Maternity Care by means of Data Mining. In A. Azevedo, & M. F. Santos (Eds.), Integration of Data Mining in Business Intelligence Systems. Hershey, PA, USA: IGI Global Book.

Portela, F., Santos, M.F., & Abelha, A., Machado, J. (2015). A Real-Time Intelligent System for tracking patient condition.

Portela, F., Aguiar, J., Santos, M. F., Silva, Á., & Rua, F. (2013). Pervasive Intelligent Decision Support System - Technology Acceptance in Intensive Care Units. In Á. Rocha, A.M. Correia, T. Wilson, & K.A. Stroetmann (Ed.), Advances in Intelligent Systems and Computing, CCIS (Vol. 206, pp. 279-292). Springer.

Portela, F., Pinto, F., & Santos, M. F. (2012). Data Mining Predictive Models For Pervasive Intelligent Decision Support. *Intensive Care Medicine.*

Portela, F., Santos, M. F., Gago, P., Silva, Á., Rua, F., Abelha, A., …. (2011). Enabling real-time intelligent decision support in intensive care. *Paper presented at the 25th European Simulation and Modelling Conference ESM'2011*, Guimarães, Portugal.

Portela, F., Vilas-Boas, M., Santos, M. F., Abelha, A., Machado, J., Cabral, A., ... (2010). Electronic Health Records in the Emergency Room. *Proceedings of the 9th IEEE/ACIS International Conference on Computer and Information Science* (pp. 195-200). 10.1109/ICIS.2010.98

Portela, F., Cabral, A., Abelha, A., Salazar, M., Quintas, C., Machado, J., Neves, J., & Santos, M. F. (2013). Knowledge Acquisition Process for Intelligent Decision Support in Critical Health Care. In R. Martinho, R. Rijo, M.M. Cruz-Cunha, & J. Verajao (Eds.), Information Systems and Technologies for Enhancing Health and Social Care (Ch. 4, pp. 55-68). Hershey, PA, USA: IGI Global.

Santos, M. F., & Portela, F. (2011). Enabling Ubiquitous Data Mining in Intensive Care - Features selection and data pre-processing. *Proceedings of the 13th International Conference on Enterprise Information Systems*, Beijing, China.

Smithson, D. S., Twohey, R., Rice, T., Watts, N., Fernandes, C. M., & Gratton, R. J. (2013). Implementing an obstetric triage acuity scale: Interrater reliability and patient flow analysis. *American Journal of Obstetrics and Gynecology*, *209*(4), 287–293. doi:10.1016/j.ajog.2013.03.031 PMID:23535239

Wang, F., & Hannafin, M. J. (2005). Design-based research and technology-enhanced learning environments. *Educational Technology Research and Development*, *53*(4), 5–23. doi:10.1007/BF02504682

ADDITIONAL READING

Murray, M., Bullard, M., & Grafstein, E. (2004). Revisions to the Canadian Emergency Department Triage and Acuity Scale implementation guidelines. *Canadian Journal of Emergency Medical Care*, *6*(6), 421–427. Retrieved from http://www.ncbi.nlm.nih.gov/pubmed/17378961 PMID:17378961

Peixoto, H., Santos, M., Abelha, A., & Machado, J. (2012). Intelligence in Interoperability with AIDA. In L. Chen, A. Felfernig, J. Liu, & Z. Raś (Eds.), *Foundations of Intelligent Systems SE - 31* (Vol. 7661, pp. 264–273). Springer Berlin Heidelberg. doi:10.1007/978-3-642-34624-8_31

Smithson, D. S., Twohey, R., Rice, T., Watts, N., Fernandes, C. M., & Gratton, R. J. (2013). Implementing an obstetric triage acuity scale: Interrater reliability and patient flow analysis. *American Journal of Obstetrics and Gynecology*, *209*(4), 287–293. doi:10.1016/j.ajog.2013.03.031 PMID:23535239

Wang, F., & Hannafin, M. J. (2005). Design-based research and technology-enhanced learning environments. *Educational Technology Research and Development*, *53*(4), 5–23. doi:10.1007/BF02504682

KEY TERMS AND DEFINITIONS

AIDA: Platform developed to ensure interoperability among healthcare information systems.

Business Intelligence: A technology that uses data analysis tools and applications to help business users make more informed decision.

Clinical Recommendation System: Combines several computational techniques to select custom items based on user interests and as the context in which they live.

Decision Support System: A computerized information system used to support decision-making process in an organization or business.

Gynaecology and Obstetrics: The medical specialty dealing with fields of through only one postgraduate training programmer. This combined training prepares the practicing Gynaecology and Obstetrics to be adept at the care of female reproductive organs' health and at the management of obstetric complications, even though surgery.

Interoperability: Autonomous ability to interact and communicate.

Maternity Care: Health institution where patients of gynaecology and obstetrics specialties are admitted.

Pre-Triage System: A triage system has as main aim to improve the quality of care in that it provides a service based on clinical characteristics and the target time.

Triage: The sorting of patients (as in an emergency room) according to the urgency of their need for care.

This research was previously published in Applying Business Intelligence to Clinical and Healthcare Organizations edited by José Machado and António Abelha; pages 64-83, copyright year 2016 by Medical Information Science Reference (an imprint of IGI Global).

Chapter 2
An Emerging Model of Pregnancy Care:
The Introduction of New Technologies in Maternal Wellbeing

Claudia Carissoli
Università Cattolica del Sacro Cuore, Italy

Daniela Villani
Università Cattolica del Sacro Cuore, Italy

Giuseppe Riva
Università Cattolica del Sacro Cuore, Italy & I.R.C.C.S. Istituto Auxologico Italiano, Italy

ABSTRACT

Pregnancy is a very special time in a woman's life, a time of important and complex step that can lead to the fall the previous personal balances and looking for new. This phase potentially critical, is often accompanied by anxiety, negative emotions, worries and stress about themselves, the couple's life, the baby. Among the many interventions available for the welfare of pregnant women, new technologies are playing an increasingly important role, thanks to its spread, the lower costs and its peculiar characteristics (interactivity, sociality, customizability, ubiquity, multimediality, velocity, etc). Smartphones and tablets in particular are proving excellent tools to accompany women on this journey toward a healthy motherhood.

DOI: 10.4018/978-1-7998-2351-3.ch002

INTRODUCTION

Pregnancy is a complex phase in a woman's life, a period in which she changes her status from daughter to mother in just a few months. Becoming a mother requires a profound reconstruction of self (Barclay et al., 1997). This process of change is not bounded by a particular time frame, and it can even happen before the end of the neo-maternal month (Rubin, 1984).

In addition to biological changes, pregnancy leads to a search for a new identity that has to be positioned at the individual, couple and social levels (Stern et al., 1998; Bibring, 1959; Ammaniti et al., 1996; Monti et al. 2006).

In this sense pregnancy is a psychologically complex period in a woman's life, and every pregnancy could be seen as a phase of potential vulnerability. Indeed, this metamorphosis is characterized by physiological and psychological changes that can enhance anxiety or other negative emotional states and favor risky behaviors, such as the lack of attention to personal hygiene and prenatal screening, poor diet, alcohol consumption, smoking and drug use (Lindgren, 2001).

A wide consensus exists about the role of maternal psychological state in influencing the development of the child and the course of the pregnancy: negative emotions, such as anxiety and stress, are often associated with a redoubt variability in the fetal cardiac frequency, greater motor activity (which can cause spontaneous abortion), various pregnancy complications, pre-term birth and low birth weight (Hoffman & Hatch, 2000; Dunkel-Schetter, 1998; Dayan et al., 2002). Davies and colleagues showed that the level of maternal cortisol, measured between 30-32 weeks of gestation, is a predictor of a difficult temperament in children at two months of age (Davis et al., 2007); it is also inversely related to scores of cognitive and motor development in children at both three and eight months (Buitelaar et al., 2003). Anxiety detected at 32 weeks gestation was predictive of severe behavioral problems in children at 4 years of age (O'Connor et al., 2002).

This situation appears even more critical in cases of anxiety or depression disorders during pregnancy that are related to postpartum depression (Grant et al., 2008; Austin et al., 2007) and to negative effects on infant mental development (Tronick, 1999). Postnatal depression has been clearly associated with negative health consequences for both women and their babies (O'Hara and Swain, 1996).

Specifically, impaired maternal-infant interactions have been linked to vulnerability in infants and children (Murray et al., 1996), to attachment insecurity and delay in cognitive and emotional development (Hipwell et al., 2000; Murray et al., 1992; Cogill et al., 1986; Cummings & Davies, 1994), and to social and interaction difficulties (Murray et al., 1999).

As well-being of the mother is critical for optimal pregnancy outcomes, it is important to regulate maternal stress and provide expecting mothers with coping strategies to increase their quality of life and to maximize infant health and development.

This chapter pursues a threefold objective. First, it aims to investigate how it is possible to enhance women's well-being during pregnancy by taking into consideration the three levels of well-being identified by positive psychology. Second, it aims to analyze how actual mothers-to-be use new technologies to meet several needs. Finally, it aims to describe the Italian mobile app "BenEssere Mamma," which was developed by the chapter's authors to support mothers' well-being during pregnancy.

HOW TO ENHANCE WOMEN'S WELL-BEING DURING PREGNANCY

Pregnancy, evoking a range of emotions from great joy and anticipation to crippling anxiety, is likely to increase several needs, including the needs for information, to share experiences with others or to be instantly connected, and to consult professionals (Tripp et al., 2014). There are several ways to meet these needs, including self-soothing techniques, psycho-education and relaxation, that are particularly important in this transitional and meaningful time (Beddoe & Lee, 2008).

According to the positive psychology perspective – which emerged as the scientific study of positive personal experience, positive individual traits, and positive institutions (Seligman, 2003; Seligman and Csikszentmihalyi, 2000) - it is critical to focus on human strengths, healthy processes, and fulfillment in order to improve quality of life, as well as to increase wellness and resilience in individuals, organizations, and societies. This is also true for pregnant women.

Keyes and Lopez (Keyes & Lopez, 2002) suggested that positive functioning could be achieved by working on three levels of well-being: (a) high emotional well-being, (b) high psychological well-being, and (c) high social well-being. This means that positive psychology identifies three characteristics of our personal experience—affective quality, engagement/actualization, and connectedness—that serve to promote personal well-being.

By following this categorization it is possible to identify three critical perspectives to take into consideration in order to improve quality of life and well-being during pregnancy.

Fostering Maternal Positive Emotional States (Hedonic Perspective)

Theoretical perspectives suggest that the experience of positive emotions may be important in helping individuals recover quickly from stress. According to the Broaden-and-Build Theory of positive emotions (Fredrickson, 2001), the form and function of positive and negative emotions are distinct and complementary. Negative emotions (e.g., fear, anger, and sadness) narrow momentary thoughts and actions to produce autonomic nervous system activation that prepares the body for specific actions that served the ancestral function of promoting survival. By contrast, positive emotions (e.g., joy, interest, and contentment) broaden an individual's momentary thought–action repertoire, which in turn can build that individual's enduring personal resources, resources that also served the ancestral function of promoting survival. One implication of the Broaden–and–Build model is that positive emotions have an undoing effect on negative emotions. In this sense, experiences of positive emotions, in turn, should broaden habitual modes of thinking and build personal resources for coping with adversity. Positive emotions are likely to be the active ingredient that energizes this upward spiral that optimizes health and well-being.

Although studies have investigated the relationship between stress/negative emotional states and delivery and neonatal complications, up to now the association of positive emotional states with these variables has been less investigated. Nevertheless, some preliminary evidence underlines the importance and beneficial effects of maternal positive affect in the context of pregnancy and birth outcomes.

Concerning the motherhood period, positive appraisal has been associated with a high level of stability in coping and less distress throughout pregnancy (Yali & Lobel, 2002). A recent study demonstrated that positive life events predicted significantly lower third-trimester maternal morning cortisol levels across the cortisol awakening response (Pluess et al., 2012). These findings suggest that positive affect dampens endocrine and psychological responses to stress in pregnancy, which may be protective for the developing fetus. Furthermore, in healthy pregnant women, Costa and colleagues (2003) examined leisure-time physical activity (LTPA) patterns during pregnancy and the association with psychological well-being. Authors found a consistent association between enhanced psychological well-being, as measured by a variety of psychosocial inventories, and LTPA participation, particularly during the first and second trimesters of pregnancy. According to this study, even low-intensity regular exercise may be a potentially effective low-cost method of enhancing psychological well-being.

Concerning the relationship between positive affective states and delivery experience, a recent study described associations of positive state of mind and emotional stability in the immediate post-partum period with having experienced a normal delivery (Hernandez-Martinez et al., 2011). However, positive affect was assessed in the immediate post-partum period, so it was not possible to state in a definite way if the positive delivery experience may have caused the higher positive affect in these women or vice versa.

Voellmin and colleagues (2013) assessed the relationship between positive affect and length of gestation and suggested that higher levels of positive affect in pregnancy are associated with longer length of gestation and with a reduced risk of delivering preterm. Specifically, the level of positive affect in the early second trimester of pregnancy, as well as the rate of increase in positive affect over the course of pregnancy, were positively associated with a longer length of gestation.

These preliminary studies suggest the importance of orienting mothers towards the cultivation of positive experiences in their lives.

Promoting Maternal Growth and Fulfillment (Eudamonic Perspective)

Supportive and educational care is provided for most women who give birth. In several countries offering health care, there are many standard interventions—both public and private—available to support women in this particular phase of life. The characteristics and duration of care vary according to the status and training of the persons providing it (Rush et al., 1991). For example, the typical intervention offered in Italy is a childbirth class designed to provide information about maternal and fetal health from pregnancy to childbirth. Although very useful and popular, these courses are begin during the sixth or seventh month of pregnancy, when a lot of changes and doubts have already happened. Furthermore, mothers-to-be often struggle to follow these courses because of inconvenient hours, lack of time or long journeys required to reach the course locations. In addition, only a few of these courses include training for developing personal skills like resilience or coping skills to deal with maternity and childbirth effectively. Thus, the psychological component is often less explored than the educational-informative one.

The focus on mind-body practices that cultivate general health, diminish distress, and increase self-awareness may be particularly effective in addressing both the physical and psycho-emotional aspects of pregnancy and labor (Beddoe and Lee, 2008). Indeed, regular and moderate physical exercise can be helpful in the management of stress and other associated conditions or symptoms accompanying pregnancy, such as gestational diabetes and hypertension (Melzer et al., 2010). As well as physical exercise during pregnancy, routine prenatal care also includes relaxation and meditation practices during, which have various notable effects (Dunn et al., 2012; Beddoe & Lee, 2008).

Both these interventions represent possible effective approaches to well-being and quality of life during pregnancy, and they can also offer good strategies to support women in labor pain management. Labor pain is a subjective and multidimensional experience that varies according to each woman's individual perceptions and reactions to nociceptive information during labor and is influenced by several psychosocial, cognitive, and physiological factors (Lowe, 2002). Relaxation and meditation interventions have become popular for pain management in labor. On one hand, women are seeking alternatives to traditional treatment approaches, including analgesics and anesthesia, which can be invasive and are sometimes associated with negative side effects for both mother and infant (Smith et al., 2011). On the other hand, it is suggested that practitioners use a multidisciplinary approach to pain management in labor and incorporate non-pharmacological approaches that can be tailored to individual preferences and needs (Jones, 2012). As maternal prenatal anxiety is negatively associated with pre-labor self-efficacy for childbirth and labor pain (Beebe and Lee, 2007), relaxation and meditation represent good practices to help women feel more competent in coping with this specific experience, to reduce complication rates, and to have an overall better experience (Dunn et al., 2012 ; Gedde-Dahl & Fors, 2012).

The effects of relaxation and meditation practices during pregnancy will be described in the following paragraphs.

Relaxation Strategies for Pregnant Women

When combined with regular exercise, relaxation techniques contribute to a reduction in preterm birth, longer gestation, increase in birth weight, and reduced risks of Caesarean section and instrumental extraction. The immediate impact of relaxation on pregnant women indicates a reduction in experienced stress or anxiety (Nickel et al., 2006; Bastani et al., 2005, 2006; Teixeira et al., 2005; Field et al., 2004, 1999; Urizar et al., 2004). Furthermore, relaxation could improve fetal health by reducing the basal fetal heart rate and increasing the number of fetal heart accelerations (Akbarzade et al., 2015).

The studies typically included a wide range of interventions like applied relaxation, massage, hypnotherapy, yoga therapy, verbal instructions, breathing instructions, progressive muscular relaxation (PMR) and guided imagery (GI). All of these techniques have shown promising results regarding a reduction in perceived stress and various physical symptoms and promotion of positive affect and well-being (Urech et al., 2010; Beddoe & Lee, 2009; Vieten & Astin, 2008; Nickel et al., 2006; Bastani et al., 2005,2006; Naredran et al., 2005; Teixera et al., 2005).

Although a variety of interventions exists, so far only a few research groups have directly evaluated whether different relaxation techniques have different impacts during pregnancy with randomized controlled trials. Thus, results obtained are heterogeneous with respect to the pattern of variables that are affected by the interventions (Field et al., 2006a, 2004, 1999; Teixeira et al., 2005).

Among the interventions, yoga therapies (Satyapriya et al., 2009; Narendran et al., 2005) and PMR over a longer period (Nickel et al., 2006; Field et al., 1999, 2004) are more likely to enhance psycho-biological well-being (Field et al., 1999) compared to massage therapy and a PMR relaxation group over 5 weeks. The massaged pregnant women showed reduced anxiety levels and stress hormones, fewer sleep disturbances, and fewer incidences of back pain and obstetric and postnatal complications. Only women in the PMR group had decreased anxiety levels after their first session.

Teixeira et al. (2005) investigated active versus passive relaxation techniques in pregnant women. Active relaxation was based on hypnotherapeutic methods, whereas women in the passive relaxation group sat quietly and read women's fashion magazines. A reduction in anxiety and heart rate, but not in stress hormones, was found in the women who participated in active relaxation. The effects of passive relaxation were comparable to those evoked by active relaxation. The outcomes of these studies indicate that different relaxation techniques can have different impacts on psycho-biological well-being in pregnant women.

Urech et al. (2010) evaluated the effects of a brief PMR and GI relaxation exercise, as well as a passive relaxation control condition, on pregnant women's psychological, endocrine and cardiovascular activity. Results indicated specific beneficial effects of the active relaxation techniques on pregnant women's psychological and/or cardiovascular state. Specifically, the GI condition was more effective for inducing relaxation than PMR. In addition, the GI, but not the PMR condition, was more effective in increasing self-reported relaxation than a passive relaxation control condition. Moreover, participants were more comfortable with GI than PMR. By including both physiological level assessment and self-reported experience, a discrepancy emerged between the two approaches. Apparently, the muscle relaxation exercises were more effective on cardiovascular arousal, whereas guided imagery achieved better results in terms of subjective relaxation measures. The implication for clinical practice is related to the importance of choosing psychological interventions that can be easily perceived as effective. Since GI is a comfortable relaxation technique and appears to be especially suitable to participants, it is likely that this technique will enhance compliance in pregnant women in a longer-term exercise program. Tragea and colleagues (2014) have recently examined the effectiveness of two relaxation techniques (progressive muscle relaxation and diaphragmatic breathing) during pregnancy. The results of the study demonstrate significant benefits from the use of the techniques in the pregnant women's psychological state. The systematic implementation of the proposed relaxation techniques contributed to a reduction in perceived stress and anxiety and increased the women's sense of internal control. Authors also found changes in many lifestyle factors to be associated with stress.

Mindfulness for Pregnant Women

Mindfulness constitutes another effective approach in symptom reduction and general health improvements in pregnancy, such as management of anxiety, depression, back pain, and stress (Kabat-Zinn, 1994). Preliminary data supporting the potential benefits of mindfulness in the perinatal period has been found by Dunn and colleagues (2012). Based on that and other recent pilot studies (Duncan and Bardacke, 2009; Vieten and Astin 2008), it is possible to suggest that women who learn mindfulness during pregnancy are likely to use those skills to manage stressful aspects of pregnancy, childbirth and parenting, resulting in reductions in psychological distress and improvements in psychological well-being. Specifically, Duncan and Bardacke (2010) found that a mindfulness-based childbirth and parenting education program led to reductions in anxiety and depression; also, positive affect increased in women during the third trimester of pregnancy (Duncan & Bardacke, 2010). Similarly, Vieten and Astin (2008) carried out a study evaluating a psychosocial mindfulness-based intervention administered in the second half of pregnancy, and they found reductions in anxiety and negative mood when compared to wait list control. Altogether these pioneer researches indicate the importance of teaching mindfulness in the perinatal period and the potential effect of improving the developmental trajectory of parents and infants by broadening women's personal repertoire of coping strategies (Dunn et al., 2012).

Enhancing Maternal Integration and Connectedness (Social Perspective)

Abundant evidence suggests that social support from family, friends, co-workers, and other social ties is associated with physical health and psychological well-being in different phases of the lifespan (House et al., 1988).

Social support plays a critical role in reducing the risk of depression and stress susceptibility and improving overall maternal well-being (Stice et al., 2004; Israel et al., 2002; Mathiesen et al., 1999). For this reason, social support may be especially important to consider as a protective factor for mothers during pregnancy (Dunkel-Schetter, 2011). It is possible to identify several persons that could contribute to the psychological well-being of future mothers. Professionals at different levels can provide information about prenatal care and assistance with daily tasks that are burdensome, as well as caring about and understanding stressors. Emotional support can also come from a husband/partner and friends, and it can be an emotional buffer that shields individuals from the negative effects of stress and depression (Campbell et al., 2009; Cooper et al., 2009; Mulsow et al., 2002).

The role of social and marital support has been extensively studied concerning antenatal depression, as documented by a recent review (Lancaster et al. 2010), while just a few studies (Roos et al., 2013; Nasreen et al., 2011) have investigated the relationship between social and marital support and antenatal anxiety.

Social support is significantly associated with psychological well-being in pregnancy (Dunkel-Schetter et al., 1996; Dunkel-Schetter, 2011). Specifically, several studies underline the association between quality of support, support satisfaction, perceived availability of support and actual receipt of support and significantly less prenatal and postpartum depression, less anxiety, fewer stressors, and improved health (e.g., Oakley et al., 1996; Collins et al., 1993; Tietjen & Bradley, 1985; Oakley, 1990, 1992; Cutrona, 1984).

INTEGRATING TECHNOLOGIES INTO MOTHER-TO-BE WELL-BEING: CURRENT SCENARIOS

E-health and m-health are becoming the new way to promote healthcare by using information and communication technologies worldwide (Watterson et al., 2015; Bert et al., 2013). The rapid expansion of web access and mobile technologies gives the opportunity to improve well-being by fostering healthy behavior, reducing risky behavior and extending prevention and care-seeking culture. Internet and mobile technologies may represent a low-cost solution to cope with some global health challenges like lack of health care providers, lack of information or limited training for health workers (Watterson et al., 2015;).

New technologies offer new strategies to achieve the United Nation Millennium Development Goals (MDGs). Mobile phones and smartphones may offer easy health information access and provide support and skills to face with a specific health condition; these devices can also be used by care providers to monitor health status, offer training, answer questions and stay in touch with their patients (Rotheram-Borus et al., 2012).

A key factor in achieving MDG5 and improving maternal health is a healthier pregnancy that implies less risk of pregnancy-related complications and lower fetal and infant mortality rates (MDG4).

Pregnancy, in fact, can be considered a unique "teachable moment" for health and wellness interventions: women in this phase of their life are willing to make significant behavioral changes to improve fetus and maternal health. According to

Peyton (2014) and Rotheram-Borus et al. (2012), although pregnant women lack pregnancy-related information, they are interested in nutrition, diet, exercise, growth stages of the fetus, gestational diseases, emotional states and fluctuation and more general information on pregnancy from the very beginning.

Internet, smartphones and mobile services are more and more being considered the best information source by pregnant women (Lagan et al., 2011) because they are able to offer new and powerful instruments to promote positive emotional states and to develop coping skills in order to let women live an aware, informed and healthy pregnancy.

The current scenario includes several technologies that will be described in the next paragraphs. First, the Internet, which is used both as a source of information and a source of social support, as well as to support self-help psychological training. Second, mobile services and mobile applications are designed to suggest correct behaviors and to meet pregnant women's different needs.

Internet as a Source of Information and Social Support

The Internet is changing our relationship with health: today we have easy access to information on diseases, treatments and healthy behavior, and we can find answers to all of our questions in a click.

Pregnancy-related websites are more and more available on the Internet and pregnancy e-health is now practiced worldwide. According to Lagan and colleagues, in 2011 there were almost 136 million websites containing pregnancy-related information online and these sites' usage by pregnant women is constantly growing (Lagan et al., 2011).

According to a recent survey, the usage rate of the Internet amongst pregnant women is massive: participants affirmed to have used the Internet at least 10 times during their pregnancy. They also stated that they were mainly interested in antenatal or intrapartum issues and complications of pregnancy (Lagan et al., 2010). The Internet is often used to obtain further information about things mentioned by health care providers, or for assistance in making conscious decisions related to pregnancy and childbirth (epidural, induction or cesarean, etc). Sixty-three percent of women are influenced by Internet content in thinking and managing their pregnancy and childbirth (Lagan et al., 2010).

E-health consultations may help women feel empowered and informed enough to become "expert patients," able to negotiate their health care in an active and proactive manner with careful research and self-education (Johnson, 2014).

According to some studies, pregnant women consider online resources one of the main sources of useful information (Hearn et al., 2014; O' Higgins et al., 2014): women regularly use the Internet to get information and consider it the third most useful source of information after family and friends (O'Higgins et al., 2014). In some cases, women stated that the Internet is the only source they used to seek information about pregnancy (Lagan et al., 2010), or that it was their second source of information after doctors (Lima-Pereira et al., 2013).

E-health represents a common practice worldwide: a U.S. survey affirms that more than 75% of pregnant women practiced pregnancy e-health (Declercq et al., 2007). In Italy, around 95% of the women in the sample were Internet users, and almost all of them used the Internet for pregnancy-related topics (Bert et al., 2013). In Spain, the 95.5% of women interviewed reported daily Internet access (Lima-Pereira et al., 2013). In Sweden, 91% of women have access to the Internet and 84% of women used the Internet as source of information on pregnancy (Larsson, 2009). In China, the data are similar to those of the Western world (Gao et al., 2013).

This new trend in managing health raises theoretical and practical issues, such as ensuring quality and trustworthiness of content and avoiding the risk of misunderstandings or incomplete comprehension by women.

Although women consider the information they retrieve online good and useful, sometimes they don't have the appropriate knowledge to evaluate the quality of online content. Nevertheless, they would like to be oriented in choosing reliable sites or online content from healthcare providers (Lagan et al., 2010; Hearn et al., 2014; Romano, 2007). Thus, healthcare professionals may play an important role in safeguarding well-being, guiding mothers in online searches and recommending high-quality websites (O'Higgins et al., 2014; Bert et al., 2013; Larsson, 2009).

The Internet doesn't just meet the need for information. The web, in fact, is becoming a new way of finding social support: pregnant women access the Internet to share information through online discussion forums and to find support from other pregnant women or new mothers. By belonging to groups, even virtual ones, women can reduce their anxiety and feelings of isolation, receive reassurances and feel helped and relieved in the decision-making process (Lagan et al., 2010).

One possible reason for seeking support online may be the decline of the extended family: in the past, extended family members accompanied women in this transition to motherhood, but now, because of frequent loss of proximity, women may feel isolated and lonely. Discussion forums, social media platforms and online communities provide places to exchange advice, information and support (Miyata, 2002, Sharf, 1997, Preece, 2001, Wellman and Frank, 2001). Generating a sense of community with other women going through similar experiences can reduce loneliness (O'Higgins et al, 2014). Thanks to online resources, mothers-to-be can find a sense of belonging to a social community and social support, both of which are so important for their psychological well-being (Dunkel-Schetter et al., 1996; 2001). Online forums can promote individual empowerment by the sharing of information, which furthers the demand for accurate data and challenges health professionals (Lima-Pereira et al., 2012)

Internet forums enable women to connect with people with the same interests or that are living the same experience. In this way virtual communities are able to offer support, comfort, answers and a space where women can vent and share their private emotions and fears (Romano, 2007).

Several advantages have contributed to make the Internet so popular in this specific phase of life: not only the anonymity and the asynchronous communication, but also the convenience and the effectiveness.

Anonymity is fundamental: women appreciate the opportunity to talk about their pregnancies and doubts anonymously before announcing their pregnancy to their families, and even after because anonymity reduces shame for sharing private matters (sex and sexuality, vaginal bleeding and discharge or emotional changes in pregnancy and early parenthood, discomfort of pregnancy, breast changes, etc.). Online it is possible to anonymously post questions and receive answers, comfort and support. Anonymity lets women feel free to ask and talk about every aspect of pregnancy or private life and enables them to receive support and suggestions for every topic. No "silly" demands exist online; everybody can feel free to ask any questions without fear of judgment.

Asynchronous communication allows mothers-to-be to get in touch with friends or other mothers when and how they prefer, especially at night in the last trimester when sleep becomes difficult.

On Facebook, one of the most famous social networks in the world, people can share information, photos and emoticons about their lives in every moment and keep in touch with friends and family members, allowing the creation of social capital, which is essential for well-being (Johnson, 2014). As Bartholomew pointed out, "Facebook serves an important function in the acquisition of social capital and social support resources, which are beneficial at the transition to parenthood" (Bartholomew et al., 2012: 464).

Immediacy, easiness, convenience, effectiveness, interactivity, clarity and control are other aspects that make surfing the Web so appealing (Lagan et al., 2010). Women can access the Internet instantly from home, the workplace or public spaces (thanks to wireless access and mobile phones) without going out, wasting time or waiting for a medical consultation (Romano, 2007).

Web-Based Training Programs

More and more people are looking for self-help programs to enhance their well-being and health, which is consistent with the rapid growth of web-based interventions and smartphone apps in behavioral healthcare (Luxton et al., 2011). Self-help programs, such as interventions that people practice individually without contact with a professional in the field, have been demonstrated to be effective in helping people enhance their quality of life (Haug et al., 2012 ; Newman et al., 2011; Cuijpers et al., 2010; Sethi et al., 2010; Van Vliet and Andrews, 2009; Williams et al., 2001).

This type of intervention is supported by technologies that enable individuals to overcome limits related to traditional support, such as time, resources, flexibility, accessibility and availability (Taylor and Luce, 2003).

Internet-based interventions have been demonstrated to be effective in reducing depression, anxiety, phobias and addictions; Web-based programs are salutary for people suffering from these diseases and successful in reaching woman with lower socio-economic status (Haga et al., 2013)

Web-based applications consist of self-help programs that are able to enhance personal empowerment and support women during pregnancy or at the beginning of motherhood. These are nowadays becoming a new strategy to promote subjective well-being and deal with pregnancy concerns, such as the risks of post-partum depression. Table 1 is a selection of some promising web-based programs.

Mobile Services

The Global Observatory for eHealth (GOe) of the World Health Organization (WHO) defines m-health or mobile health as the "medical and public health practice supported by mobile devices, such as mobile phones, patient monitoring devices, personal digital assistants (PDAs), and other wireless devices." According to the World Health Organization (WHO), m-health can play an important role in promoting healthier pregnancy not only in developing countries, but also in lower income populations in developed states.

M-health may represent a booster for healthier pregnancy management. As a part of the "continuum of care" of the modern clinic and community, it can be useful to encourage correct behavior (physical exercise and weight control), provide clear and focused health information and help women become competent and learn skills to cope with physical and emotional changes in pregnancy (Peyton et al., 2014; Tamrat et al, 2012).

Mobile communication makes quick, low-cost and widespread healthcare services feasible; text SMS, voice call or IVR (Interactive Voice Response) offer the opportunity to reach a big part of the target population (including those living in rural and poor areas).

Mobile devices enable efficient perinatal education campaigns. Thanks to advice and personalized "tips" sent by text or voice-recorded messages, it is possible to suggest correct behaviors and make mothers more aware of information pertaining to pregnancy, dangerous symptoms, proper nutrition and risky behavior. Free vouchers for healthcare providers are a further well-being booster (Lund et al., 2014).

Table 1. Examples of Web-based programs for the well-being of pregnant women and new mothers

Name and Location	Description	Technical Features	Clinical Approach/ Results
Mamma Mia (Haga et al., 2013) Norway	This is a free, Web-based self-help intervention designed to reduce the risk of postpartum depression and to promote subjective well-being in pregnant women or new mothers with mild-to-moderate symptoms of depression. The program consists of 44 sessions over a period of 11 months: for each session, the user receives an email with a hyperlink; by activating the link, the user gains access to Mamma Mia and proceeds in a predetermined sequence of Web pages.	• Free • Self-help intervention • Compatible with different operating systems • English language • Attractive content and interfaces • Discussion forum	• Assessment of depressive symptoms, metacognitive therapy, positive psychology, couples therapy, breastfeeding, and psycho-education • First trial feedback is positive both in terms of acceptability and effectiveness by women and their partners
MomMoodBooster (Danaher et al., 2013) Australia	This is a free web-based program to help new mothers deal with postpartum depression. The program consists of sox sessions (Getting Started, Managing Mood, Increasing Pleasant Activities, Managing Negative Thoughts, Increasing Positive Thoughts and Planning for the Future) introduced by a video explaining the session goal. Participants can complete the program in 6-12 weeks (every session can be completed in 2 weeks) with 6-12 coach calls. It proposes different interactive activities designed to encourage participant engagement and behavioral change.	• Free • Self-help intervention • Compatible with different operating systems • English language • Attractive and interactive content and interfaces • Discussion forum • Coach calls	• Based on Milgrom's adaptation of the Coping With Depression Course (CWDC) for postpartum depression as well as an adaptation of the CWDC for Web-based delivery • A pilot study tested the efficacy with a clinical sample of 53 women recruited from the United States and Australia. Women were very engaged with the program and showed significant clinical improvements.
MODIAB-web (Adolfsson et al., 2014) Sweden	This is a web-based support for pregnant women and new mothers with type 1 diabetes mellitus that aims to promote well-being and diabetes management. It consists of three parts: 1) evidence-based information (being pregnant, labor and childbirth, and life as a new mother); 2) a self-care diary for self-reported monitoring; and 3) a discussion forum for peer support moderated by the research group.	• Free • Self-help intervention • Compatible with different operating systems • Swedish language • Discussion forum	• Based on a holistic approach • Provides person-centered support in addition to usual care • The first trial is supposed to be completed in February 2016

The "text4baby" (Parker et al., 2012) program is an effective and successful example of mobile phone education training. In the United States, future moms can sign up for the "text4baby" service by sending a text message with their child's expected birth date and postal code. They will receive three messages a week offering evidence-based information relevant to the stage of pregnancy they are in; each message includes a toll-free telephone number linked to low-cost services related to the message topic that are consistent with the mother's location.

The IVR system (Interactive Voice Response) is an alternative tool to provide similar interventions for illiterate or less educated people. "Aponjon" is a Voice (IVR) and SMS mobile health service that provides weekly text and voice health messages to pregnant women, mothers with newborn babies and their family members in Bangladesh. Aponjon gives reliable and accurate messages about pregnancy symptoms, nutrition and obstetric danger signs congruent with the week of pregnancy or the age of the baby (Ahsan & Raihan, 2013).

Mobile Apps

New intervention areas are continuously emerging thanks to smartphones and mobile applications. In 2012, according to global research and consulting firm Strategy Analytics (2014), the number of active smartphone users worldwide was 1 billion; another billion will become smartphone users by 2015.

Smartphones and apps have significantly expanded healthcare possibilities. According to research2guidance reports, 500 million smartphone users worldwide will use at least one mHealth app by 2015. By 2018 it is forecasted that more than 50% of smartphone and tablet users will have downloaded m-health applications (Research2guidance 2014 and 2015 report).

According to the European Commission's Green Paper on mobile health (2014), mobile health covers medical and public health practice supported by mobile devices, such as mobile phones. It also includes applications (''apps'') that are primarily intended to maintain or improve healthy behaviors, quality of life and the well-being of individuals directly or indirectly. Mobile apps can encourage adherence to a healthy lifestyle, resulting in more personalized treatments.

These new media may be capable of providing educational and training content that can help future mothers satisfy their need of communication, information and connection with others (Tripp et al., 2014; Romano, 2007).

According to some researchers, smartphones are the most common devices used by pregnant women who are active Internet users. Further, the mobile versions of websites are preferred to static resources because of their ubiquitous accessibility (Hearn et al., 2014; Waring et al., 2014).

These new devices have features capable of enabling pregnant women to communicate, track the progress of their pregnancy and alleviate their anxiety thorough interactive professional and private consultation (Tripp et al., 2014).

According to Rotheram-Borus and colleagues, there are six foundational functions for m-health interventions for pregnant women (Rotheram-Borus et al., 2014):

1. Informing about health, behaviors and resources;
2. Training, sending text messages, calls, pictures, or even videos that recommend the desired behaviors;
3. Monitoring behavior in real time to help people in adopting new habits;
4. Shaping healthy behaviors thanks to feedback, prompts, alerts, reminders, encouragement, and rewards provided at the right moment;
5. Supporting development and maintenance by linking women to peers, friends, family, or healthcare workers for social support and instrumental support services;
6. Linking to hospitals, clinical or emergency services to better manage critical situations.

Jihye and Iftekahr (Jihye and Iftekhar, 2016) analyzed some international pregnancy apps according to the framework created by Rotheram-Borus and colleagues and pointed out that apps generally contain more than one function (e.g., informing, training, monitoring, shaping and linking).

According to Jihye and Iftekahr's study, the informing function is important for users but not critical to app adoption because of the availability of other information services and online materials.

It is well known that pregnancy increases the need for information and that women surf the Web to find rapid and complete answers to their questions (Lagan et al., 2010, Lagan et al., 2011). Additionally, as the months pass, women show different informational needs. At an early stage they want information about indicators of pregnancy or dietary concerns, food aversion, banned food and, advice for vomiting and nausea. Then in the second trimester they desire to know more about unusual symptoms, and during the last trimester they are more and more focused on childbirth events (premature birth, epidural, hospital quality) or newborn parenting questions (Peyton et al., 2014).

This deep need for information does not seem satisfied by printed material. Brochures and leaflets are perceived as too general and lacking details, and they are often lost or discarded; books are considered expensive, difficult to search in, and limited in view.

Pregnancy apps are able to provide an appropriate, positive and effective response to these problems. Informative apps are the most common and usually provide a large range of general information about pregnancy, fetus development, maternal nutrition, advice and information on diseases such as gestational diabetes.

Among informative apps, women show a clear preference for interactive ones, which allow women to enter their personal information and then get recommendations and suggestions "tailor-made".

The users receive advice and information related to their specific gestational week, which helps them experience a new level of awareness of the responsbilities of pregnancy (Johnson, 2014). These apps often show 3D images of a developing fetus, reminders for healthcare appointments, pregnancy milestones, timely advice about pregnancy symptomatology, info on foods and weight and exercises to engage in, all of which have the possibility to invoke behavioral change as a result (monitoring and shaping functions).

Monitoring and shaping functions are crucial in keeping people using apps. It has been demonstrated that mobile phones may be acceptable for monitoring or self-monitoring by much of the population. Their behaviors—reminders, alarms, warnings and supportive messages—effectively promote healthy behavior including cessation of smoking, managing diabetes, engaging in physical activities and weight control (Rotheram-Borus et al., 2014). Some apps, for example, include a "bump photos" section, a feature which allows women to create a gallery of images of their growing baby bump. This capability may be a way to develop more awareness of pregnancy and to promote healthy behaviors and bonding (Johnson, 2014).

Supporting functions include features that enable women to obtain social support thanks to mobile online communities.

An interesting example of peer-to-peer support promoted by SMS contact is the Diabetes Buddy project. The Diabetes Buddies program is a pilot project to promote a healthy lifestyle and better management of diabetes thanks to reciprocal support among women in South Africa. During the course of 12 weeks, women were able to contact each other outside of the group sessions by a mobile phone; this allowed ongoing support between buddies. Furthermore, one SMS (or probe) was sent daily to each participant with the goal of helping the women gather information to use in the management of their disease (Rotheram-Borus et al., 2012).

The linking function is the least developed feature at the moment, but it is the one that can become the real "killer" capability. This function allows the app to be integrated into the overall system of healthcare and make a quick connection between women and health professionals. Thanks to the development of wireless sensors, apps can monitor physiological data (heartbeat, breathing, fetus hearth rate, glucose levels) and transmit them instantly to medical centers to get immediate support or medical contact.

Many apps providing data on fetus well-being (such as Baby Heart Monitors and Pregnancy Calculator) already exist, but without a direct connection or supervision with medical personnel, they are likely to become a source of anxiety rather than help (Tripp et al., 2014).

Smartphone technologies and apps, thanks to their always being in our pockets, may offer a new strategy to promote self-health practices more effectively than other existing material (Jihye and Iftekhar, 2016; Johnson, 2014). They are not simply an extension of traditional static forms of self-help, but a new way of using resources through a device in a variety of locations and even whilst multitasking.

Apps and social media are not simply sources of information; they also operate as performative devices in that they push women to act on and through their bodies via these devices (Johnson, 2014). They enable interactive and customized use more effective in promoting change in behavior than usual self-help tools (Hearn et al., 2014).

Last but not least, finding a pregnancy-related app on the Web is simple, low-cost and accessible to everyone. A quick Internet search with basic words (pregnancy, antenatal parent education, fetus, etc.) can be sufficient to find an app, and people can install these apps on their mobile devices without hassle and sometimes even for free.

In Table 2 we reported some examples of popular international pregnancy-related apps.

Apps and online resources may also play an important role in promoting psychological well-being of pregnant women. The availability of high-quality health information can decrease feelings of anxiety and stress born from the doubts and uncertainties that pregnancy naturally generates and increase a sense of control and self-efficacy in women. These new interactive and tailor-made tools are more likely to persuade women to change their lifestyles than are traditional tool kits. Training, monitoring and shaping functions can become a "good coach" in causing change.

Apps are becoming a guide for pregnant women, and for this reason it is important to guarantee content quality and reliability to avoid increases in anxiety or misleading interpretation of data.

E-health and m-health still have great potential available to exploit, but healthcare professionals are fundamental in supporting this process. It would be good if care providers became an integral part of this system; they could protect women from e-health practice risks and promote e-health and mobile e-health both by filling the information gap and guiding women in online searches (Tripp et al., 2014; Bert et al., 2013; Romano, 2007).

Table 2. Examples of mobile apps for pregnancy well-being

App/Developer	Main Features	Informing	Training	Monitoring	Shaping	Supporting	Linking
My Pregnancy Today – BabyCenter	• Free • For IoS and Android • Customizable • English language	√	√	√	√	√	
I'm Expecting – pregnancy app - MedHelp, Inc	• Free • For IoS and Android • Customizable • English language	√		√	√	√	
Dr. Miriam Stoppard Pregnancy - Dorling Kindersley	• Paid • For IoS and Android • Customizable • English language • Antenatal bonding functions	√	√	√	√	√	
Healthy you, healthy baby - Ngala Organization	• Free • For IoS (Android not available) • Customizable • English language • Activities during pregnancy to the first 18 months of motherhood	√		√	√	√	
Happy Pregnancy Ticker – Softcraft system and solutions private limited	• Free • For IoS and Android • Customizable • English language	√	√	√	√	√	√
I'm Pregnant - Kolsoft	• Free • For IoS and Android • Customizable • English language	√	√		√		√

BenEssere Mamma, The Application

In recent years, many mobile apps for mental health have been developed and have demonstrated good potential for stress and anxiety management (Preziosa et al., 2009; Villani et al., 2012; Villani et al., 2013; Repetto et al., 2013). Typically they include several relaxation training approaches, but recently meditation has also been successfully included in self-help interventions supported by new technologies (Warnecke et al., 2011; Sharma et al., 2012; Cavanagh et al., 2013; Ahtinen et al., 2013; Chittaro and Vianello, 2014; Ly et al., 2014).

Nowadays, thanks to new mobile technologies like the Internet, social networks and mobile applications, it is possible to reach more and more mothers-to-be than through traditional methods. Pregnant women's ability to easily find information, give suggestions and tips and support each other in this delicate and magical life phase has helped reduce risks and dangers for them and for their unborn children.

Starting from these premises, the app BenEssere Mamma was developed to help pregnant women better manage anxiety and stress, especially in the last trimester of pregnancy, and better cope with childbirth.

BenEssere Mamma consists of a brief self-help protocol containing mindfulness meditation and guided imagery exercises delivered through a smartphone to reduce stress during pregnancy and to restore levels of energy and well-being. The creators of the app intend it to be a response to the desire of pregnant women to promote their wellness without investing too much time in courses that sometimes barely fit into working life (women are entitled to maternity leave starting two months prior to the expected date of delivery). The app aims to help women recognize, bring out and use their resources that are designed to promote awareness of their potential in addressing problems and difficulties related to pregnancy and childbirth. It is a personal empowerment app: a four-week self-help program that includes daily relaxation exercises to reduce anxiety and perceived stress level of pregnant women.

Reducing anxiety and negative mood can reduce the risk of postnatal depression. The application includes activities and materials that can be divided into the following areas:

- An *informative area*, to increase knowledge about stress, relaxation and its salutary effects:
    - The "Good to Know" section, containing explanations about stress, pregnancy and relaxation practices;
    - "Other practices," (see Figure 1) consisting of first-hand descriptions of the relaxation exercises and explanations about how they function;
- An *emotional awareness area*, called the "mood journal:" in this section it is possible to record notes on emotional state, thoughts and events to become aware of what influences mood and thus develop confidence in one's own ability to change negative emotional states and the correlated physiological activation. Expectant mothers are guided with positive emoticons (see Figure 1) to recognize and assess their mood day-by-day to improve awareness of their emotional state and what affects it. This daily practice allows women to recognize when their negative moods subside and to identify possible events, feelings, thoughts and emotions that influence it. The objective is to develop a different way of thinking about their minds. Thanks to meditation exercises and daily mood mapping, pregnant women can realize the variability of

their moods and consciously accept and recognize the link between mood, emotions and thoughts, sometimes unwanted. In this way it is possible to start breaking the usual and automatic routine that perpetuates difficulties and issues. Discovering what affects women's state of mind allows them to avoid behaviors and automatic thoughts that lead to a recurrence of the disorder; for example, focusing attention on the present moment rather than keeping minds on the past or the future. Awareness can help expectant mothers recognize early symptoms of post-partum or pregnancy depression and ask for support as soon as possible.

- An *experiential area*, called "your path:" a set of 20 daily exercises, each lasting about 10 minutes (5 days a week for 4 weeks), such as breath meditation, visualizations and listening to music/natural sounds. Several types of exercises are proposed to allow users to experiment with different practices and find the one they like best.
    - **Breathing Meditation:** These practices invite users to sit in a calm and peaceful location and focus their attention on breath and bodily movement (particularly of the chest and belly). When the mind wanders, the mother-to-be is invited to notice what distracted her and then return to observing her breathing. This practice consists of mindful breathing and thought distancing. In terms of mindful breathing, participants learned how to direct their attention to the sensations of breathing and to notice when their mind wandered away; in terms of thought distancing, participants had to try to perceive thoughts as ''events'' in their minds, simply observing the process of thought.
    - **Body Scan Exercises:** To strengthen the connection between the mind and the body, which is essential in facilitating childbirth. Body scan meditation is a form of Vipassana meditation that helps to expand mind/body awareness, release tension and quiet the mind. It is an effective meditation technique for strengthening concentration, focusing attention, relaxing the breath and making body-mind connection stronger.
    - **Imagery and Positive Visualizations:** Which can be considered a way the mind uses to communicate with the body (in some way this represents the biological connection between mind and body). It is really important for pregnant women to recover their body-mind connection so they will be able to cope with fear, pain and fatigue during childbirth. Different typologies of visualizations are proposed within the app:
        - **Safe Place Visualizations:** That invite a pregnant woman to imagine herself in a quiet, peaceful and secure place to rest and to release anxieties, worries and thoughts, allowing her to come out of this imagery with a sense of comfort and refreshment. For

example, mothers-to-be were encouraged to imagine "a luminous sphere" and visualize the image's form, color and flow, and to focus attention on how they are feeling. The voice guide suggested desired psychological states and emotions (e.g., "You feel calm, You feel relaxed, Your body is calm and relaxed, also your baby is relaxed") to induce them. These images may mediate the communication between perception, emotion and physiological change and may induce a positive physiological process such as reducing the stress reaction and related stress symptoms (Schaub et al., 1995)

- **Baby in Womb Meditations:** Are exercises designed to create particular imagery during a state of direct connection with the baby to strengthen the relationship between mother and child. This connection can prepare mother and child for the childbirth, an event that marks the end of one past (pregnancy) and the beginning of a new one (motherhood).
- **Inner Smile Meditations:** Are designed to start a developed, healthy and loving relationship with themselves. These exercises create a strong mind-body connection and can relax both the body and and mind. The aim of constant practice is to improve the ability to accept oneself, exactly as one is, to promote self-esteem as well as love and acceptance for others.

- A *professional support link*, to take care of questions or doubts, is provided through the button "SOS" (the "contact me" section). Women can send an e-mail asking for information or psychological orientation to a psychologist, in addition to a range of information about stress, pregnancy and techniques for mental and physical relaxation.

Social support functions at the moment have not been implemented to avoid the risk of increased anxiety due to emotional contagion, which is common in mom-to-be communities. In the future, the app could be enhanced by including a virtual community that would be constantly monitored and supervised by health professionals (midwives, psychologists, doctors, etc.).

The app BenEssere Mamma strives to be a complement to existing courses in childbirth preparation, offering techniques to manage anxiety, stress and fear of childbirth and to allow future moms to better enjoy the experience of becoming mothers without forcing them to attend a course with fixed times and places.

Through practice, mothers-to-be can increase awareness of the present moment and of thoughts, feelings and body sensations. Mindfulness can help them, both during pregnancy and during labor, to deal with their feelings in a conscious way and to avoid reacting automatically on the basis of habits and rigid behavioral patterns.

Daily practice is critical to transform mindfulness meditation in a real habit, a way of being and living, and pregnant users will become able to relax more and more quickly and on demand.

Thanks to BenEssere Mamma, expectant mothers can practice meditation when and where they want, acquiring day-by-day familiarity with meditation and their constant changes, increasing confidence in their abilities and developing greater awareness of their own emotional states and confidence in their ability to generate positive emotional states.

BenEssere Mamma aims to help mothers-to-be develop critical skills useful in promoting the health of women and their children. Greater emotional awareness and confidence in personal abilities can help women accept their emotional state. It is fundamental to change the Western culture model that considers it unacceptable for pregnant women and new mothers to be sad, angry, unhappy, worried and distressed. Sadness, anxiety, and distress are often a part of the transition to motherhood, and women have to live these emotional experiences and ask for help if they need to be supported. Women who are more aware of their psychological status can accept their supposedly "inadequate" emotions and thus feel comfortable asking for professional help without waiting for months. Thanks to this app, emotions, both good and bad, can become familiar and acceptable as a part of this special time.

Additionally, emotional awareness and self-confidence can make depressive symptoms more recognizable and thus reduce depression risk. Postnatal depression is the most frequent complication occurring after pregnancy and affects about 10–15% of new mothers in Western countries; it can even evolve into puerperal psychosis, with an incidence of 0.2%, usually in the first weeks after childbirth but also after a few months.

Some studies have affirmed that symptoms of depression can be common and severe during pregnancy. Watson et al. declared that 23% of women with postnatal depression showed symptoms during pregnancy (Watson et al., 1984). Thus, it is important to understand, recognize and treat antenatal depression (Evans et al., 2001).

By increasing their mindfulness about their capabilities and self-esteem, women will be able to more quickly recognize the symptoms of depression and deal with them from the beginning, thereby avoiding negative consequences on the bond between mother and newborn. BenEssere Mamma can make women familiar with mood variability and help them to manage anxiety and negative emotions during pregnancy, reducing the risk of ante- and post-natal depression.

Figure 1. App home page, the other relaxing practices menu and mood diary emoticons

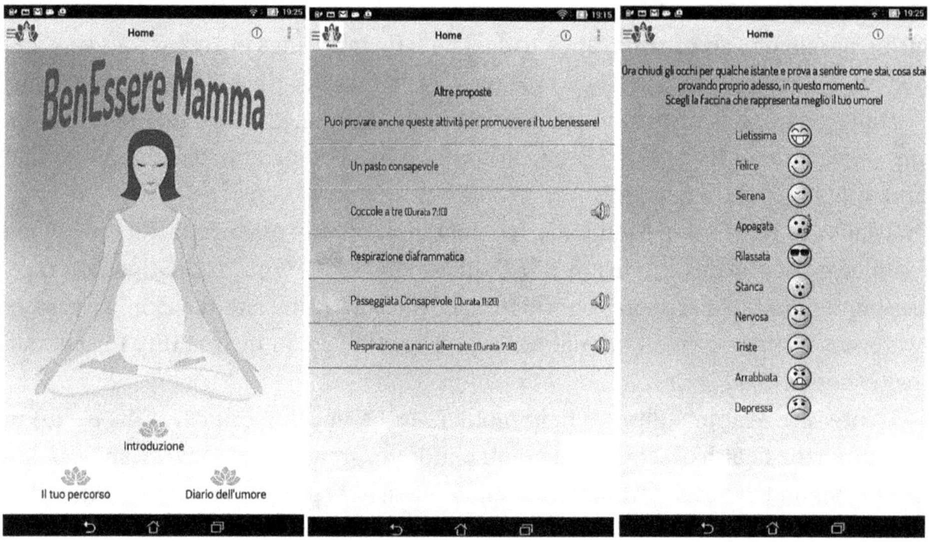

FUTURE RESEARCH DIRECTIONS

Despite the growing recent literature about the emergency model of pregnancy care, wherein technologies are included and the scientific rationale of this approach seems to confirm the potentialities, to our knowledge very few studies have investigated the outcomes of many websites and pregnancy-related apps.

Given the paucity of contributions in this field, future research should use controlled studies to test the short-term and long-term outcomes of these services to well-being during pregnancy and to specific disease prevention, particularly for depression. Furthermore, research about possible inconveniences and negative effects of online and mobile services should be considered.

Thus, BenEssere Mamma at the moment represents a good proposal that has been tested to verify its effectiveness in promoting psychological well-being and positive affective state and in reducing anxiety, stress, negative mood and post-natal depression risk through controlled trials.

CONCLUSION

Pregnancy is a complex phase in a woman's life characterized by physiological and psychological changes that can enhance anxiety or negative emotional states and favor risky behaviors (Lindgren, 2001).

Women's well-being during pregnancy is important for them as well as for the development of the child and the course of the pregnancy (Dayan et al., 2002; Hoffman & Hatch, 2000; Dunkel-Schetter, 1998; Austin et al., 2007; Grant et al., 2008).

By following the three levels of well-being identified by Keyes and Lopez (2002)—high emotional well-being, high psychological well-being, and high social well-being—this chapter proposes three critical aspects to take into consideration in order to improve quality of life and well-being during pregnancy. These aspects include the importance of positive affective states, the need to enhance the psychological skills of mothers in regulating their affective states through relaxation and meditation protocols, and the role of social support given by several persons (professionals as well as family, friends, co-workers and others).

Today, new technologies are becoming emergent tools to meet these needs. Thanks to their ubiquity, multimodality, interactivity, ease of use and sociality, new technologies allow pregnant women to communicate with each other and with health professionals, to share information, to constantly monitor their pregnancy status, to assume and maintain correct and healthy behaviors and to develop personal skills to better deal with impending childbirth and motherhood; they can even learn to relieve their stress in an interactive and fast way (Tripp et al., 2014; Peyton et al., 2014).

Many websites and pregnancy-related apps are already available in the market, and the popularity of these services amongst pregnant women indicates a shift towards patient empowerment within maternity care provision.

Although the Internet and mobile devices offer several advantages, up to now very few self-help interventions have been tested. Thus, it is not possible at the moment to come to a conclusion about the effectiveness of this approach.

At the end of the chapter, an Italian app (BenEssere Mamma) developed by the authors and intended to help pregnant women promote and take care of their well-being was described. Specifically, the app proposes an intervention based on the three levels of well-being. The goal of this app, which includes a four-week self-help intervention based on daily relaxation and meditation exercises, is to increase women's confidence in their abilities to generate positive emotional states and help them to develop new coping skills and a greater awareness of their own emotional states.

Making women better informed and more self-efficacious in managing their psychological state and their behavior represents an important goal. Prompted by positive technologies, mothers-to-be can become more engaged in care. This emerging model of pregnancy care will make the lives of pregnant women easier and more fulfilling and could also be critical in reducing possible healthcare and social costs.

ACKNOWLEDGMENT

This work was partially supported by the Italian funded project "VRehab. Virtual Reality in the Assessment and TeleRehabilitation of Parkinson's Disease and Post-Stroke Disabilities" - RF-2009-1472190.

REFERENCES

500m people will be using healthcare mobile applications in 2015. (2015). Research2guidance. Retrieved from http://research2guidance.com/500m-people-will-be-usinghealthcare-mobile-applications-in-2015/

Adolfsson, A., Linden, K., Sparud-Lundin, C., Larsson, P. G., & Berg, M. (2014). A web-based support for pregnant women and new mothers with type 1 diabetes mellitus in Sweden (MODIAB-Web): Study protocol for a randomized controlled trial. *Trials, 15*(1), 513. doi:10.1186/1745-6215-15-513 PMID:25543854

Ahsan, A., & Raihan, A. (2013, December). Understanding m-health impact among Aponjon (MAMA Bangladesh) subscribers through a phone survey in Bangladesh. *Proceedings of the Sixth International Conference on Information and Communications Technologies and Development: Notes* (*Vol. 2*, pp. 1-4). ACM.

Ahtinen, A., Mattila, E., Välkkynen, P., Kaipainen, K., Vanhala, T., Ermes, M., & Lappalainen, R. (2013). Mobile mental wellness training for stress management: Feasibility and design implications based on a one-month field study. *JMIR mHealth and uHealth, 1*(2).

Akbarzade, M., Rafiee, B., Asadi, N., & Zare, N. (2015). The Effect of Maternal Relaxation Training on Reactivity of Non-Stress Test, Basal Fetal Heart Rate, and Number of Fetal Heart Accelerations: A Randomized Controlled Trial. *International journal of community based nursing and midwifery, 3*(1), 51.

Ammaniti, M. (1996). *Maternità e gravidanza: studio delle rappresentazioni materne*. Raffaello Cortina.

Austin, M. P., Tully, L., & Parker, G. (2007). Examining the relationship between antenatal anxiety and postnatal depression. *Journal of Affective Disorders, 101*(1), 169–174. doi:10.1016/j.jad.2006.11.015 PMID:17196663

Barclay, L., Everitt, L., Rogan, F., Schmied, V., & Wyllie, A. (1997). Becoming a mother—an analysis of women's experience of early motherhood. *Journal of Advanced Nursing, 25*(4), 719–728. doi:10.1046/j.1365-2648.1997.t01-1-1997025719.x PMID:9104667

Bartholomew, M. K., Schoppe-Sullivan, S. J., Glassman, M., Kamp Dush, C. M., & Sullivan, J. M. (2012). New parents' Facebook use at the transition to parenthood. *Family Relations, 61*(3), 455–469. doi:10.1111/j.1741-3729.2012.00708.x PMID:23671354

Bastani, F., Hidarnia, A., Kazemnejad, A., Vafaei, M., & Kashanian, M. (2005). A randomized controlled trial of the effects of applied relaxation training on reducing anxiety and perceived stress in pregnant women. *Journal of Midwifery & Women's Health, 50*(4), e36–e40. doi:10.1016/j.jmwh.2004.11.008 PMID:15973255

Bastani, F., Hidarnia, A., Montgomery, K. S., Aguilar-Vafaei, M. E., & Kazemnejad, A. (2006). Does relaxation education in anxious primigravid Iranian women influence adverse pregnancy outcomes?: A randomized controlled trial. *The Journal of Perinatal & Neonatal Nursing, 20*(2), 138–146. doi:10.1097/00005237-200604000-00007 PMID:16714913

Beddoe, A. E., & Lee, K. A. (2008). Mind-Body Interventions during Pregnancy. *Journal of Obstetric, Gynecologic, and Neonatal Nursing, 37*(2), 165–175. doi:10.1111/j.1552-6909.2008.00218.x PMID:18336440

Beebe, K. R., Lee, K. A., Carrieri-Kohlman, V., & Humphreys, J. (2007). The Effects of Childbirth Self-Efficacy and Anxiety during Pregnancy on Prehospitalization Labor. *Journal of Obstetric, Gynecologic, and Neonatal Nursing, 36*(5), 410–418. doi:10.1111/j.1552-6909.2007.00170.x PMID:17880311

Bert, F., Gualano, M. R., Brusaferro, S., De Vito, E., de Waure, C., La Torre, G., ... & Carubia, L. (2013). Pregnancy e-health: a multicenter Italian cross-sectional study on Internet use and decision-making among pregnant women. *Journal of epidemiology and community health*, jech-2013.

Bribing, G. (1959). Some considerations of the psychological process in pregnancy. *The Psychoanalytic Study of the Child, 14*, 113–119.

Buitelaar, J. K., Huizink, A. C., Mulder, E. J., de Medina, P. G. R., & Visser, G. H. (2003). Prenatal stress and cognitive development and temperament in infants. *Neurobiology of Aging, 24*, S53–S60. doi:10.1016/S0197-4580(03)00050-2 PMID:12829109

Campbell, S. B., Morgan-Lopez, A. A., Cox, M. J., & McLoyd, V. C. (2009). A latent class analysis of maternal depressive symptoms over 12 years and offspring adjustment in adolescence. *Journal of Abnormal Psychology*, *118*(3), 479–493. doi:10.1037/a0015923 PMID:19685946

Cavanagh, K., Strauss, C., Cicconi, F., Griffiths, N., Wyper, A., & Jones, F. (2013). A randomised controlled trial of a brief online mindfulness-based intervention. *Behaviour Research and Therapy*, *51*(9), 573–578. doi:10.1016/j.brat.2013.06.003 PMID:23872699

Chittaro, L., & Vianello, A. (2014). Computer-supported mindfulness: Evaluation of a mobile thought distancing application on naive meditators. *International Journal of Human-Computer Studies*, *72*(3), 337–348. doi:10.1016/j.ijhcs.2013.11.001

Cogill, S. R., Caplan, H. L., Alexandra, H., Robson, K. M., & Kumar, R. (1986). Impact of maternal postnatal depression on cognitive development of young children. *BMJ*, *292*(6529), 1165–1167. doi:10.1136/bmj.292.6529.1165 PMID:3085767

Collins, N. L., Dunkel-Schetter, C., Lobel, M., & Scrimshaw, S. C. (1993). Social support in pregnancy: Psychosocial correlates of birth outcomes and postpartum depression. *Journal of Personality and Social Psychology*, *65*(6), 1243–1258. doi:10.1037/0022-3514.65.6.1243 PMID:8295121

Cooper, P. J., Tomlinson, M., Swartz, L., Landman, M., Molteno, C., Stein, A., ... Murray, L. (2009). Improving quality of mother-infant relationship and infant attachment in socioeconomically deprived community in South Africa: Randomised controlled trial. *BMJ (Clinical Research Ed.)*, *338*(Apr. 14), b974. doi:10.1136/bmj.b974 PMID:19366752

Costa, D. D., Rippen, N., Dritsa, M., & Ring, A. (2003). Self-reported leisure-time physical activity during pregnancy and relationship to psychological well-being. *Journal of Psychosomatic Obstetrics and Gynaecology*, *24*(2), 111–119. doi:10.3109/01674820309042808 PMID:12854395

Cuijpers, P., Donker, T., van Straten, A., Li, J., & Andersson, G. (2010). Is guided self-help as effective as face-to-face psychotherapy for depression and anxiety disorders? A systematic review and meta-analysis of comparative outcome studies. *Psychological Medicine*, *40*(12), 1943–1957. doi:10.1017/S0033291710000772 PMID:20406528

Cummings, E. M., & Davies, P. T. (1994). Maternal depression and child development. *Journal of Child Psychology and Psychiatry, and Allied Disciplines*, *35*(1), 73–112. doi:10.1111/j.1469-7610.1994.tb01133.x PMID:8163630

Cutrona, C. E. (1984). Social support and stress in the transition to parenthood. *Journal of Abnormal Psychology, 93*(4), 378–390. doi:10.1037/0021-843X.93.4.378 PMID:6512084

Danaher, B. G., Milgrom, J., Seeley, J. R., Stuart, S., Schembri, C., Tyler, M. S., ... Lewinsohn, P. (2013). MomMoodBooster web-based intervention for postpartum depression: Feasibility trial results. *Journal of Medical Internet Research, 15*(11), e242. doi:10.2196/jmir.2876 PMID:24191345

Davis, E. P., Glynn, L. M., Schetter, C. D., Hobel, C., Chicz-Demet, A., & Sandman, C. A. (2007). Prenatal exposure to maternal depression and cortisol influences infant temperament. *Journal of the American Academy of Child and Adolescent Psychiatry, 46*(6), 737–746. doi:10.1097/chi.0b013e318047b775 PMID:17513986

Dayan, J., Creveuil, C., Herlicoviez, M., Herbel, C., Baranger, E., Savoye, C., & Thouin, A. (2002). Role of anxiety and depression in the onset of spontaneous preterm labor. *American Journal of Epidemiology, 155*(4), 293–301. doi:10.1093/aje/155.4.293 PMID:11836191

Declercq, E. R., Sakala, C., Corry, M. P., & Applebaum, S. (2007). Listening to Mothers II: Report of the Second National US Survey of Women's Childbearing Experiences: Conducted January–February 2006 for Childbirth Connection by Harris Interactive® in partnership with Lamaze International*. *Journal of Perinatal Education, 16*(4), 9–14. doi:10.1624/105812407X244769 PMID:18769512

Dover, S. (2012). Study: Number of smartphone users tops 1 billion. *CBSNews*. Retrieved from http://www.cbsnews.com/8301-205_162-57534583/study-numberof-smartphone-users-tops-1-billion

Duncan, L. G., & Bardacke, N. (2010). Mindfulness-based childbirth and parenting education: Promoting family mindfulness during the perinatal period. *Journal of Child and Family Studies, 19*(2), 190–202. doi:10.100710826-009-9313-7 PMID:20339571

Dunkel-Schetter, C. (1998). Maternal stress and preterm delivery. *Prenatal and Neonatal Medicine, 3*, 39–42.

Dunkel Schetter, C. (2011). Psychological science on pregnancy: Stress processes, biopsychosocial models, and emerging research issues. *Annual Review of Psychology, 62*(1), 531–558. doi:10.1146/annurev.psych.031809.130727 PMID:21126184

Dunkel-Schetter, C., Sagrestano, L. M., Feldman, P., & Killingsworth, C. (1996). Social support and pregnancy. In Handbook of social support and the family (pp. 375-412). Springer US. doi:10.1007/978-1-4899-1388-3_16

Dunn, C., Hanieh, E., Roberts, R., & Powrie, R. (2012). Mindful pregnancy and childbirth: Effects of a mindfulness-based intervention on women's psychological distress and well-being in the perinatal period. *Archives of Women's Mental Health*, *15*(2), 139–143. doi:10.100700737-012-0264-4 PMID:22382281

Field, T., Diego, M., & Hernandez-Reif, M. (2006). Prenatal depression effects on the fetus and newborn: A review. *Infant Behavior and Development*, *29*(3), 445–455. doi:10.1016/j.infbeh.2006.03.003 PMID:17138297

Field, T., Diego, M. A., Hernandez-Reif, M., Schanberg, S., & Kuhn, C. (2004). Massage therapy effects on depressed pregnant women. *Journal of Psychosomatic Obstetrics and Gynaecology*, *25*(2), 115–122. doi:10.1080/0167482041233128223 1 PMID:15715034

Field, T., Hemandez-Reif, M., Hart, S., Theakston, H., Schanberg, S., & Kuhn, C. (1999). Pregnant women benefit from massage therapy. *Journal of Psychosomatic Obstetrics and Gynaecology*, *20*(1), 31–38. doi:10.3109/01674829909075574 PMID:10212885

Field, T., Hernandez-Reif, M., Diego, M., Schanberg, S., & Kuhn, C. (2006). Stability of mood states and biochemistry across pregnancy. *Infant Behavior and Development*, *29*(2), 262–267. doi:10.1016/j.infbeh.2005.12.009 PMID:17138281

Fredrickson, B. L. (2001). The role of positive emotions in positive psychology: The broaden-and-build theory of positive emotions. *The American Psychologist*, *56*(3), 218–226. doi:10.1037/0003-066X.56.3.218 PMID:11315248

Gao, L. L., Larsson, M., & Luo, S. Y. (2013). Internet use by Chinese women seeking pregnancy-related information. *Midwifery*, *29*(7), 730–735. doi:10.1016/j.midw.2012.07.003 PMID:22958935

Gedde-Dahl, M., & Fors, E. A. (2012). Impact of self-administered relaxation and guided imagery techniques during final trimester and birth. *Complementary Therapies in Clinical Practice*, *18*(1), 60–65. doi:10.1016/j.ctcp.2011.08.008 PMID:22196576

Grant, K. A., McMahon, C., & Austin, M. P. (2008). Maternal anxiety during the transition to parenthood: A prospective study. *Journal of Affective Disorders*, *108*(1), 101–111. doi:10.1016/j.jad.2007.10.002 PMID:18001841

Green Paper on mobile-health (mHealth). (2014, June). Brussels, Belgium.

Haga, S. M., Drozd, F., Brendryen, H., & Slinning, K. (2013). Mamma mia: a feasibility study of a Web-based intervention to reduce the risk of postpartum depression and enhance subjective well-being. *JMIR research protocols, 2*(2).

Haug, T., Nordgreen, T., Öst, L. G., & Havik, O. E. (2012). Self-help treatment of anxiety disorders: A meta-analysis and meta-regression of effects and potential moderators. *Clinical Psychology Review*, *32*(5), 425–445. doi:10.1016/j.cpr.2012.04.002 PMID:22681915

Hearn, L., Miller, M., & Lester, L. (2014). Reaching perinatal women online: The Healthy You, Healthy Baby website and app. *Journal of Obesity*, 2014. PMID:24872891

Hernández-Martínez, C., Val, V. A., Murphy, M., Busquets, P. C., & Sans, J. C. (2011). Relation between positive and negative maternal emotional states and obstetrical outcomes. *Women & Health*, *51*(2), 124–135. doi:10.1080/03630242.2010.550991 PMID:21476173

Hipwell, A. E., Goossens, F. A., Melhuish, E. C., & Kumar, R. (2000). Severe maternal psychopathology and infant–mother attachment. *Development and Psychopathology*, *12*(02), 157–175. doi:10.1017/S0954579400002030 PMID:10847622

Hoffman, S., & Hatch, M. C. (2000). Depressive symptomatology during pregnancy: Evidence for an association with decreased fetal growth in pregnancies of lower social class women. *Health Psychology*, *19*(6), 535–543. doi:10.1037/0278-6133.19.6.535 PMID:11129356

Israel, B. A., Farquhar, S. A., Schulz, A. J., James, S. A., & Parker, E. A. (2002). The relationship between social support, stress, and health among women on Detroit's East Side. *Health Education & Behavior*, *29*(3), 342–360. PMID:12038743

Jihye, H., & Iftekhar, S. N. Comparison on the Use of Smartphone Application between International and Korean Pregnant Women.

Johnson, S. A. (2014). "Maternal Devices", Social Media and the Self-Management of Pregnancy, Mothering and Child Health. *Societies*, *4*(2), 330–350. doi:10.3390oc4020330

Jones, L. (2012). Pain management for women in labour: An overview of systematic reviews. *Journal of Evidence-Based Medicine*, *5*(2), 101–102. PMID:22419342

Kabat-Zinn, J. (1994). *Wherever you go, there you are: Mindfulness meditation in everyday life*. New York: Hyperion.

Keyes, C. L. M., & Lopez, S. J. (2002). Toward a science of mental health: positive direction in diagnosis and interventions. In C. R. Snyder & S. J. Lopez (Eds.), *Handbook of Positive Psychology*. New York: Oxford University Press.

Lagan, B. M., Sinclair, M., & George Kernohan, W. (2010). Internet Use in Pregnancy Informs Women's Decision Making: A Web-Based Survey. *Birth (Berkeley, Calif.)*, *37*(2), 106–115. doi:10.1111/j.1523-536X.2010.00390.x PMID:20557533

Lagan, B. M., Sinclair, M., & Kernohan, W. G. (2011). What Is the Impact of the Internet on Decision-Making in Pregnancy? A Global Study. *Birth (Berkeley, Calif.)*, *38*(4), 336–345. doi:10.1111/j.1523-536X.2011.00488.x PMID:22112334

Lancaster, C. A., Gold, K. J., Flynn, H. A., Yoo, H., Marcus, S. M., & Davis, M. M. (2010). Risk factors for depressive symptoms during pregnancy: A systematic review. *American Journal of Obstetrics and Gynecology*, *202*(1), 5–14. doi:10.1016/j.ajog.2009.09.007 PMID:20096252

Larsson, M. (2009). A descriptive study of the use of the Internet by women seeking pregnancy-related information. *Midwifery*, *25*(1), 14–20. doi:10.1016/j.midw.2007.01.010 PMID:17408822

Lima-Pereira, P., Bermúdez-Tamayo, C., & Jasienska, G. (2012). Use of the Internet as a source of health information amongst participants of antenatal classes. *Journal of Clinical Nursing*, *21*(3-4), 322–330. doi:10.1111/j.1365-2702.2011.03910.x PMID:22093043

Lindgren, K. (2001). Relationships among maternal–fetal attachment, prenatal depression, and health practices in pregnancy. *Research in Nursing & Health*, *24*(3), 203–217. doi:10.1002/nur.1023 PMID:11526619

Lowe, N. K. (2002). The nature of labor pain. *American Journal of Obstetrics and Gynecology*, *186*(5), S16–S24. doi:10.1016/S0002-9378(02)70179-8 PMID:12011870

Lund, S., Nielsen, B. B., Hemed, M., Boas, I. M., Said, A., Said, K., & Rasch, V. (2014). Mobile phones improve antenatal care attendance in Zanzibar: A cluster randomized controlled trial. *BMC Pregnancy and Childbirth*, *14*(1), 29. doi:10.1186/1471-2393-14-29 PMID:24438517

Luxton, D. D., McCann, R. A., Bush, N. E., Mishkind, M. C., & Reger, G. M. (2011). mHealth for mental health: Integrating smartphone technology in behavioral healthcare. *Professional Psychology, Research and Practice*, *42*(6), 505–512. doi:10.1037/a0024485

Ly, K. H., Trüschel, A., Jarl, L., Magnusson, S., Windahl, T., Johansson, R., ... Andersson, G. (2014). Behavioural activation versus mindfulness-based guided self-help treatment administered through a smartphone application: A randomised controlled trial. *BMJ Open*, *4*(1), e003440. doi:10.1136/bmjopen-2013-003440 PMID:24413342

Mathiesen, K. S., Tambs, K., & Dalgard, O. S. (1999). The influence of social class, strain and social support on symptoms of anxiety and depression in mothers of toddlers. *Social Psychiatry and Psychiatric Epidemiology*, *34*(2), 61–72. doi:10.1007001270050113 PMID:10189811

Melzer, K., Schutz, Y., Soehnchen, N., Othenin-Girard, V., de Tejada, B. M., Irion, O., ... Kayser, B. (2010). Effects of recommended levels of physical activity on pregnancy outcomes. *American Journal of Obstetrics and Gynecology*, *202*(3), 266–e1. doi:10.1016/j.ajog.2009.10.876 PMID:20022583

mHealth App Developer Economics 2014: The State of the Art of mHealth App. (2014). Research2guidance. Retrieved from http://research2guidance.com/r2g/mHealth-App-Developer-Economics-2014.pdf

mHealth: New Horizons for Health through Mobile Technologies: Based on the Findings of the Second Global Survey on eHealth (Global Observatory for eHealth Series, Volume 3) (2011). World Health Organization.

Miyata, K. (2002). Social support for Japanese mothers online and offline. *The internet in everyday life*, 520-548.

Monti, F., Fagandini, P., Agostini, F., Vettori, D., & La Sala, G. B. (2006). *La complessità della nascita: genitorialità e modalità di parto. La Sala GB, Iori V., Monti F., Fagandini P.(a cura di), La "normale" complessità del venire al mondo.* Milano: Guerini Studio.

Mulsow, M., Caldera, Y. M., Pursley, M., Reifman, A., & Huston, A. C. (2002). Multilevel factors influencing maternal stress during the first three years. *Journal of Marriage and the Family*, *64*(4), 944–956. doi:10.1111/j.1741-3737.2002.00944.x

Murray, L. (1992). The impact of postnatal depression on infant development. *Journal of Child Psychology and Psychiatry, and Allied Disciplines*, *33*(3), 543–561. doi:10.1111/j.1469-7610.1992.tb00890.x PMID:1577898

Murray, L., Fiori-Cowley, A., Hooper, R., & Cooper, P. (1996). The impact of postnatal depression and associated adversity on early mother-infant interactions and later infant outcome. *Child Development*, *67*(5), 2512–2526. doi:10.2307/1131637 PMID:9022253

Murray, L., Sinclair, D., Cooper, P., Ducournau, P., Turner, P., & Stein, A. (1999). The socioemotional development of 5-year-old children of postnatally depressed mothers. *Journal of Child Psychology and Psychiatry, and Allied Disciplines*, *40*(08), 1259–1271. doi:10.1111/1469-7610.00542 PMID:10604404

Narendran, S., Nagarathna, R., Narendran, V., Gunasheela, S., & Nagendra, H. R. R. (2005). Efficacy of yoga on pregnancy outcome. *Journal of Alternative and Complementary Medicine (New York, N.Y.)*, *11*(2), 237–244. doi:10.1089/acm.2005.11.237 PMID:15865489

Nasreen, H. E., Kabir, Z. N., Forsell, Y., & Edhborg, M. (2011). Prevalence and associated factors of depressive and anxiety symptoms during pregnancy: A population based study in rural Bangladesh. *BMC Women's Health*, *11*(1), 22. doi:10.1186/1472-6874-11-22 PMID:21635722

Newman, M. G., Szkodny, L. E., Llera, S. J., & Przeworski, A. (2011). A review of technology-assisted self-help and minimal contact therapies for anxiety and depression: Is human contact necessary for therapeutic efficacy? *Clinical Psychology Review*, *31*(1), 89–103. doi:10.1016/j.cpr.2010.09.008 PMID:21130939

Nickel, C., Lahmann, C., Muehlbacher, M., Pedrosa Gil, F., Kaplan, P., Buschmann, W., ... Nickel, M. (2006). Pregnant women with bronchial asthma benefit from progressive muscle relaxation: A randomized, prospective, controlled trial. *Psychotherapy and Psychosomatics*, *75*(4), 237–243. doi:10.1159/000092894 PMID:16785773

O'Connor, T. G., Heron, J., & Glover, V. (2002). Antenatal anxiety predicts child behavioral/emotional problems independently of postnatal depression. *Journal of the American Academy of Child and Adolescent Psychiatry*, *41*(12), 1470–1477. doi:10.1097/00004583-200212000-00019 PMID:12447034

O'Hara, M. W., & Swain, A. M. (1996). Rates and risk of postpartum depression-a meta-analysis. *International Review of Psychiatry (Abingdon, England)*, *8*(1), 37–54. doi:10.3109/09540269609037816

O'Higgins, A., Murphy, O. C., Egan, A., Mullaney, L., Sheehan, S., & Turner, M. J. (2013). The use of digital media by women using the maternity services in a developed country. *Irish Medical Journal*, *107*(10), 313–315. PMID:25556255

Oakley, A. (1992). Social support in pregnancy: Methodology and findings of a 1-year follow-up study. *Journal of Reproductive and Infant Psychology*, *10*(4), 219–231. doi:10.1080/02646839208403955

Oakley, A., Hickey, D., Rajan, L., & Rigby, A. S. (1996). Social support in pregnancy: Does it have long-term effects? *Journal of Reproductive and Infant Psychology*, *14*(1), 7–22. doi:10.1080/02646839608405855

Oakley, A., Rajan, L., & Grant, A. (1990). Social support and pregnancy outcome. *BJOG: An International Journal of Obstetrics & Gynaecology*, *97*(2), 155–162. doi:10.1111/j.1471-0528.1990.tb01741.x PMID:2317466

Parker, R. M., Dmitrieva, E., Frolov, S., & Gazmararian, J. A. (2012). Text4baby in the United States and Russia: an opportunity for understanding how mHealth affects maternal and child health. *Journal of health communication, 17*(sup1), 30-36.

Peyton, T. (2014, November). Pregnancy Ecologies As Teachable Moments For The Lifecourse: Changing The mHealth Design Paradigm. *Proceedings of the 18th International Conference on Supporting Group Work* (pp. 269-271). ACM. 10.1145/2660398.2660438

Peyton, T., Poole, E., Reddy, M., Kraschnewski, J., & Chuang, C. (2014, June). Every pregnancy is different: designing mHealth for the pregnancy ecology. *Proceedings of the 2014 conference on Designing interactive systems* (pp. 577-586). ACM. 10.1145/2598510.2598572

Pluess, M., Wurmser, H., Buske-Kirschbaum, A., Papousek, M., Pirke, K. M., Hellhammer, D., & Bolten, M. (2012). Positive life events predict salivary cortisol in pregnant women. *Psychoneuroendocrinology*, *37*(8), 1336–1340. doi:10.1016/j.psyneuen.2012.01.006 PMID:22309824

Preece, J. (2001). Online communities: Usability, sociabilty, theory and methods. In *Frontiers of human-centered computing, online communities and virtual environments* (pp. 263–277). Springer London. doi:10.1007/978-1-4471-0259-5_18

Preziosa, A., Grassi, A., Gaggioli, A., & Riva, G. (2009). Therapeutic applications of the mobile phone. *British Journal of Guidance & Counselling*, *37*(3), 313–325. doi:10.1080/03069880902957031

Repetto, C., Gaggioli, A., Pallavicini, F., Cipresso, P., Raspelli, S., & Riva, G. (2013). Virtual reality and mobile phones in the treatment of generalized anxiety disorders: A phase-2 clinical trial. *Personal and Ubiquitous Computing*, *17*(2), 253–260. doi:10.100700779-011-0467-0

Riva, G., Banos, R. M., Botella, C., Wiederhold, B. K., & Gaggioli, A. (2012). Positive technology: Using interactive technologies to promote positive functioning. *Cyberpsychology, Behavior, and Social Networking*, *15*(2), 69–77. doi:10.1089/cyber.2011.0139 PMID:22149077

Romano, A. M. (2007). A changing landscape: Implications of pregnant women's Internet use for childbirth educators. *Journal of Perinatal Education, 16*(4), 18–24. doi:10.1624/105812407X244903 PMID:18769519

Roos, A., Faure, S., Lochner, C., Vythilingum, B., & Stein, D. J. (2013). Predictors of distress and anxiety during pregnancy. *The African Journal of Psychiatry, 16*(2), 118–122. PMID:23595531

Rotheram-Borus, M. J., Tomlinson, M., Gwegwe, M., Comulada, W. S., Kaufman, N., & Keim, M. (2012). Diabetes buddies peer support through a mobile phone buddy system. *The Diabetes Educator, 38*(3), 357–365. doi:10.1177/0145721712444617 PMID:22546740

Rotheram-Borus, M. J., Tomlinson, M., Swendeman, D., Lee, A., & Jones, E. (2012). Standardized functions for smartphone applications: Examples from maternal and child health. *International Journal of Telemedicine and Applications, 2012*, 21. doi:10.1155/2012/973237 PMID:23304136

Rubin, R. (1984). Maternal Identity and the Maternal Experience. *AJN The American Journal of Nursing, 84*(12), 1480. doi:10.1097/00000446-198412000-00030

Rush, J., Chalmers, I., & Enkin, M. (1991). Care of the new mother and baby. In I. Chalmers, M. Enkin, & M. Kierse (Eds.), *Effective Care in Pregnancy and Childbirth* (Vol. 2, pp. 1333–1346). Oxford: Oxford University Press.

Satyapriya, M., Nagendra, H. R., Nagarathna, R., & Padmalatha, V. (2009). Effect of integrated yoga on stress and heart rate variability in pregnant women. *International Journal of Gynaecology and Obstetrics: the Official Organ of the International Federation of Gynaecology and Obstetrics, 104*(3), 218–222. doi:10.1016/j.ijgo.2008.11.013 PMID:19110245

Schaub, B. G. (1995). Imagery in health care: Connecting with life energy. *Complementary Health Practice Review, 1*(2), 113–115.

Seligman, M. E. (2003). Fundamental assumptions. *The Psychologist, 16*(3), 126.

Seligman, M. E., & Csikszentmihalyi, M. (2000). Positive psychology: An introduction: Vol. 55. *No. 1* (p. 5). American Psychological Association.

Sethi, S., Campbell, A. J., & Ellis, L. A. (2010). The use of computerized self-help packages to treat adolescent depression and anxiety. *Journal of Technology in Human Services, 28*(3), 144–160. doi:10.1080/15228835.2010.508317

Sharf, B. F. (1997). Communicating breast cancer on-line: Support and empowerment on the Internet. *Women & Health, 26*(1), 65–84. doi:10.1300/J013v26n01_05 PMID:9311100

Sharma, V., Bauer, B., Prasad, K., Sood, A., & Schroeder, D. (2012). P02.197 Self help intervention to decrease stress and increase mindfulness: A pilot trial. *BMC Complementary and Alternative Medicine, 12*(Suppl. 1), 253. doi:10.1186/1472-6882-12-S1-P253 PMID:23237355

Smith, C. A., Levett, K. M., Collins, C. T., & Crowther, C. A. (2011). Relaxation techniques for pain management in labour. *The Cochrane Library*. PMID:22161453

Stern, D. N., Bruschweiler-Stern, N., & Freeland, A. (1998). *The birth of a mother*. London: Bloomsbury.

Stice, E., Ragan, J., & Randall, P. (2004). Prospective relations between social support and depression: Differential direction of effects for parent and peer support? *Journal of Abnormal Psychology, 113*(1), 155–159. doi:10.1037/0021-843X.113.1.155 PMID:14992668

Tamrat, T., & Kachnowski, S. (2012). Special delivery: An analysis of mHealth in maternal and newborn health programs and their outcomes around the world. *Maternal and Child Health Journal, 16*(5), 1092–1101. doi:10.100710995-011-0836-3 PMID:21688111

Taylor, C. B., & Luce, K. H. (2003). Computer-and Internet-based psychotherapy interventions. *Current Directions in Psychological Science, 12*(1), 18–22. doi:10.1111/1467-8721.01214

Teixeira, J., Martin, D., Prendiville, O., & Glover, V. (2005). The effects of acute relaxation on indices of anxiety during pregnancy. *Journal of Psychosomatic Obstetrics and Gynaecology, 26*(4), 271–276. doi:10.1080/01674820500139922 PMID:16457423

Tietjen, A. M., & Bradley, C. F. (1985). Social support and maternal psychosocial adjustment during the transition to parenthood. *Revue canadienne des sciences du comportement [Canadian Journal of Behavioural Science], 17*(2), 109.

Tragea, C., Chrousos, G. P., Alexopoulos, E. C., & Darviri, C. (2014). A randomized controlled trial of the effects of a stress management programme during pregnancy. *Complementary Therapies in Medicine, 22*(2), 203–211. doi:10.1016/j.ctim.2014.01.006 PMID:24731890

Tripp, N., Hainey, K., Liu, A., Poulton, A., Peek, M., Kim, J., & Nanan, R. (2014). An emerging model of maternity care: Smartphone, midwife, doctor? *Women and Birth; Journal of the Australian College of Midwives*, *27*(1), 64–67. doi:10.1016/j.wombi.2013.11.001 PMID:24295598

Tronick, E. Z., & Weinberg, K. (1999). *Le madri depresse ei loro bambini: l'insuccesso nella formazione degli stati di coscienza diadici. Murray, L., Cooper, P.(a cura di). Depressione del post-partum e sviluppo del bambino*. Roma: CIC Edizioni Internazionali.

Urech, C., Fink, N. S., Hoesli, I., Wilhelm, F. H., Bitzer, J., & Alder, J. (2010). Effects of relaxation on psychobiological wellbeing during pregnancy: A randomized controlled trial. *Psychoneuroendocrinology*, *35*(9), 1348–1355. doi:10.1016/j.psyneuen.2010.03.008 PMID:20417038

Urizar, G. G. Jr, Milazzo, M., Le, H. N., Delucchi, K., Sotelo, R., & Muñoz, R. F. (2004). Impact of stress reduction instructions on stress and cortisol levels during pregnancy. *Biological Psychology*, *67*(3), 275–282. doi:10.1016/j.biopsycho.2003.11.001 PMID:15294386

Vieten, C., & Astin, J. (2008). Effects of a mindfulness-based intervention during pregnancy on prenatal stress and mood: Results of a pilot study. *Archives of Women's Mental Health*, *11*(1), 67–74. doi:10.100700737-008-0214-3 PMID:18317710

Villani, D., Grassi, A., Cognetta, C., Toniolo, D., Cipresso, P., & Riva, G. (2013). Self-help stress management training through mobile phones: An experience with oncology nurses. *Psychological Services*, *10*(3), 315–322. doi:10.1037/a0026459 PMID:23937091

Villani, D., & Riva, G. (2012). Does interactive media enhance the management of stress? Suggestions from a controlled study. *Cyberpsychology, Behavior, and Social Networking*, *15*(1), 24–30. doi:10.1089/cyber.2011.0141 PMID:22032797

Vliet, H. V., & Andrews, G. (2009). Internet-based course for the management of stress for junior high schools. *The Australian and New Zealand Journal of Psychiatry*, *43*(4), 305–309. doi:10.1080/00048670902721145 PMID:19296285

Voellmin, A., Entringer, S., Moog, N., Wadhwa, P. D., & Buss, C. (2013). Maternal positive affect over the course of pregnancy is associated with the length of gestation and reduced risk of preterm delivery. *Journal of Psychosomatic Research*, *75*(4), 336–340. doi:10.1016/j.jpsychores.2013.06.031 PMID:24119939

Waring, M. E., Simas, T. A. M., Xiao, R. S., Lombardini, L. M., Allison, J. J., Rosal, M. C., & Pagoto, S. L. (2014). Pregnant women's interest in a website or mobile application for healthy gestational weight gain. *Sexual & Reproductive Healthcare*, *5*(4), 182–184. doi:10.1016/j.srhc.2014.05.002 PMID:25433828

Warnecke, E., Quinn, S., Ogden, K., Towle, N., & Nelson, M. R. (2011). A randomised controlled trial of the effects of mindfulness practice on medical student stress levels. *Medical Education*, *45*(4), 381–388. doi:10.1111/j.1365-2923.2010.03877.x PMID:21401686

Watterson, J. L., Walsh, J., & Madeka, I. (2015). Using mHealth to Improve Usage of Antenatal Care, Postnatal Care, and Immunization: A Systematic Review of the Literature. *BioMed Research International, 2015.*

Wellman, B., & Frank, K. (2001). Network capital in a multilevel world: Getting support from personal communities. *Social capital: Theory and research* (pp. 233-273).

Williams, C., & Whitfield, G. (2001). Written and computer-based self-help treatments for depression. *British Medical Bulletin*, *57*(1), 133–144. doi:10.1093/bmb/57.1.133 PMID:11719913

Yali, A. M., & Lobel, M. (2002). Stress-resistance resources and coping in pregnancy. *Anxiety, Stress, and Coping*, *15*(3), 289–309. doi:10.1080/1061580021000020743

KEY TERMS AND DEFINITIONS

E-Health: A general term for the use of information and communications technologies (ICT) in the healthcare promotion and medical fields.

Empowerment: Consists of a process of increasing personal resources and awareness of them to promote individual wellbeing and environment adaptation.

Guided Imagery/Visualization: A relaxation technique used to induce positive mental images, feelings and thoughts. Guided Imagery can be used by everyone: it is able to overcome barriers of education, class, race, gender and age. Because it involves all senses (not just sight) it is perceived as more pleasant and efficient. This practice is particularly powerful, as well as simpler than mindfulness meditation for most beginners.

M-Health: This term indicates the use of mobile and wireless technologies in health fields.

Mindfulness: A type of meditative technique that emphasizes an observant and nonreactive stance toward one's thoughts, emotions and body states. It involves purposeful attention to daily activities (e.g., mindfulness of eating).

Mobile Application: Software developed to be installed and run on mobile devices such as smartphones, PDAs or tablets. They can be both fun and useful, and they can be executed (run) on a mobile platform.

Progressive Muscular Relaxation: A relaxation technique of stress management developed by Edmund Jacobson in 1934, based on tensing and releasing tensions in the 16 different muscle groups. PMR (progressive muscular relaxation) programs include four sets of exercises: arms relaxation; face and shoulders relaxation; bust and legs relaxation. All exercises are based on two principles: contraction and relaxation, with the aim being to achieve a profound and aware state of calm.

Smartphone: An advanced mobile phone that includes mobile communication, a camera, a video camera, GPS system, a music player, Internet access, sensors and a range of multimedia capabilities in a single device. Several accessories are being developed to transform smartphones into "medical machines." They can become meters of blood glucose level, blood rate of oxygen, blood pressure and so on.

Web-App: This term is used to indicate any program stored on a remote server and delivered over the Internet through a browser interface. They are usable only with an Internet connection and use HTTP as communication protocol.

This research was previously published in Integrating Technology in Positive Psychology Practice edited by Daniela Villani, Pietro Cipresso, Andrea Gaggioli, and Giuseppe Riva; pages 162-192, copyright year 2016 by Information Science Reference (an imprint of IGI Global).

Chapter 3
The MAMICare Project:
Monitoring Maternal and Child Health in Rural Areas

Juan C. Lavariega
Tecnológico de Monterrey, Mexico

Gustavo Córdova
Tecnológico de Monterrey, Mexico

Lorena G. Gómez
Tecnológico de Monterrey, Mexico

Alfonso Avila
Tecnológico de Monterrey, Mexico

ABSTRACT

This chapter is an updated version of a previous work about the authors' project on monitoring pregnancy progress in rural areas and/or areas with poor support of medical services. The project is based on an information technology solution based on mobile devices and health sensors such as electrocardiogram, stethoscope, pulse-oximeter, and blood-glucose meter to automatically collect relevant health data for monitoring pregnancy. In this chapter, the authors provide a detailed description of the software architecture of the system. They include a description of the test they have been performing and the difficulties they have faced for the complete implementation of their system.

DOI: 10.4018/978-1-7998-2351-3.ch003

INTRODUCTION

United Nations launched in 2000 the eight Millennium Development Goals (MDGs), which define the roud to follow for the correct implementation of the UN general objectives for Peace, Security, Development and Human Rights. There are eight MDGs to be reached by 2015 ideally. One of those is to provide correct maternal and pre-natal health in the world. The lack of appropriate maternal and child health in rural areas results in an alarming number of maternity and infant deaths (World Health Organization, UNICEF, UNFPA and The World Bank, 2012). In Mexico, although the infant and maternal mortality has been declining (maternal mortality fell from 89.0 to near 50 per 100 000 live births between 1990 and 2010), the states of Chiapas, Oaxaca, and Guerrero have high rates, with mortality rates highest among indigenous children. The leading causes of death continue to be associated with hypertension, hemorrhages, and other complications of delivery (World Health Organization, 2006) that could be avoided. It has been demonstrated in other countries that by means of an information technology approach several medical conditions such as maternity care can be intelligently monitored, managed and treated on a long term (Blank et al., 2013; Mougiakakou et al., 2010).

Current health conditions in Mexico present a downward trend in overall maternity and infant mortality. However, it is highly remarkable that unequal access to healthcare services still prevail as a challenge in the country (World Health Organization, 2006). More specifically rural areas are the ones lacking the high-quality services needed to reduce maternal and infant mortality in the whole region. According to Jennert et al (Jennett, Yeo, Scott, Hebert, & Teo, 2005) health services and human health resources are more valuable for rural communities, thus the delivery of these services remotely using accessible technology could help to level up the unequal access to health services.

We based our work on the actual situation of rural communities in some regions of Mexico. Further, in the article we present a case scenario that reflect the reality of such communities with respect to medical services. In the scenario, the characters are fictions to protect the identity of people. Our objective is to highlight the improvement of healthcare quality and accessibility using wireless technology in a rural area.

We came to identify the need of better health services in that region, due to a demographic study that colleagues from the Social Sciences in our institution performed in the area. From that study several projects were identified; some related to rainwater harvesting; dignified dwelling; reforestation and better use of natural resources; and of course, heath improvement. For health improvement we have identified as the key problem maternal and infant care

Since we first describe our work in the International Journal of Healthcare Information Systems and Informatics in 2014, we have developed a complete information technology solution that we describe in this chapter. However, due externa factors such as changes in the political regulations in the region and an aggressive reduction in the programs that the Ministry of Health supports in the same region, we have not been able to conduct the field test, as we desired.

Our project MAMICare's objective is to reduce maternal and child mortality rates in rural areas. MAMiCare uses information and communication technology (ICT) to strengthen the current health delivery practices for both the mother and child during pregnancy. During the last three years we have been working in our IT solution for proper health monitoring during pregnancy considering the proper technological limitations that prevail in rural areas.

This chapter is organized as follows, Section 2 presents related work relevant to our solution approach, Section 3 describes the software architecture for our project. Section 4 briefly discuss the current stage of our work with respect to usability in rural areas. Section 5 discuss on the limitations we have faced and the current status for MAMICare. Finally, Section 6 concludes the chapter.

RELATED WORK

In the past 10 years Information technology (IT) has been used to improve the accuracy of patient records, and health monitoring. Benefits and challenging unsolved problems continue to be the outcomes of such attempts (Bates, 2003), such as electronic health records, remote monitoring, telehealth, health data collection and processing, and clinical decision support systems, to name a few. Groups interested in the IT-Healthcare efforts have gathered and exchanged opinions to identify technological areas with the highest benefits. These groups integrated by members of the public, health care provider and private sectors selected tele-health and electronic health records, in this order, as the most valuable IT approaches. The groups of interest also identified as a disadvantage the changes in the current practices and processes in the delivery of health services (Jennet et al., 2005).

The use of electronic health records (EHR) is one of the most successful examples of the application of IT to support health care services. Research efforts state that EHR is a solution with great potential as EHR strengthens the collaboration between public and primary care (Calman et al 2012). Electronic health records offer additional benefits such as improving public health surveillance by documenting patient data, real-time guiding of the physician interventions using statistical data to generate clinical alerts, improving surveillance and management of a communicable disease, etc. (Calman et al., 2012).

Other research effort focuses in supporting the treatment of patients with type 1 diabetes mellitus. This decision support system (Mougiakakou et al., 2010) provides risk assessment for long-term complications. Data exchange between a unit for the patient and a unit for the management of the patient occurs, and data is also stored in a web server. By combining database technologies, simulation algorithms and data mining, the system provides an advanced processing of the stored data to support the decision making for the physician. Although a study to evaluate the user requirements satisfaction, the cost and the effectiveness of the solution is needed, this work has allowed a proper risk assessment for long-term diabetes mellitus complications. Other risk-assessment technologies have been developed allowing the physician to do a smart diagnosis of the patient.

In Ghana, a software solution was designed in response to the rapid expansion of community health workers in Africa and Asia. This was made taking as an advantage the proliferation of mobile devices. The Mobile Technology for Community Health (MoTeCH) offers features such as calculating the schedule for each patient; and notifying both patient and community workers when care is due. The system automates the delivery of information for routine reports and integrates with existing software applications for mobile data collection. The presented project is the initial part of an iterative process and still requires advanced software development skills, attention to standards and configurable design to make it more readily available to groups of interest within the research (Macleod, Phillips, Stone, Walji & Awoonor-Williams, 2012).

From Brazil and Peru, a Windows-based application called "TeleConsult" proposes to reduce the high mortality on rural areas in Latin America. TeleConsults proposes the establishment of a medical network that communicates using satellite. The system acquires images from ultrasound examinations, electrocardiogram and blood imaging and pretends to cover disciplines such as cardiology, gynecology pediatrics and infections from the region (Sachpazidis, Rizou & Menary, 2008).

An effort in the maternity and prenatal care is the 'Prenatal Risk Calculation (PRC)'. PCR is a software solution based on a previously introduced system known as JOY. PCR and JOY work using chromosome data information (aneuploidies), through this analysis prenatal risk could detect symptoms such as Down syndrome and potential cancer cells on the product. The test performance between PCR and JOY gave higher significant results while detecting aneuploidies in the first trimester trial; testing alone, the test performance results of JOY were better than the results of PRC. PRC demonstrated to be a good tool to detect prenatal risk but it still needs to be improved (Hörmansdörfer et al., 2008).

A clinical decision support system on maternal care field was created and implemented for rural healthcare centers in Africa. The QUALMAT CDSS provides guidance for antenatal, delivery and post-delivery care. This guidance is possible by incorporating features such as an orientation process based on set of routinely actions, algorithms to detect situations of concern, and electronic tracking of perinatal and postnatal care. CDSS is a java-based application that incorporates the World Health Organization (WHO) guidelines for pregnancy and childbirth care. The CDSS was first developed in English for the use in Ghana and consist of four parts: a user interface; an XML-database for patient data, a set of algorithms to screen entered values; and a set of training documents. Decision support is implemented by offering guidance through routine action in maternal and perinatal care, detection of critical situations using clinical data and electronic partograph for observation on the progress of delivery up to 24 hours. This system requires an equipped site with a laptop computer. Staff members in charge receive general software and QUALMAT training and are left in charge of user administration. The implementation presented limitations in complex medical environments leading to a different conclusion than expected. Another challenging issue was the implementation of the system in a resource-poor environment, leading to hardware insufficiencies and user frustration (Blank et al., 2013).

Medical and health systems have incorporated new technological advances, such as a wide use of smart phones' apps, biosensors and data analytics. These improved systems result in a more pleasant and satisfactory experience for patients with a personalized monitoring and treatment. Patients are taking a more active role in their own overall well-being (Weaver & Bryce. 2015). Body sensor networks similar to our approach will continuously report personal health data to other medical systems for recording, analysis and prediction. (Velikova & van der Hijden, 2015). Most of these advances are targeted for environments with some degree of technological support such as hospitals, urban areas with connectivity, and users with smart phones in developed countries.

In our case, the lack of connectivity (wifi, 3G, 4G or any communication technology) support in rural areas, remains as a problem we have to deal with. Also the heterogeneity of the data sources that feed these systems put additional constraints for supporting better and integrated health services. Health data integration has been addressed in Bahga and Madisetti (2015).

Population groups in rural areas continue to be underserved even though technological advances are incorporated into health systems and applications.

In general, as we have seen in this section, a great deal of effort in applying IT to health systems is based on keeping records and monitoring patients through a network. However, little effort has been set to use mobile technologies for a better diagnostic in remote areas. One example of applying mobile and wireless computing in health remote health assistance is ERPHA (Emergency Remote Pre-Hospital Assistance) a work by Muñoz, Avila, Lavariega, González, and Grote (2012). ERPHA is a IT solution based on mobile technologies to improve remote monitoring under emergency situations. ERPHA enhances the pre-hospital care quality by allowing early intervention of specialist physicians with key data such as video, audio and visualization of patient's vital signs. ERPHA collects key health data from patient using body sensors that transfer their data to a mobile device (usually a smartphone) creating a body-sensor-network (BSN). The mobile device processes, displays and forwards the collected data to a hospital or medical center where a specialist physician can remotely assist paramedics in the diagnosis. Additionally, at the medical center the data sent by de mobile device is stored into a database for maintaining historical records of the patient. These records can be later used for identifying patterns for a more effective treatment or for classifying the severity of injuries.

DESCRIPTION OF THE PROJECT

Existing healthcare support systems have been proved to be efficient in the improvement of medical services. Most of these systems are applied in controlled environments like hospitals. Other systems are implemented to be used at home, where patients have access to such technologies and can follow the health recommendations that an expert or experts provide remotely. Also, as shown in the related work, aiming the healthcare problem in rural areas seems to be a growing concern, particularly in less developing countries such as Mexico, Peru, or Brazil in Latin America or Ghana in Africa. However, direct application of similar technologies would result in an inefficient solution for the Mexican communities included in the scope of this proposal. This is mainly because of the limited communication technology to which those rural areas have access. Our project is focused on the Magdalena Peñasco community, a rural area in the state of Oaxaca, Mexico. In that region, the communities lack of current communication systems such as Internet or Cellular Networks. Most of the time, the only communication service to which they have access is civil band radio communication.

Background

The current process for maternity-infant care attention in the community of Magdalena de Peñasco is a manual process. Because primary attention is performed by volunteers, enough documentation exists about the attention protocols to follow. However, it is hard to identify if everyone involved has a full knowledge of the steps to follow when immediate attention is required. Medical assistance, in particular Maternity-Infant assistance, is based in a hierarchy of levels of attention. Attention levels range from the most elemental home visit performed by a social worker (called Rural Volunteer Promoter or PRV) to the most equipped but expensive trip to the Zone Hospital at the capital of the state. In between the PRV and the Zone Hospital there are the Health House, the Rural Medical Unit (UMR), the Basic Services Hospital(HSB) and the Rural Hospital.

In order to understand what those levels of attention represent for anyone in the community a brief description of each level is given. The Social worker has a basic follow up equipment, accordingly to the Mexican Social Security Institute (IMSS). Health houses are a base for the social workers, vaccine campaigns, and have access to a basic medical kit. The UMR is conformed by a medicine practitioner or a general physician as well as an auxiliary worker. The HSB is considered to be fairly similar to an UMR with some additional equipment such as an ambulance and a delivery room, although much of the information is not clearly defined. Only the Rural Hospital and Zone Hospital have all the basic services (pediatric, internal medicine, general surgery, and gynecology) with the difference that the Zone Hospital in Oaxaca also has more special services. However, Oaxaca´s Zone Hospital gives services to patients from the whole state and most of the time is over capacity.

In general terms, attention in the rural communities, in particular in Magdalena de Peñasco is very limited. Health services are hard to reach, personnel are sometimes under trained and most of the time hospitals or health centers are over capacity or can't cover the full needs of the community. In order to provide a better understanding, a case scenario is described.

Original Situation Scenario

This scenario illustrates in a fair amount the current state of maternity-infant attention in the community of Tlaxiaco. Names and fictitious characters have been developed to illustrate the case.

Maria is a voluntary Social Worker (or PVR) in the region of Chalcatongo; Rosa is a mixtec woman that lives in a settlement 700m far from Chalcatongo. Rosa is 7 month pregnant, this is her fourth pregnancy; her children are 7, 4 and 2 years old. She is a healthy 36 years old woman. Her husband left 3 months ago to continue working in Los Angeles, California (USA); Maria lives 500m away from Rosa's home.

A Health House is 3 km. away from Rosa's home. UMR is 6km away from the Health House and 12km away from Rosa's. The closest HSB is 48 km. away. The orography of the zone makes travelling really slow and hard for all those distances.

As part of her duties as rural promoter, Maria performs a home visit to Rosa to check her pregnancy evolution. Maria following her basic training takes the recommended vital signs from Rosa such as blood pressure, cardiac rhythm, and belly size. However, Maria does not remember how to properly use the sphygmomanometer and is hard for her to interpret the attached instructions. Maria skips some measurements, mainly because the form where data is registered does not indicate them. Also, Rosa has been working hard at home moving some heavy objects, and Maria does not know about that. Maria fills the form with normal data and proceeds to finish the evaluation. At that moment, Rosa begins to feel pain in her belly and turns pale. Maria interprets those symptoms as abnormal and proceeds to make Rosa rest while she seeks for help. Rosa's older son runs to the nearest home (100m away). A neighbor goes to the nearest Health House seeking for help, 20 minutes passed, and the place is closed. The neighbor goes to the nearest UMR, an extra 40min passed. Meanwhile, Rosa is feeling worse. People in the community find the kid and decide to help him by driving him to Rosa's home in order to take her to the nearest UMR. 1 hour and 15 min. has passed since the first symptom appeared on Rosa; she has not gotten any sort of expert medical attention yet. As situations gets worse, they decide to go straight to the HSB looking for better facilities and the possibility of having an ambulance. Thirty minutes of traveling hurt on Rosa's situation because of the ground conditions. Rosa's evaluation takes longer than expected because the doctor was not notified on time about the emergency. He wasn't ready to receive Rosa. Maria stayed and did not travel with Rosa, moreover the forms with information of Rosa's evaluation were missing. Therefore, there is no information that allows the doctor to make a smart decision. Rosa's critic situation forces her to be transferred to the hospital in Tlaxiaco. Fortunately, the ambulance was in good conditions, but still it takes 1.5 hours to take Rosa to Tlaxiaco. It was too late by then; unfortunately, both Rosa and her baby die on arrival.

This case scenario illustrates that failing to communicate fast and efficiently is a critical factor to solve any emergency of this type on time and effectively. Also the incomplete information is a really big factor in the final outcome of the maternity-infant attention.

MAMICare System Description

It is believed that by using information technology, the above-described problem could be mitigated. The e-Health solution that was developed aims to generate a positive impact in the community by improving the communication channels and offering the possibility of having reliable information about the patients at the time when it is most needed.

There are special characteristics in the highest needed rural areas that challenge the implementation of a simple healthcare solution. Currently, most of the monitoring is done by social workers without any special preparation and that belong to the same community. In the zone, there is no telecommunication infrastructure (Wi-Fi or cellular networks) - the most advanced technology is civil band radio. Due to the lack of sufficient communication technologies, the developed solution is an asynchronous support system to assist the social workers in the monitoring process and the physician with reliable information. Also the system works as a data center for patient's information.

MAMICare is a system that covers three major setbacks currently present over rural communities in Mexico. First, the proper monitoring and control of the patient's evolution by storing adequate information and following up data required in basic maternity-infant care; second, the failure to detect risk situations on-time due to the lack of a proper knowledge under those circumstances; and finally, the communication gap within the rural communities in relation to the healthcare problem. Those three issues are covered by MAMICare under different use conditions. The eventual availability in the future of communication infrastructure in the different rural areas would make possible to extend the MAMICare functionalities to forward the recorded information in a live stream fashion to the nearest hospital or medical facility. This functionality provides an additional tool for the social worker by allowing a health professional to check on the patient and a remote physician to give complete feedback on time. Data in the MAMICare is locally stored and used to properly follow up the patient's record. At the same time and when available, data is shared to a centralized database via an API, this database should ideally be accessible in the community center to be properly analyzed for statistics and in-depth knowledge of the illness under medical treatment. MAMICare also has a risk-condition assessment algorithm that identifies the situation and alerts the social worker of critical conditions.

MAMICare is integrated by two parts: MAMITa and MAMI Server, as illustrated in Figure 1, each will handle part of the previously described functionality. The first part (MAMITa) is a tablet device that will be used by the social worker or physician to record, store and analyze information of the patient. The MAMI Server is a system that allows wireless communications between the tablet (MAMITa) and the community center in which a database system will be implemented for the storage and administration of the data. This paper focuses in the MAMITa part of the project; although MAMI Server may be briefly discussed it is only considered to be part of the long-term solution.

MAMITa Overview

Following ERPHA architecture as a reference, the MAMITa system is a software solution that integrates different sensor devices (as shown in Figure 1) such as pulse-oximeter, ECG, Doppler, and glucometer. MAMITa keeps valid track records of patients by aiding the social worker in her job through a visual interface. Such interface includes a step-by-step process to be followed in order to avoid any missing information. MAMITa will also include support video on how to use the sensors

Figure 1. MAMICare overall architecture

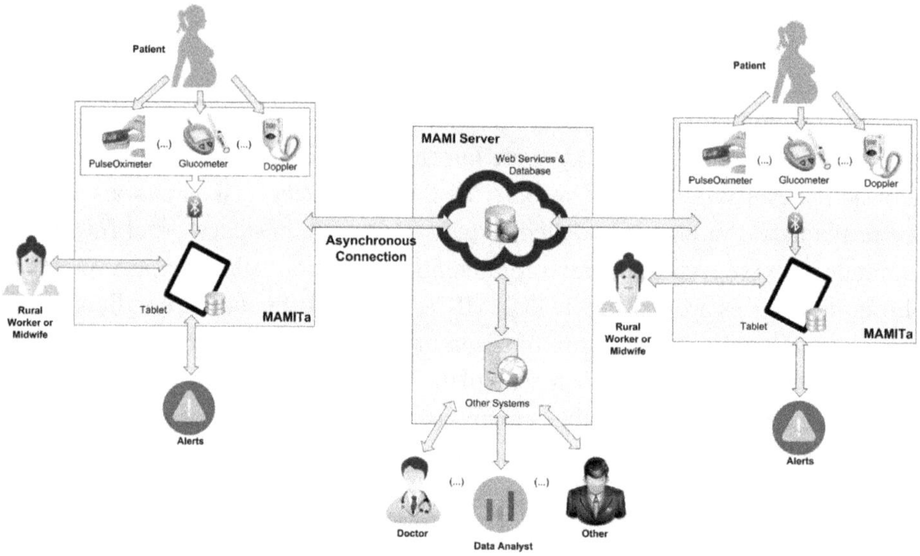

and follow the exploration protocols in order to avoid missing critical information. MAMITa consists of a risk assessment algorithm that will alert if measurements are out of a healthy range and possibly become a risk situation for the patient. The application incorporates the definition of system priorities to alert the social worker of any maternity-infant risk such as hypertension following norms and standards as the Mexican Official Norm NOM-007-SSA2-1993. This Mexican norm specifies prenatal, during and after labor attention for women and newborn children (Secretaria de Salud del Gobierno Mexicano, 1995). Also the WHO "Pregnancy, childbirth, postpartum and newborn care - A guide for essential practice" provides recommendations to guide health-care professionals in the treatment and management of women during their pregnancy, childbirth, postpartum period or any complications that may arise (World Health Organization, Department of Making Pregnancy Safer, 2006). When the system has been input with some conditions and considers a risk situation, MAMITa gives feedback to the PRV for what's best to do. In an ideal scenario, MAMITa gives feedback to the PRV to communicate with and pass the system to the physician or to tell the patient to visit the nearest hospital. The doctor can get access to the system to be informed by the system on the patient's current condition allowing him/her to make a smart decision by fully knowing all the details. As described in the original situation scenario, the patient, the social worker and the doctor are the ones that should be in direct contact with MAMITa system.

The MAMITa solution keeps track of different measurements such as weight, blood pressure, blood-glucose, and contractions. It includes a bluetooth integration with a pulse-oximeter, and blood-glucose meter and will eventually be extended to support other medical devices such as an ECG (electrocardiogram), or a stethoscope. Integrated devices sync with the tablet and are used for the proper monitoring of the patient vitals. The mentioned devices are considered part of the basic medical kit and should be included with the tablet; other devices will be selected in order to fulfill the requirements in the rural communities. Devices properly synched with MAMITa system allow the system to keep track of the patient's situation and at the same time to keep an electronic record of patient's health. Figure 2 illustrates the way in which MAMITa reads the patient measurements through the devices. Also it shows the way in which interaction occurs between the Social Worker, the patient and the device (D). System allows the social worker to input data as well as to receive readings and instructions from the system in order to aid in the process of recording information.

MAMITa interface interacts with multiple devices (D´s in Figure 2 and Figure 3). It uses the mobile device database as well as an internal control layer that interacts with the view layer. View layer is in charge of communications and the tablet to be used requires to have at least one of the Wi-Fi/3G/4G communication protocols that will be used for some external communication activities in a further stage of the project. All these are shown graphically in Figure 3.

While readings are being stored locally in the MAMITa, MAMITA Server complements the functionality by allowing communications between tablets and a data center. Local MAMITa data is synched in the cloud to be accessed by the community center via Wi-Fi whenever communication is allowed or connection is achieved. This scenario happens locally within a single health community center such as the Rural Hospital. MAMITa will be later extended to a wireless environment, when communications are allowed between medical centers. By allowing having patient's information centralized in one place the doctors or other social workers

Figure 2. Social worker, patient interactions with the MAMITa through the use of devices

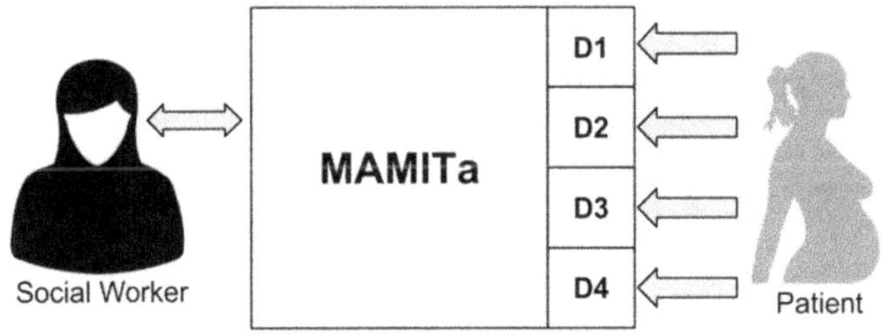

will have better accessibility to the patient's information without the original social worker or the tablet being required to travel. Storing the data will also allow further data processing for having statistics or applying algorithmic solutions that allow improving the risk assessment evaluation process.

Figure 4 illustrates the whole MAMICare system interactions. First, the MAMI Server in which different tablets from different patients are being synchronized and data is being centralized in the cloud in order to be accessible from any workstation. Secondly, the MAMITa system in which medical measurements are input and stored locally in the tablet device.

Figure 3. Shows the MAMI tablet (MAMITa) internal interface and communications

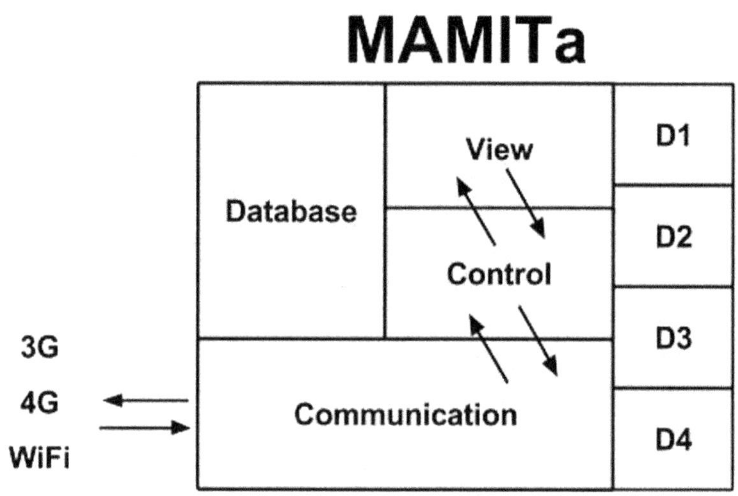

Figure 4. Full 2-part functionality of MAMI care project

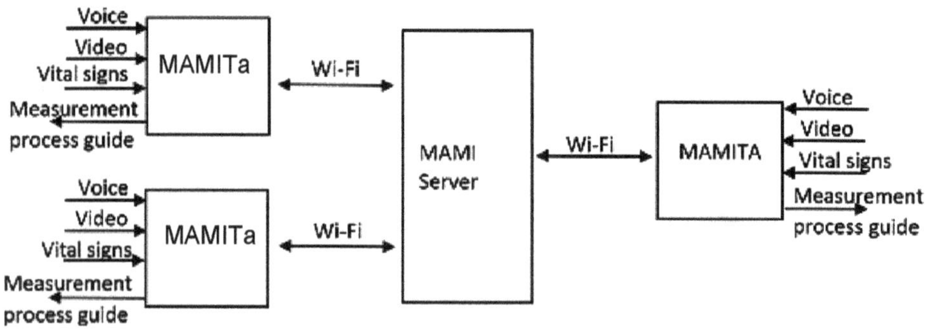

For the short-term, the Denis cheap CDMA 450/800 Mhz 7 inches Android 4.0 CDMA tablet was used as a base development environment due to its inclusion of the CDMA450 communications protocol which has been chosen by Mexican telephone company TELMEX (2008) to be used for expanding the communications services to the rural areas since 2007. However at the moment or writing this paper, there are no communication services yet in the rural area of our attention. The Denis CDMA tablet also enables a later process of syncing the data with a cloud database, which will help to keep track records of the patient's evolution.

It is important to highlight, that even though MAMICare is a full solution, having only MAMITa available does help to reduce the problems of data accuracy and risk assessment. MAMITa implements a risk assessment flow and algorithm that allows the device to provide recommendations to the Social Worker and the patient. The main risk assessment flow and algorithm will be discussed in detail next.

MAMITa Risk Assessment Algorithm

MAMITa covers a limited list of use cases that go from patient registration, periodic assessment, diagnosis and recommendations, and cloud sync (Figure 5). The risk assessment algorithm leverages the information recovered during the patient registration, and periodic assessment to provide with an informed diagnosis and a set of recommendations or actions to take. The MAMITa algorithm follows a set of rules that dictate the type of measurements and data that is required from the patient.

The risk assessment algorithm can be broken down in three main parts: (1) Medical history, (2) Periodic Screening, and (3) Diagnosis and recommendation. A description of each of these parts is included:

1. During the patient registration, a set of guided questions need to be answered about the patient, also the periodic screening information is tracked and considered part of the medical history.
2. The periodic screening will use the medical history follow through a set of questions and request for specific medical measurements. The answer to each question, the patient measurements and the medical history will directly affect the next step in the assessment.
3. Diagnosis and recommendations will not provide a full medical diagnosis, but will rather provided a green, yellow, red status and a list of recommendations such as taking folic acid, or aspirins in cases of hypertensions. This diagnosis will also refer the patients to the nearest hospital in case of elevated risk.

Figure 5. MAMITa use cases

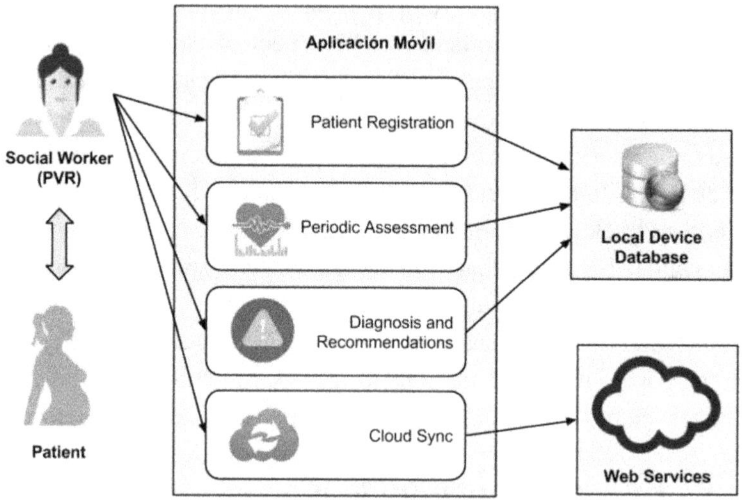

As it was mentioned earlier, MAMICare aims to provide a full mobile and cloud solution, and it is limited by the current rural area accesibility to the internet. However, MAMITa still keeps valid track records of patients information and uses an algorithm to detect risk. While MAMI Server may be unavailable, it is expected that MAMITa will be transported with the patient in case of an emergency; this allows the physician to have access to the patient's information and a proper assessment of conditions and a quick decision-making. In order to have a better understanding of the expected impact of this system, our original use-case situation will be exposed next, this time under the assumption that the MAMITa system is already implemented in the community.

Expected Impact of Health Information Technology Scenario

Considering the same characters, distances, orography and characteristics originally described in the original situation scenario. This time Maria has her full kit including the sensor devices and the MAMITa system.

During her scheduled visit to Rosa's home, Maria activates the MAMITa system. MAMITa guides her thoroughly during the metrics process. Maria uses the stethoscope as required by the system and data is stored in the system using wireless communication. MAMITa shows Maria a set of images/video on how to use the sphygmomanometer properly, the system receives the data and detects an abnormality in Rosa's health. MAMITa asks Maria to write down the anomaly in the form. Maria is asked by the system to make some follow up questions such as what her activities have been during the past days. MAMITa uses a microphone to record and store Rosa's description. Using a Doppler ultrasound, MAMITa stores data being sent by the device, in that moment the system detects another anomaly and asks the social worker to use her radio communication system to notify the Health House, UMR and HSB that a patient in critical situation has to be transferred to the HSB. One of the neighbors with vehicles comes to help move Rosa. Eight minutes later, Rosa is at the HSB, the physician practitioner in charge makes her diagnosis based on the tablet information. Data allows him to decide to move her to Tlaxiaco Hospital. In Tlaxiaco Rosa is timely attended; both Rosa and her baby are safe.

Expected Impact

As shown in the previous use cases, expected impact of implementing MAMICare in the rural areas include having truthful information and thus reducing diagnostic errors. The PVR will be better prepared to act under any circumstance. Another great advantage is the preservation of data. At the UMR, data could remain active from a few hours up to three days. In the Rural Hospital, data could remain relevant from one up to four days. Also inside the Hospital, communication and data transfer occurs immediately between tablets and workstations. MAMITa expects to reduce the time of capturing the medical records by giving proper instructions, as well as by having available truthful information that allows physicians and social workers to have the best possible scenario for decision-making and even highlighting any considered risk situation.

USABILITY FOR RURAL AREAS

Research demonstrates that MAMICare is a viable solution to the maternity-infant problem that is currently present among the rural community areas in the states of Chiapas, Oaxaca, and Guerrero. However, given the low-literacy context to which the project is aimed, it was expected that the solution would present many challenges related to usability, and user interfaces. For MAMITa User Experience and User Interface Design was defined as a critical part of the design and development. For this, the most common design guidelines for health care Systems in rural areas were selected and analyzed on the context of the problematic. Specifically, the five design principles provided by Medhi, Sagar and Toyama (2006) were taken as a reference for the design of this solution. Some modifications had to be made regarding Speech-Inputs, the use of color and navigation.

The following are the five selected principles with the mentioned modifications that were applied to the solution: (a) avoid text inputs (Numbers may be okay, Use Speech-Inputs when possible), (b) Use of colors, semi-abstracted graphics, and increase photorealism with deeper interaction, (c) Reduced use of Scrolling and Hierarchical Navigation, (d) Provide voice feedback for all functional units, (e) Provide "help" on all screens.

We have conducted an initial set of usability tests (focus groups, cognitive walkthroughs and interviews) with doctors and students from the associated School of Medicine of our University. This audience is technologically and with a strong medical science background, but our initial approach has been to verify the accuracy of the procedures and protocols implemented in MAMICare, and also verify that that the application is intuitive enough for people familiarized with the use of mobile devices.

The findings of the conducted assessment worked as a guideline for defining the path in which the application development of health care systems for rural areas should be taken, in particular the MAMITa prototype. However, further work is required to better adequate the prototype for rural areas. Also, it is required to properly test the application with Doctor, in the mentioned community of Magdalena de Peñasco, and continue to improve the application upon users feedback. By doing this, it is expected to provide a solution that makes a positive impact in the rural areas in Mexico.

RESEARCH LIMITATIONS AND FUTHER STUDY ISSUES

As we mentioned before our work is based on the population needs identified in a demographic study in rural areas, therefore there exists some limitations which we have to deal with and eventually reduce our expected impact. First of all the communication issue: the lack of proper communication means is consider in the initial phase of MAMICare, but further versions depend on the availability of communication technologies in the region (WiFi, 3G, or 4G). Availability communication technology depends of federal agencies and findings, which are out of scope of influence. In addition, the adoption or rejection of MAMICare depends of the approval of the state and federal health agency. This approval however is not only based on the technical merit of our project, sometimes, political reasons have more impact that technical benefits. As we mentioned before, our technical solution is ready and fully functional but political and economical changes have limited deployment of MAMICare in the area.

CONCLUSION

MAMICare System is a solution that is expected to make a positive impact once it is implemented in any of the rural areas in Mexico. Research demonstrates that MAMICare is a viable solution to the maternity-infant problem that is currently present among the rural community areas in the states of Chiapas, Oaxaca, and Guerrero. Also the use of electronic healthcare services makes possible to reduce attention issues associated with the main causes of death (hypertension, hemorrhages, and other complications of delivery) that are much higher in maternity-infant care. The MAMICare System is a two-part system MAMITa and MAMIServer, that combined provided an integral solution for monitoring pregnancy progress and help to reduce the overall maternal-infant mortality rate in rural areas of Mexico. MAMITa – a tablet system to aid the social workers in the patient's assessment process. MAMI Server consolidates the electronic health records of patients with data captured by the social works using MAMITa. Such consolidated information is available at the Medical Centers in the region.

We continue our effort to obtain the required resources and support of the local leaders and authorities to make MAMICare and mortality ratio reduction a reality in underserved communities.

REFERENCES

Bahga, A., & Madisetti, V. (2015, February). Healthcare Data Integration and Informatics in the Cloud. IEEE Computer, 50-57.

Bates, D., & Gawade, A. (2003). Improving safety with information technology. *The New England Journal of Medicine*, *348*(25), 2526–2534. doi:10.1056/NEJMsa020847 PMID:12815139

Blank, A., Kaltschmidt, J., Krings, A., Sukums, F., Mensah, N., Haefeli, W., & Gustafsson, L. (2013). "Quality of prenatal and maternal care: Bridging the know-do gap" (QUALMAT study): An electronic clinical decision support system for rural Sub-Saharan Africa. *BMC Medical Informatics and Decision Making*, *13*(1), 44. doi:10.1186/1472-6947-13-44 PMID:23574764

Calman, N., Hauser, D., Lurio, J., Wu, W. Y., & Pichardo, M. (2012). Strengthening Public Health and Primary Care Collaboration Through Electronic Health Records. *American Journal of Public Health*, *102*(11), e13–e18. doi:10.2105/AJPH.2012.301000 PMID:22994274

Hörmansdörfer, C., Hillemanns, P., Schmidt, P., Scharf, A., Golatta, M., Vaske, B.. (2008). Preliminary analysis of the new 'Prenatal Risk Calculation (PRC)' software. *Archives of Gynecology and Obstetrics*, *279*(4), 1-5.

Jennett, P., Yeo, M., Scott, R., Hebert, M., & Teo, W. (2005). Delivery of rural and remote health care via a broadband Internet Protocol network - views of potential users. *Journal of Telemedicine and Telecare*, *11*(8), 419–424. doi:10.1177/1357633X0501100808 PMID:16356317

Macleod, B., Phillips, J., Stone, A., Walji, A., & Awoonor-Williams, J. (2012). The Architecture of a Software System for Supporting Community-based Primary Health Care with Mobile Technology: The Mobile Technology for Community Health (MoTeCH) Initiative in Ghana. *Online Journal of Public Health Informatics*, *4*(1). doi:10.5210/ojphi.v4i1.3910 PMID:23569631

Medhi, I., Sagar, A., & Toyama, K. (2006). Text-Free User Interfaces for Illiterate and Semi-Literate Users. In *2006 International Conference on Information and Communication Technologies and Development*. IEEE. 10.1109/ICTD.2006.301841

Mougiakakou, S. G., Bartsocas, C. S., Bozas, E., Chaniotakis, N., Iliopoulou, D., Kouris, I., & Nikita, K. S. (2010). SMARTDIAB: A communication and information technology approach for the intelligent monitoring, management and follow-up of type 1 diabetes patients. *IEEE Transactions on Information Technology in Biomedicine*, *14*(3), 622–633. doi:10.1109/TITB.2009.2039711 PMID:20123578

Muñoz, D., Avila, A., Lavariega, J., González, A., & Grote, W. (2012). *Emergency Remote Pre-Hospital Asssitance (ERPHA)*. Project Final Report at Latin America and Caribbean Collaborative ICT Research Federation. Retrieved from www.laccir.org

Sachpazidis, I., Rizou, D., & Menary, W. (2008). *Broadband Health Care Network in Brazil and Peru*. Retrieved from Scopus database.

Secretaria de Salud del Gobierno Mexicano. (1995). *Norma Oficial Mexicana NOM-007-SSA2-1993, Atención de la mujer durante el embarazo, parto y puerperio y del recién nacido. Criterios y procedimientos para la prestación del servicio*. Retrieved from www.salud.gob.mx/unidades/cdi/nom/007ssa23.html (in Spanish)

Teléfonos de México, S. A. B de C. V. (TELMEX). (2008). *Comunicados 2008: Boletín Informativo*. Retrieved from www.telmex.com/mx/corporativo/salaPrensa_ComPrensa2008_080117.89.html (in Spanish)

Velikova, M., Lucas, P., & van der Hijden, M. (2015, February). Intelligent Disease Self-Management with Mobile Technology. IEEE Computer, 32-39.

Weaver, A., & Bryce, R. (2015, February). Technological Advances in Medicine:Its Personal. IEEE Computer, 21-23.

World Health Organization, Department of Making Pregnancy Safer. (2006). *Pregnancy, childbirth, postpartum and newborn care - A guide for essential practice*. Retrieved from www.who.int/reproductivehealth/publications/

World Health Organization, UNICEF, UNFPA, & The World Bank. (2012). *Trends in maternal mortality: 1990 to 2010 WHO, UNICEF, UNFPA and The World Bank estimates*. Retrieved from www.who.int/reproductivehealth/publications

World Health Organization (WHO). (2006). *Country Cooperation Strategy: at a glance – Mexico*. Retrieved from www.who.int/countryfocus/cooperation_stratefy/briefs

This research was previously published in the Handbook of Research on Emerging Perspectives on Healthcare Information Systems and Informatics edited by Joseph Tan; pages 483-497, copyright year 2018 by Medical Information Science Reference (an imprint of IGI Global).

Chapter 4
Cyber-Moms Facing Motherhood:
Holding Functions and Regressive Movements in Parenting Websites

Valentina Boursier
University of Naples Federico II, Italy

Francesca Gioia
University of Naples Federico II, Italy

Valentina Manna
Association for Social Promotion Roots in Action, Italy

Federica Coppola
University of Naples Federico II, Italy

Noemi Venosa
University of Naples Federico II, Italy

ABSTRACT

Mothers and mothers-to-be often become e-health users because of their need for sharing emotional and practical parental experiences. In this sense, web forums seem to positively contribute to parenting skills and transition to motherhood. This study aims at exploring how 379 Italian mothers use two Italian forums, the manifest and latent contents of their interactions, and the emotional connections between their own maternal experiences and the e-group dynamics. The qualitative analysis of 7433 comments pointed out five main themes, describing how mothers make sense of their experiences through the online dimension: the group; I am; personal experience; perspective knowhow; tech-moms. This study confirms that parenting experience represents a big challenge for rising mothers. Moreover, it shows that the e-groups can alternatively reproduce a peer group functioning and a feeding breast, a reassuring container with holding functions, or a "toilet breast", encouraging progressive as well as regressive movements.

DOI: 10.4018/978-1-7998-2351-3.ch004

INTRODUCTION

Pregnancy and the transition to parenthood represent some of the biggest life challenges, which need support. As Albrecht and Adelman (1984) highlighted, social support allows people to manage the uncertainty related to the stress and improve the sense of personal control or efficacy over their environments. Web communities offer a great opportunity to create online groups and receive necessary and appropriate experiences of social support and comparison. Probably, for this reason, parents and parents-to-be represent a large category of *e-health* users, as they can express and satisfy online their need for sharing emotional and practical experiences. For example, a recent multicenter Italian cross-sectional study (Bert et al., 2013) revealed that around 20% of pregnant women use online forums to share information and to experience support from other pregnant women. It has been demonstrated that pregnant women frequently use the internet to search for pregnancy-related information (Scaioli et al., 2005).

Furthermore, the increasing role of the Internet in everyday life has changed the meaning of what a community is. Indeed, on the Web, parents can create communities based on shared interests (Kirk & Milnes, 2015), setting up groups composed of different individuals who offer different perspectives, experiences, opinions and sources of information (Brady & Guerin, 2010), and, lastly, to receive Internet-based peer support, despite the geographical distance or time constraints (Niela-Vilén et al., 2014). Thus, what the parents and parents-to-be are searching for on the *e*-communities? How and why they are using them? The reason for participating in e-parents' groups should be investigated, taking into account the underlying meanings and psychological dynamics which possibly characterize an identity and role transition.

Background

Overall, future parents have to face changes with a number of adaptive and transformative tasks (Stern & Bruschweiler-Stern, 1998) to successfully transit from the couple dyad to the family triad (Montigny, Lacharité, & Amyot, 2006), crossing an important adulthood crisis (Cadei & Simeone. 2011). Moreover, they are required to transform their roles and identities, integrating new parental functions (Deave, Johnson, & Ingram, 2008; Slade, Cohen, Sadler, & Miller, 2009; Widarsson, Kerstis, Sundquist, Engström, & Sarkadi, 2012; Spinelli et al., 2016). Particularly, the psychodynamic literature strongly highlighted how much these challenges influence in a specific way the mothers rather than the fathers, due to the cultural stereotype of the "perfect mother", socially established and internalized by women, thus becoming a kind of phantasy (Chodorow & Contratto, 1989), not present in the same vein among fathers. Indeed, during pregnancy women undergo a physical and psychological transformation in preparing to become a mother. From a psychodynamic perspective, the *birth of a mother* (Stern & Bruschweiler-Stern, 1998) involves a reorganization of the woman's inner world and the creation of a mental space to host both the ideas of the child and herself as a parent (Bibring, 1959; Ambrosini & Stanghellini, 2012). Moreover, assuming that motherhood is both a site of social and identity change (Thomson, 2011), the process of becoming a mother includes a deep psychological *re-negotiation* of several aspects of the woman's life and identity as a woman, partner, daughter, and mother. On the one hand, internal conflicts and ambivalence (in a psychodynamic sense, i.e. the coexistence of disparate feelings at the same time), also fostered by prior movements of identification and parental representations above mentioned, need solution and integration (Slade et al, 2009), passing through an interpersonal and a transgenerational[1] dimension (Grienenberger & Slade, 2002; Kelly, Slade, & Grienengerger, 2005). On the other hand, these movements have now increased due to modifications of maternal involvement in the society: the maternal identity and role construction cover a difficult *self-balancing*, for example involving work and family issues as the Work-Family Conflict perspective profusely argues (Hammer & Thompson, 2003). All these topics basically represent mothering tasks, thus the ways mothers respond to the inner role and identity conflicts affect parenting styles (Greenberger, O'neil, & Nagel, 1994; Repetti & Wood, 1997; Crouter & Bumpus, 2001; Costigan, Cox, & Cauce, 2003; Anderson 2007), revealing peculiarities of the mother-child functioning or the adoption of a specific model of what being a mother means to that woman. Indeed, following Brown's reasoning (2010), the modern female identity is a social phenomenon which stems from the relationship that mothers entertain with the social institution of motherhood, and with the social expectations of the maternal role. For example, according to Blair-Loy (2003) and Ridgeway and Correll (2004), the cultural normative of idealized sacrificial motherhood (McCormick, 2010), consistent with the ideology of intensive mothering (Hays, 1996), usually requires an exclusive attentive focus on child rearing in order to be an excellent mother (Stuart, 2007). Consequently, working women often feel guilty because they are not conforming to the societal standard of what a good mother is deemed to be (Guendouzi, 2006), facing the truth that they cannot be both a good worker and a good mother at the same time (Williams & Segal, 2003). Thus, ambivalence about motherhood, choices, and time frequently appears (Chodorow, 2003; Hewlett, 2002).

The informal and professional support and the family's encouragement appear extremely important for mothers and mothers-to-be, helping them to face stressful events like the transition to parenthood (Montigny et al., 2006), the body changes, the baby birth, and their life with a newborn or a growing child.

MAIN FOCUS OF THE CHAPTER

Issues, Controversies, Problems

As Parks (2011) explained, there are two conceptualizations of the term "community": one usually restrict it to groups of people who share physical space, are relatively self-sufficient within that space, and who are linked by ties that include kinship. The second one had lost the geographical trait, becoming stands for culture, a set of ideas and interpersonal sentiments rather than as a physical place (Bender, 1978; Calhoun, 1980). Within this framework, a virtual community is a social group that has the psychological and cultural qualities of a strong community without physical proximity (Willson, 2006). Every group, also virtual, can be defined a community if it acts collectively, thinks of itself as a community and the members identify with the community, sharing and exchanging information and exhibiting attachments to one another and to the community more generally (Willson, 2006; Parks, 2011). Thus, web communities offer a great opportunity to create online groups and receive necessary and appropriate experiences of social support and comparison (Gibson & Hanson, 2013; Niela-Vilén, Axelin, Salanterä, & Menelnder, 2014), as an alternative to face-to-face ones. Due to the increased geographical mobility of people and families, also according to work and career plans, parents, especially mothers, feel more isolated and they are losing daily support from their own family networks (Litt, 2000; Plantin & Daneback, 2009; Gibson & Hanson, 2013). Moreover, grandparents' experiences result in more "out of date" than in the past (they become grandparents at older age than before), thus new parents' requirements are mainly directed to the experience-based source of information, i.e. other "modern" parents in similar situations (Litt, 2000; Niela-Vilén et al., 2014). For example, during postpartum hospital recovery *strangers* become *confidants* because hospitalized new mothers share similar parenting doubts (Oakley & Roberts, 1981), and the parental website offers the opportunity to recreate the hospital scenario (Madge & O'Connor, 2004). Thus, new parents and parents-to-be represent a large category of users (Bartholomew, Schoppe-Sullivan, Glassman, Kamp Dush, & Sullivan, 2012; Morris, 2014), and the *e-health* communities have some advantages for them, especially mothers (Mo, Malik, & Coulson, 2009; Moorhead et al., 2013), in particular when they are socially and geographically isolated.

Sundstrom (2016) underlined how social attachments in online communities may facilitate associations despite the anonymity of members. Several studies describe the reasons for and benefits of the online support group participation (i.e. emotional and instrumental support, community connections and protection, anonymity which allow to express itself candidly) (Drentea & Moren-Cross, 2005; Hall & Irvine, 2009; Brady & Guerin, 2010; Jang, Dworkin, & Connell, 2012; Palmén, Korpela, & Saranto, 2012).

New mothers use the Internet for sharing their baby stories by posting photos or text messages, and reporting special events in their family life (Jomhari, Gonzalez, & Kurniawan, 2009); moreover, they enjoy social communities satisfying their desire of social interactions (Gibson & Hanson, 2013). Indeed, online communities can be considered an important medium in the communication process, serving the function of personal influence and promoting direct interpersonal connection through forum and blogs (Sundstrom, 2016). Particularly, it seems that blogs and forums' participation increase the well-being of mothers, as they receive support in return, more than on the social networks sites (McDaniel, Coyne, & Holmes, 2012). Furthermore, future mothers using online forums declare to be more likely to change their own behavior (for example, concerning the breastfeeding and childcare) according to their online findings. Overall, the time spent on motherhood specific sites seem to have a greater impact on maternal intentions and behaviors despite normative pressures (McKeever & McKeever, 2017).

According to Rogers (2003), interpersonal communication channels can lead the social change more than mass media and, as Tangherlini et al. (2016) highlighted, the persuasive nature of a personal storytelling can catalyze the decision-making process. Additionally, the internet anonymity allows personal disclosure (Suler, 2004; Quian & Scott, 2007; Jordan, 2010) through a direct or an indirect participation in the conversation (Kraut et al., 2004): it reduces inhibitions, and facilitates the users to be honest about their own opinions and feelings (O'Connor & Madge, 2001). As Ley (2007) showed, sites' design influences members' commitment (including loyalty, obligation, attachment, respect, encouragement), developing a sense of security and safety regarding the site because of their evolving and active nature based on shared cultural values, practices, and collective identity that improve support and trust within the online group's boundaries. As Sundstrom (2016) demonstrate, mothers prefer texting as form of communication because of flexibility that text messages offer, because of their easy access, and the possibility to delete it either save it as a future reference or forward it. Thus, writing or replying to posts on the Internet, mothers can create virtual relations through an open and interactive writing; moreover, they can share personal thoughts and feelings, disclosing parental concerns (McDaniel et al., 2012), and experiencing ways of self-expression (Gibson & Hanson, 2013; Morris, 2014), which can or cannot reveal something about the author's identity (Cadei & Simeone. 2011).

At a personal level, people in cyberspace seem to be influenced by the online disinhibition effect, which involves six factors: dissociative anonymity, invisibility, solipsistic introjections, dissociative imagination, and minimization of status and authority. It is not a mere representation of a "true self" but a complex process of "working through" as a shift among deeper aspects of intrapsychic structure (Suler, 2002, 2004). At a relational level, as highlighted by Walther (2007), in a hyperpersonal perspective the computer mediated communication can facilitate desired relationships: the users' self-presentation takes advantage of the written interface and the extra time to edit and re–write the messages before sending them. In this way, this communication channel contributes to greater intimacy and desirability. Thus, from a psychodynamic perspective, *e*-parents may become a protective community and a source of emotional, formal, informal and instrumental support (Drentea & Moren-Cross, 2005), performing a "holding" function[2], and normalising mothers' *in*experience (Madge & O'Connor, 2004; Brady & Guerin, 2010). In this sense, they may provide a safe space for mothers who need to escape from a romanticized motherhood model (Mungham & Lazard, 2011), space where they can admit that they are not "perfect". Moreover, these communities allow parents to transition from being passive containers of information towards actively searching for different perspectives, experiences, and information (Brady & Guerin, 2010; Jang et al., 2012). Indeed, the online peer support groups represent an endless source of medical data and social assistance (Plantin & Daneback, 2009), characterized by instant responses and low costs (Madge & O'Connor, 2004), even though they cannot constitute an alternative to high-quality professional websites (Reichow et al., 2012) because of the risk of sharing inaccurate information (Madge & O'Connor, 2004; Jordan, 2010).

Furthermore, despite the geographical distances or time constraints (Niela-Vilén et al., 2014), online peer support groups are a rich source of comparison and practical advice. They make a positive contribution to parents and parenting (Nieuwboer, Fukkink, & Hermanns, 2013), for example: satisfying mothers' needs when they suffer from postpartum depression (Dennis et al., 2009; Dennis, 2010); helping new mothers to feel more connected with others through the Internet (McDaniel et al., 2012); and committing mothers practically to online activities, thus helping them to be awake during the night while feeding (Gibson & Hanson, 2013). Thus, e-groups seem to make a positive contribution to parenting skills and transition to motherhood. Recently, an Italian study on families of patients with rare diseases (Tozzi et al., 2013) showed that 66% of parents participate in an online forum on health and demonstrated that Italian parents of children with rare diseases are active Internet users (searching for information and/or joining online communities), confirming that the information management is an important component of coping with illness and illness-related uncertainties (Brashers, Goldsmith, & Hsieh, 2002). What about parents not specifically involved with child's diseases? And what about mothers-to-be? The Italian context is lack of studies on this issue, i.e. on if, how and why mothers and mothers-to-be use the web communities. Two Italian studies (Bert et al., 2013; Scaioli et al., 2015) carried out a multicentre survey to assess the sociodemographic and geographic differences existing in a sample of pregnant women searching for information on the web. These studies also explored the factors influencing the choices of childbirth after the Internet consultation and investigated potential differences between primiparous and multiparous women in the Internet use. Moreover, Tozzi et al. (2013) conducted an online survey among Italian parents of patients with rare diseases to describe their Internet user profile and to explore how Internet use affects their health decisions. Nevertheless, there is a lack of Italian studies about the use of web forums dedicated to mothering and about motivations for its use by mothers, *mothers-to-be*, and women trying to have a baby.

SOLUTIONS AND RECOMMENDATIONS

Aims

From a psychodynamic perspective, the aim of the present study is to explore the Italian e-mothers context -specifically focusing on the rising maternity- questioning *whether*, *why*, and *how* they use specific online forums. The analysis of the manifest and latent contents of the mothers' interactions and of the emotional connections between their own maternal experiences and their online group belonging represents a specific task.

Methods

Data Collection

According to Kraut et al. (2004), although conducting online research can potentially affect data quality, researchers' actions, and human subjects, it does not involve more risks than traditional research. Rather, it changes the nature of the risks and investigators' ability is required to evaluate them. First, the online research entails serious sampling problems, especially for traditional quantitative studies. Indeed, recruiting a random or representative sample and verifying the identity of online participants is not possible (Madge & O'Connor, 2002). Moreover, possible risks to subjects participating in internet-based interviews and surveys regard their direct participation, for example, emotional reactions or experimental manipulations, and harm resulting from a breach of confidentiality (Kraut et al., 2004). The issues relating to anonymity, informed consent, boundaries, and the difference between public and private behaviors have still not been clarified and the debate is far from over.

However, internet-based methodologies offer new and many opportunities. They allow researchers to interact with participants in innovative ways, to use different sampling strategies, to conduct qualitative research (Mann & Stewart, 2000; Madge & O'Connor, 2002; Hooley, Wellens, & Marriott, 2011), to explore the online and offline experience in everyday life, and to involve marginalized populations (Sparks, Collins, & Kearns, 2016). Moreover, as Kraut et al. (2004) explained, the use of the Internet in psychological research allows researchers to recognize psychological phenomena that would be much more difficult to identify in traditional settings. It is very difficult to chase the evolution of groups because of the difficulties and costs of tracking many individuals for a long time. In this regard, the Internet represents a valuable tool for long-term research on groups.

Data for this study were extracted on the Internet by searching for Italian websites with forums about maternity. Forums were searched on Google search engine using few representative Italian keywords, descriptive of this study interest: forum, mothers, children. Two forums specifically directed to mothering and raising maternity, with mothers coming from all over Italy, were selected because of their users' daily activity and the variety of themes discussed. From these two forums, 231 relevant threads were extracted. They have been written in a time frame of three years (2013-2016).

After a first summary reading of posts and personal users' account, threads were selected using following criteria:

- written or active from January 1, 2013, to December 31, 2016;
- written by mothers-to-be and mothers of young children (0-3 years).

The data collection focused on women who were having their first child as the study focused on the maternity process, assuming that pregnant women and mothers experiencing maternity with very young children could specifically face with similar topics (different from mothers of adolescents for example). Moreover, it was not possible to select only a specific target of mothers, as mothers of young children often participate in forum discussions about pregnancy, presenting their quite close experience. On the contrary, it was improbable to find a mother of an adolescent.

Finally, a total number of 7433 comments were collected. Each thread was extracted by copying and printed into a document for a pencil on paper analysis.

To protect forum members' real identity (Kraut et al., 2004), all the identifying data in the text were omitted, such as the Internet forum name, names or pseudonyms of the writers, or references to places. Also, the usernames or URLs for any specific threads were omitted. Therefore, it is not possible to identify any single forum user in our final results.

Sample

In the collected data, 379 Italian writers were included: mothers of young children and 57 declared mothers-to-be. The gender and the geographical origin of users were explicitly declared on their personal forum profile. Being a mother, pregnant or trying to have a baby were determined by information explicitly provided by the authors (i.e., in profiles) or inferred from the content of comments (for example, "my baby is 20 months old", "I and my husband are trying to have a baby"). On the personal forum profile, nobody had explicitly declared her age.

Data Analysis

According to the guidelines described by Braun and Clarke (2006), a Latent Thematic Analysis was realized to identify, analyze, and report themes from a qualitative source of data. Taking into account the psychodynamic epistemological authors' background, an inductive data-driven (not theory-driven) analysis was conducted through an analytic process, which moves from the data description to the interpretation. Indeed, thematic analysis entails research across the data set to find repeated patterns of meaning, mainly in the latent thematic analysis the development of the themes themselves involves an interpretative work. Specifically, a line by line thematic analysis at a latent level "goes beyond the semantic content of the data, and starts to identify or examine the *underlying* ideas, assumptions, and conceptualizations" (Braun & Clarke, 2006, p. 13).

According to Braun and Clarke (2006), the Latent Thematic Analysis is not a linear process from one phase to the next. Rather, it is a recursive process and consists of different phases, where the researcher move back and forth as needed, throughout them (Table 1). First, two researchers independently and simultaneously read all the material to familiarize with the data corpus, and after a "repeated reading" of the data in an active way, searching for meanings, patterns and so on, they wrote notes on the margins to record interesting contents. The codes could refer to semantic or latent contents that appear interesting to the analysts. Gradually, from these contents, they created a preliminary list of codes, writing notes in the text, using highlighters or colored pens to indicate potential patterns or to identify segments of data. Later, the researchers started to analyze the codes matching them up with data extracts, consider how different codes may combine to form an overarching theme, and think about the relationship between codes, between themes, and between different levels of themes. Following Braun and Clarke (2006), they discussed the findings searching for the meanings beyond the surface, unraveling the reality. Through the comparison among the researchers, a critical revision of proposed themes was conducted to guarantee internal homogeneity and external heterogeneity (data within themes should cohere together meaningfully, while there should be clear and identifiable distinctions between themes). Finally, searching for themes that work in relation to the coded extracts and the entire data set, five main themes emerged and it was possible to determine which features of data was captured by each theme, generating clear definitions and names for each of them and a "thematic map" of the analysis. In this way, it was possible to make sense of patterns of meaning (Braun & Clarke, 2013).

Table 1. Phases of thematic analysis (Braun & Clarke, 2006)

Phase	Description of the Process
1. Familiarising yourself with your data:	Transcribing data (if necessary), reading and re-reading the data, noting down initial ideas.
2. Generating initial codes:	Coding interesting features of the data in a systematic fashion across the entire data set, collating data relevant to each code.
3. Searching for themes:	Collating codes into potential themes, gathering all data relevant to each potential theme.
4. Reviewing themes:	Checking in the themes work in relation to the coded extracts (Level 1) and the entire data set (Level 2), generating a thematic 'map' of the analysis.
5. Defining and naming themes:	Ongoing analysis to refine the specifics of each theme, and the overall story the analysis tells; generating clear definitions and names for each theme.
6. Producing the report:	The final opportunity for analysis. Selection of vivid, compelling extract examples, final analysis of selected extracts, relating back of the analysis to the research question and literature, producing a scholarly report of the analysis (eventually including a thematic map).

RESULTS

Five main themes emerged from the thematic analysis, resulting from the final identification of 41 codes and 12 subthemes. These 5 themes and their connections describe the complexity of the relations among the e-mothers and (a) their on-going parental experience, (b) their identities under construction, (c) their worries and fantasies, and (d) the online group. In our interpretation, all these topics shape how mothers make sense of their experiences through the online dimension. (Figure 1)

Themes were so called: *the group* (53.06%); *I am* (17.93%); *personal experience* (14.82%); *perspective knowhow* (8.92%); *tech-moms* (5.27%) (Table 2).

On the total frequency of the codes, it has been calculated the percentage of the sub-themes and, consequently, the percentage of the themes. The first theme is the biggest one, including a little more than half of the entire corpus of data. Even though Latent Thematic Analysis does not take care of statistics and invites researchers to consider the emotional value it can be captured beyond the data description (Braun & Clarke, 2006), this amount should be considered as it refers to "the weight" the online group dynamics and functioning have in this context.

Figure 1. The map of themes connected to the categories and related codes

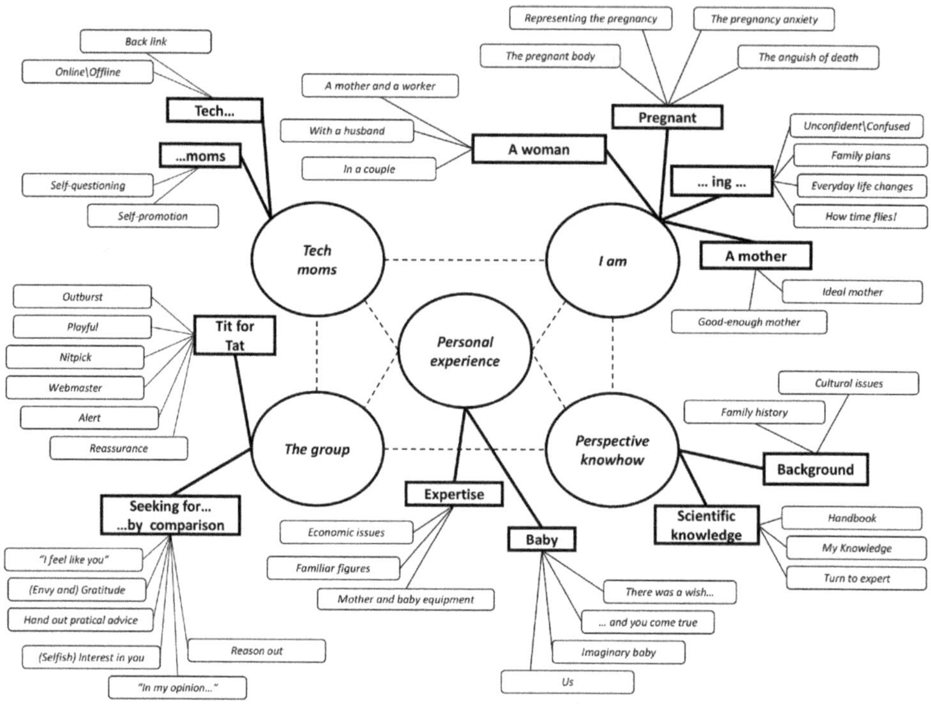

The Group

This theme seems to well describe the group functioning, how and why the members use the community. On these parenting websites, mothers can share personal experiences and knowledge with people interested in the same issue, receiving information and practical advice. The e-group interactions, as the face-to-face group, are often characterized by a *tit for tat* functioning, a back and forth communication. Moreover, as in a typical face-to-face group, both the *nitpicks* (i.e. conflicts and arguments) and *playful* moments (i.e. jokes and complicity) are unavoidable and seem to reinforce cohesion and intimacy among members. For example:

Your nickname is awesome... So funny!!!!! (Playful)

There are topics full of venom against your mothers. Has anybody ever told you to shut up?!

Seriously, what kind of speeches are these? (Nitpicks)

Table 2. Codes frequency on 7433 messages; subthemes % on total codes frequency and related themes %

THEMES (% On Total Sub Themes)	SUB THEMES (% On Total Frequency)	CODES (Frequency)
THE GROUP (53.06)	Tit for tat (20.61)	Playful (2260) Nitpick (1023) Reassurance (843) Alert (265) Outburst (227) Webmaster and censorship (155)
	Seeking for… By comparison (32.45)	"In my opinion" (2605) "I feel like you" (2239) Hand out practical advice (1233) (Selfish) Interest in you (925) (Envy and) Gratitude (389) Reason out (131)
I AM (17.93)	A mother (5.65)	Ideal mother (734) Good enough mother (575)
	A woman (3.9)	In a couple (442) A mother and a worker (250) With a husband (211)
	Pregnant (5)	The anguish of death (445) The pregnant body (377) Representing the pregnancy (171) The pregnancy anxiety (165)
	… ing … (3.38)	Unconfident/Confused (471) Everyday life changes (158) Family plans (98) How time flies! (58)
PERSONAL EXPERIENCE (14.82)	Baby (11.78)	… And you come true (1667) There was a wish … (847) Imaginary baby (191) Us (23)
	Expertise (3.04)	Mother and baby equipment (372) Familiar figures(192) Economic issues (138)
PERSPECTIVE KNOWHOW (8.92)	Background (1.21)	Cultural issues (226) Family history (54)
	Scientific knowledge (7.71)	Turn to expert (1027) My knowledge (720) Handbook (40)
TECH-MOMS (5.27)	Tech … (1.29)	Back link (263) Online/Offline (35)
	… Moms (3.98)	Self-promotion (608) Self-questioning (314)

Maybe... the first childbirth was too hard for your husband, and maybe HE doesn't want to repeat that experience!!!!!!!!!!!! (Nitpicks)

However, in the specific online context, a *webmaster* mediates the members' exchanges.

I covered the bad word you used with asterisks... Just be careful, please!!!

Through their interactions, sometimes *e*-mothers seem to verbalize their worries, anxiety, and the *alert* they undergo about their first experiences with children and/or pregnancy, transmitting it to the other members and evacuating it in the group that can contain these feelings. Thus, the e-group seems the place in which concerns and *Outbursts* (releases of negative and strong emotions) are permitted, accepted and held back by *Reassurances*. For example:

I am so irate, I know I could be egoistic, but I'm tired and I was very patience! I am very irritated! (Outburst)

Girls, thank you so much for your reassuring words, but I am so worried. Even if he is growing, the pediatrician told me that growth parameters are not good... I am so worried... The chow time is a fight, he cries and doesn't open his mouth. It's become too much for me... I need a solution! (Reassurance and Outburst)

Furthermore, the sub-theme named *comparison* includes comparative experiences reported by mothers with someone who feels the same feelings (*"I feel like you"*), *hands out practical advice*, offers a personal opinion (*"In my opinion..."*), and expresses attention and interest in other people (*Interest in you*), helping grateful mothers (*Gratitude*) to make decisions (*Reason out*).

Thank you very much for your valuable suggestion... I will take your advice! (Gratitude and Reason out)

I like so much these threads! When someone asks a question, each of us answers based on personal experiences, therefore we have a number of completely different replies. So, there are no well-specific guidelines with regard to children, only common sense (In my opinion... and Interest in you)

Indeed, the group is also the virtual place in which *selfish*ness and *envy* can be expressed, for example towards who is living actual maternity experience or pregnancy, caring their baby, while other women are trying to get pregnant.

Girls, I don't know if it's the same for you, but every day pregnant friends pop up around me. Obviously, I am happy for them, but I wish the same to me, possibly getting over the first trimester.

Sometimes it seems an obstacle course of enthusiasms and falls, often with the unpleasant feeling of seeing so many women who make it, while we keep running, falling and rising up after all this trouble, may we will be in good shape mothers.

Last year, when I started to try, all the women around me caught the stork, everyone but me. I brought good luck to many women, but now, I really would want some fortune!

I Am

The "I am" dimension involves transformations in the feminine identity the woman is experiencing. Forums about maternity seem to include hints and variations of women's identity, according to how the on-going maternity implicates a revolution in women's sense of be-*ing*: they are constantly in changing, their new lives and identities are in progress, and these transformations connect past to present and future, involving *everyday life changes, family plans*, and *unconfident* feelings. The personal identity, as *a woman* and as *a mother*, needs to become gradually and deeply integrated and balanced.

Hello, moms! This morning, drinking my coffee, I enjoyed the sunrise and the silence... Amazing! I was thinking about the need to have our own space, despite the family, where we could seek shelter from everyday life routine and problems. Have you a place to find your thoughts and yourself again? Have you a place to collect your thoughts and to process your problems and feelings?

We are first of all women, as well as mothers... Delicate souls subjected to a lot of sacrifices and continuous trials... No one of us is better than others: we are amazing women that are trying to best manage our own lives.

Mothers need to resolve a difficult mix: the job's responsibilities (as *a mother and a worker)* need to match with the woman *in a couple*, and with the mothering that implies children's requests and maternal duty; such as the idealized image of maternity (*the ideal mother*) needs to encounter reality boundaries (*the good enough mother)*.

I lasted two months... I hardly saw her because of my office hours.

In the morning I took her to the nest, during the lunch break I brought back her at home where my mother was waiting for us. I went back to work, and then I returned at home no earlier than 8 p.m., when she was already asleep. I asked for the part-time, but it was denied me. So I decided to fire me. After a while, my husband and I tried to have another child. I came back at work when my second baby was 3 years old and the first daughter started primary school

Despite my breast pain, I fed my daughter until 14 months, but I want, to be honest... I'm not sure what my strong motivation was, whether it was the love for my baby or the fear of being accused of being a bad mother

She would be labeled as a bad mother because that's how it works. In sorrow shall thou bring forth children»; you will feed them and you will forget yourself!!!

Nobody will ever tell you how you can be a parent. Being a parent means to learn from the children, reviewing themselves and the relationship with own parents.

There is no right or wrong: the important thing is the harmony you establish with your child.

All these aspects discuss an identity under construction and evolution, as it refers to the first years of the child life and to the *mother-to-be* dimension when the woman faces *body* transformations:

Your body is preparing for the event, and your mind should do the same.

How long after the childbirth can I dress in my old jeans again? I mean, how long will it take to get back in shape? I miss my favorite jeans...

... inner fantasies, and fears as the pregnancy anxiety, and the anguish of death.

I use the Angel Care, a sensor that you put under the mattress of the child, which sounds in case of absence of breath.

Today I had some slight blood losses... Hey, you [the baby] please settle at the right place!

When you are pregnant you have a thousand thoughts, even about trivial things. So you are troubled by so many doubts: « This will hurt him? Can I use, eat, do such a thing?»

Personal Experience

Digital writers often share with the *e*-group an event occurred in their everyday life. Moreover, the baby's birth implies the constitution of an "*us*" dimension that activates emotional and practical issues.

I haven't been apart from her since we checked out of the hospital... We are always together! I know that moment will come, but for now, she is so tiny!!!

Mothers narrate their experiences with the *baby*: the *imaginary* one…

I am not afraid that he might be disabled.

…the desired one *(there was a wish ...)*…

I simply felt that this was the right moment for me to realize the desire of having a child.

Just remember: you are a mother now and forever. You are a mother for this angel who lived for a too short time inside of you, bringing a lot of happiness. You will be a mother for your future babies. When the desire of a baby touch a woman's heart she is already a mother: a mother in the making.

…and the real one (... *and you come true)*. However, mothers also provide for the construction of a personal *expertise* focusing on the *mother and baby equipment,* the *familiar figures'* support and the *economic issues*. For example:

I found a great offer on e-bay, I paid 9€, it was great, wasn't it?

We bought: two baby bottles, thermos, diapers, napkins, dummy, clothes, towels, beach chair, toys, and stroller. is there something missing? What kind of ointment have I to use when I will change his diaper? Have I to buy physiological saline for his nose?

Sharing personal experiences seems to reinforce women's belonging to a new on-going dimension, facing fantasies and reality. Emotional and practical issues proceed simultaneously like two dimensions which sometimes cover and discover each other.

Perspective Knowhow

Parenting challenges and desires encourage mothers to work hard improving their own capabilities as a caregiver. The experiences they had as children basically imprint their own parental style. Indeed, a personal and cultural *background* transmitted across generations *(family history, cultural issues)* give the mothers a first direction equipping them deeply and a guide to an initial approach to mothering. This cultural background is often discussed and criticized by mothers in the *e*-group especially about themes as breastfeeding, job and gender role.

All women in my family have fed the children. For me, there can be no other kind

In my family, everybody has breastfed, maybe I didn't want to be outdone...it influenced my decision of course...

S*cientific knowledge* certainly can solve parenting doubts and dull pain, representing an important task for mothers. By reading *handbook*s or (positively or negatively) referring *to the experts*, mothers can build a personal portfolio *(my knowledge)* they can share with the other e-parents and proudly show them.

In my opinion, some good reading is necessary ... You cannot start the parental adventure without adequate training!

I was so scared before of the childbirth! But I remember a paper about this and how to get over it. It was very useful to me.

My pediatrician wrote to me the feed schedule...

Unfortunately, most pediatricians do not consider the newborns' pain as a relevant issue to be faced.

But I would like to know... why the pediatricians have to psychologically terrorize the parents?

I beg to tell you that the 10-minute-feed method is greatly exceeded: scientific studies highlighted that the first milk is lighter and more thirst-quenching than the second one. The second milk is fatter and more filling: it allows to your child to grow up. Feeding your baby 10 minutes for breast, she sucks just the first, lighter and digestible milk, so she will be hungry sooner.

Anguishes can decrease through the knowledge. Although online forums do not always represent high-quality sources of information, the Internet and the social networks offer a great opportunity to an instant access to scientific information to learn, and experiences to compare with the personal one. Sometimes this immediacy becomes more successful than the experience transmitted through generations by other family members which, on the contrary, often feed anguishes and ideals, not always useful for an identity under construction.

Tech-Moms

This theme refers to the relation between mothers and the technological medium: mothers seem to use the *e*-groups to express their style of motherhood and improve their technology-related capabilities. Within and through the safe online forum, the mothers have the opportunity to share and discuss common experiences. Moreover, moms' competencies are conveyed in the forum group as *self-promotion* (a tendency to give value to their maternal roles, experiences, and decisions) or as *self-questioning* (due to the uncertainty linked to their new roles, experiences, and decisions as a mother). For examples:

I really laughed for your expensive stroller... My 3 wheels one is perfect and costs less (Self-promoting)

I don't know, they are just messy thoughts of a mother who wants to do the best and sometimes she mess up! (Self-questioning)

Have you ever heard of guilt? Sometimes you have to seriously decide (I couldn't sleep and after a long day of struggles was too hard) but you don't know if you are right: you are tortured by self-doubt and fear, especially about your baby (Self-questioning)

The *e-group* allows promoting and improving mother's *tech*-skills: knowledge and experiences can be easier transmitted online through the *back link* or supporting them through photos or video records.

I sent you the link!

Please, share the video with us

What kind of stroller do you suggest? [Two links]

Often, thanks to the online medium, relations among mothers also become a bridge to an offline meeting and an occasion to build a close friendship, connecting the *online* to the *offline* dimensions.

Wow, where do you live exactly? I think we are very close!

I read you live in Milan, if you need the stroller, please contact me

FUTURE RESEARCH

This study confirms that parenting experience represents a big challenge for new mothers and mothers-to-be. Turning to online forums and e-groups, mothers express their need for communication, sharing emotional and practical support. Learning through shared experiences seems to have a key role in the e-group functioning.

Naturally, this qualitative and explorative study presents some limits that could direct future research: exploring how other digital device work or focusing on possible differences between mothers and fathers in regards to how they use online groups, and analyzing their subjective experiences also taking care of gender and role differences. It was not possible to delineate the specificity of the primiparous vs multiparous women through the forum's threads, but it could be very interesting to analyze whether and how experiencing e-groups diverges. Furthermore, it would be very interesting to compare these e-parents outcomes with other countries and cultures, and with other e-communities of parents facing different developmental diseases, i.e. adolescence for example, or parents facing their children special needs. Future research could provide answers to these curiosities.

CONCLUSION

The group, the *I am* dimension, *personal experience, perspective knowhow* and *tech-moms* represent the emotional core issues of the e-mothers whose forum's participation has been analyzed. The e-group functioning and the identity dimension arising from the group's dynamics are two main aspects which need to be discussed. On the one hand, it seems that the e-group membership (*the group*) can reproduce an offline peer group functioning (Parks, 2011), allowing members to identify each other, and to reshape the personal identity (*I am*) (Suler, 2002, 2004) thanks to the comparison among *personal experience*s and knowledge (*perspective knowhow*) through the technological medium (*Tech-moms*) (Kirk & Milnes, 2015). It seems to be confirmed the greater impact of the time spent on motherhood-dedicated web sites on maternal intentions, behaviors, and decisions (Rogers, 2003; McKeever & McKeever, 2017), and mothers' self-presentation (Walther, 2007) and experiences can take advantages through the online forum medium (Sundstrom, 2016).

Thus, the e-group functioning allows members' personal growth, through essential mirroring functions the woman often need during the transitional periods of life, such as the on-going experience of maternity. Indeed, rising maternity naturally implies the re-definition of personal and relational dimensions (Stern & Bruschweiler-Stern, 1998). Internal conflicts and ambivalence can characterize this condition such as a crisis of woman's identity, and this represents a social and a psychological matter. According to literature, people in difficult stages of life and experiences, need to be sustained by a social network (Montigny et al., 2006), that increasingly means a virtual plot of relationships, able to guarantee an emotional and concrete support even though in a potential space (Bert et al., 2013; Gibson & Hanson, 2013; Niela-Vilén et al., 2014). Sharing the same experiences with peers, the mothers seem to reinforce progressively their own identity, often "under construction". On the other hand, taking into account the emotional needs the rising maternity experience elicits, the e-group virtually become a breast with feeding, holding and reassuring functioning, responding to these necessities. The online community represent a source of social personal that helps mothers to face and manage the stress (Albrecht & Adelman, 1984) related to their new lives, roles, and identities. Into the large e-group container, mothers and *mothers-to-be* seem to throw up the pain they feel and through the e-group emotional functioning they can collect pieces of experiences, memories, knowledge, identity. Sometimes a reassuring container with holding functions, or a "toilet breast" (Meltzer, 1967) for evacuated anguishes, sometimes a source of rejection which can badly raise overwhelming emotions or a source of reparation for guilty parents, the e-group can also encourage regressive movements and dependence.

Thus, regressive and progressive movements seem to characterize the e-group experience as well as the developmental experiences of life and, naturally, the individual and psychic functioning. Therefore, sharing experiences and opinions the e-group empower mothering through a kind of self-promotion and self-questioning, which sustain the women's identity and the representation of a *good-enough* mother (Winnicott, 1951), frequently against an ideal image of maternity deeply and culturally ratified. Indeed, the Italian culture confers principally to mothers the responsibility to organize children's daily activities, to integrate parenting and jobs duties (Saraceno, 2003), to face with the idealization of a role - "The Mother" - and a practice that not easily allows women to feel negative feelings toward maternity and children. Just like in face-to-face communities, also in online contexts mothers can find supportive interactions and relationships which play a major role in all aspects of people's lives, such as in physical health, emotional well-being, and work performance (Albrecht & Halsey, 1992).

A new competence seems to raise from the e-group: the tech-mom through the technological medium improves her expertise and *tech*-skills. Then, encouraging women's self-questioning and self-improvement, and new mother's proficiency, the *e*-group can alternatively increase a perfect model, this time not generated by cultural issues but by the e-identity it-self.

We are parents who wonder about their own role. We believe in the importance of sharing that makes us more aware, safer and comfortable, and overcomes stereotypes and prejudices. We propose a model of curious and informed parenting, careful above all to the needs of all children. This is a place where we can repair us as parents, by working together to become of course not perfect but simply more careful parents. (From the main forum issues)

This study tried to fill the gap about *e*-motherhood and to demonstrate that maternal identity and role constructions, with all entailed processes, are played also online, especially on peer *e*-groups. Indeed, the online forums appear to be privileged "places" for the definition of these "under construction" identities. Finally, the experts should take into account the new mothers' and mothers-to-be' needs of practical advice and comparison with peers, and not just of scientific knowledge.

REFERENCES

Albrecht, T. L., & Adelman, M. B. (1984). Social support and life stress. *Human Communication Research*, *11*(1), 3–32. doi:10.1111/j.1468-2958.1984.tb00036.x

Albrecht, T. L., & Halsey, J. (1992). Mutual support in mixed-status relationships. *Journal of Social and Personal Relationships*, *9*(2), 237–252. doi:10.1177/0265407592092005

Ambrosini, A., & Stanghellini, G. (2012). Myths of motherhood: The role of culture in the development of postpartum depression. *Annali dell'Istituto Superiore di Sanita*, *48*(3), 277–286. doi:10.4415/ANN_12_03_08 PMID:23007052

Ammaniti, M., & Trentini, C. (2009). How new knowledge about parenting reveals the neurobiological implications of intersubjectivity: A conceptual synthesis of recent research. *Psychoanalytic Dialogues*, *19*(5), 537–555. doi:10.1080/10481880903231951

Anderson, O. A. (2007). Linking work stress, parental self-efficacy, ineffective parenting, and youth problem behavior. *Journal of Family Studies*, *13*(1), 119–120.

Bartholomew, M. K., Schoppe-Sullivan, S. J., Glassman, M., Kamp Dush, C. M., & Sullivan, J. M. (2012). New parents' Facebook use at the transition to parenthood. *Family Relations*, *61*(3), 455–469. doi:10.1111/j.1741-3729.2012.00708.x PMID:23671354

Bender, T. (1978). *Community and social change in America*. New Brunswick, NJ: Rutgers University Press.

Bert, F., Gualano, M. R., Brusaferro, S., De Vito, E., De Waure, C., La Torre, G., ... Torregrossa, M. V. (2013). Pregnancy e-health: A multicenter Italian cross-sectional study on Internet use and decision-making among pregnant women. *Journal of Epidemiology and Community Health*, *0*, 1–6. PMID:24072743

Bibring, G. L. (1959). Some considerations of the psychological processes in pregnancy. *The Psychoanalytic Study of the Child*, *14*, 113–121.

Blair-Loy, M. (2009). *Competing devotions: Career and family among women executives*. Cambridge, MA: Harvard University Press.

Brady, E., & Guerin, S. (2010). "Not the romantic, all happy, coochy coo experience": A qualitative analysis of interactions on an Irish parenting web site. *Family Relations*, *59*(1), 14–27. doi:10.1111/j.1741-3729.2009.00582.x

Brashers, D. E., Goldsmith, D. J., & Hsieh, E. (2002). Information seeking and avoiding in health contexts. *Human Communication Research*, *28*(2), 258–271. doi:10.1111/j.1468-2958.2002.tb00807.x

Braun, V., & Clarke, V. (2006). Using thematic analysis in psychology. *Qualitative Research in Psychology*, *3*(2), 77–101. doi:10.1191/1478088706qp063oa

Braun, V., & Clarke, V. (2013). Successful qualitative research: A practical guide for beginners. *Sage (Atlanta, Ga.)*.

Brown, I. (2010). Ambivalence of the motherhood experience. In A. O'Reilly (Ed.), *Twenty-first-century motherhood: Experience, identity, policy, agency* (pp. 121–139). New York, NY: Columbia University Press.

Cadei, L., & Simeone, D. (2011). Tra il chiaro e lo scuro. Riflessioni pedagogiche sul ruolo dell'ecografia ostetrica nel processo di transizione alla genitorialità. In E. Catarsi & J. P. Pourtois (Eds.), *Educazione familiare e servizi per l'infanzia. Education familiare et services pour l'enfance* (pp. 184–187). Firenze: University Press.

Calhoun, C. J. (1980). Community: Toward a variable conceptualization for comparative research. *Social History*, *5*(1), 105–129. doi:10.1080/03071028008567472

Chodorow, N. J. (2003). "Too late": Ambivalence about motherhood, choice, and time. *Journal of the American Psychoanalytic Association*, *51*(4), 1181–1198. doi:10.1177/00030651030510040701 PMID:14713010

Chodorow, N. J., & Contratto, S. (1989). The Fantasy of the Perfect Mother. In N. J. Chodorow (Ed.), *Feminism and Psychoanalytic Theory* (pp. 79–96). New Haven: Yale University Press.

Costigan, C. L., Cox, M. J., & Cauce, A. M. (2003). Work-parenting linkages among dual-earner couples at the transition to parenthood. *Journal of Family Psychology*, *17*(3), 397–408. doi:10.1037/0893-3200.17.3.397 PMID:14562463

Crouter, A. C., & Bumpus, M. F. (2001). Linking parents' work stress to children's and adolescents' psychological adjustment. *Current Directions in Psychological Science*, *10*(5), 156–159. doi:10.1111/1467-8721.00138

Deave, T., Johnson, D., & Ingram, J. (2008) Transition to parenthood: The needs of parents in pregnancy and early parenthood. *BioMed Central pregnancy and Childbirth*, *8*(30), 1-11.

Dennis, C. L. (2010). Postpartum depression peer support: Maternal perceptions from a randomized controlled trial. *International Journal of Nursing Studies*, *47*(5), 560–568. doi:10.1016/j.ijnurstu.2009.10.015 PMID:19962699

Dennis, C. L., Hodnett, E., Kenton, L., Weston, J., Zupancic, J., Stewart, D. E., & Kiss, A. (2009). Effect of peer support on prevention of postnatal depression among high risk women: Multisite randomised controlled trial. *British Medical Journal*, *338*, 280–284. PMID:19147637

Drentea, P., & Moren-Cross, J. L. (2005). Social capital and social support on the web: The case of an internet mother site. *Sociology of Health & Illness*, *27*(7), 920–943. doi:10.1111/j.1467-9566.2005.00464.x PMID:16313523

Ferraro, F., & Nunziante Cesàro, A. (1985). *Lo spazio cavo e il corpo saturato. La gravidanza come "agire" tra fusione e separazione*. Milano: Franco Angeli Editore.

Gibson, L., & Hanson, V. L. (2013). Digital motherhood: How does technology help new mothers? In J. A. Konstan, & K. Höök (Eds.), *Proceedings of the SIGCHI conference on human factors in computing systems* (pp. 313-322). ACM. 10.1145/2470654.2470700

Greenberger, E., O'neil, R., & Nagel, S. K. (1994). Linking workplace and homeplace: Relations between the nature of adults' work and their parenting behaviors. *Developmental Psychology*, *30*(6), 990–1002. doi:10.1037/0012-1649.30.6.990

Grienenberger, J., & Slade, A. (2002). Maternal reflective functioning, mother-infant affective communication, and infant attachment: Implications for psychodynamic treatment with children and families. *Psychologist-Psychoanalyst*, *22*(3), 1–8.

Guendouzi, J. (2006). "The guilt thing": Balancing domestic and professional roles. *Journal of Marriage and the Family*, *68*(4), 901–909. doi:10.1111/j.1741-3737.2006.00303.x

Hall, W., & Irvine, V. (2009). E-communication among mothers of infants and toddlers in a community-based cohort: A content analysis. *Journal of Advanced Nursing*, *65*(1), 175–183. doi:10.1111/j.1365-2648.2008.04856.x PMID:19016925

Hammer, L., & Thompson, C. A. (2003) Work-family role conflict. In *An encyclopedia entry for the Sloan Work and Family Research Network*. Retrieved March 18, 2017, from www.bc.edu/wfnetwork

Hays, S. (1996). *Cultural Contradictions of Motherhood*. New Haven, CT: Yale University Press.

Hewlett, S. A. (2002). *Creating a Life. Professional Women and the Quest for Children*. New York: Talk Miramax Books.

Hooley, T., Wellens, J., & Marriott, J. (2011). *What is Online research?: Using the Internet for social science research*. A&C Black.

Jang, J., Dworkin, J., & Connell, J. (2012). Babycenter. com: New parent behavior in an online community. The Forum for Family and Consumer Issues.

Jomhari, N., Gonzalez, V. M., & Kurniawan, S. H. (2009). See the apple of my eye: Baby storytelling in social space. In *Proceedings of the 23rd British HCI Group Annual Conference on People and Computers: Celebrating People and Technology* (pp. 238-243). British Computer Society.

Jordan, C. J. (2010). Evolution of autism support and understanding via the World Wide Web. *Intellectual and Developmental Disabilities*, *48*(3), 220–227. doi:10.1352/1934-9556-48.3.220 PMID:20597733

Kelly, K., Slade, A., & Grienenberger, J. F. (2005). Maternal reflective functioning, mother–infant affective communication, and infant attachment: Exploring the link between mental states and observed caregiving behavior in the intergenerational transmission of attachment. *Attachment & Human Development, 7*(3), 299–311. doi:10.1080/14616730500245963 PMID:16210241

Kirk, S., & Milnes, L. (2015). An exploration of how young people and parents use online support in the context of living with cystic fibrosis. *Health Expectations, 19*(2), 309–321. doi:10.1111/hex.12352 PMID:25691209

Kraut, R., Olson, J., Banaji, M., Bruckman, A., Cohen, J., & Couper, M. (2004). Psychological research online: Report of Board of Scientific Affairs' Advisory Group on the Conduct of Research on the Internet. *The American Psychologist, 59*(2), 105–117. doi:10.1037/0003-066X.59.2.105 PMID:14992637

Ley, B. L. (2007). Vive les roses!: The architecture of commitment in an online pregnancy and mothering group. *Journal of Computer-Mediated Communication, 12*(4), 1388–1408. doi:10.1111/j.1083-6101.2007.00378.x

Litt, J. S. (2000). *Medicalized Motherhood: Perspectives from the Lives of African-American and Jewish Women.* New Brunswick, NJ: Rutgers University Press.

Madge, C., & O'Connor, H. (2002). On-line with e-mums: Exploring the internet as a medium for research. *Area, 34*(1), 92–102. doi:10.1111/1475-4762.00060

Madge, C., & O'Connor, H. (2004). Online methods in geography educational research. *Journal of Geography in Higher Education, 28*(1), 143–152. doi:10.1080/0309826042000198710

Mann, C., & Stewart, F. (2000). Internet communication and qualitative research: A handbook for researching online. *Sage (Atlanta, Ga.).*

McCormick, A. (2010). Supermothers on Film, or Maternal Melodrama in the 21st Century. In A. O'Reilly (Ed.), *Twenty-first-century motherhood: Experience, identity, policy, agency* (pp. 140–157). New York, NY: Columbia University Press.

McDaniel, B. T., Coyne, S. M., & Holmes, E. K. (2012). New mothers and media use: Associations between blogging, social networking, and maternal well-being. *Maternal and Child Health Journal, 16*(7), 1509–1517. doi:10.100710995-011-0918-2 PMID:22094592

McKeever, R., & McKeever, B. W. (2017). Moms and Media: Exploring the Effects of Online Communication on Infant Feeding Practices. *Health Communication, 32*(9), 1059–1065. doi:10.1080/10410236.2016.1196638 PMID:27484216

Meltzer, D. (1967) *The Psycho-Analytical Process*. Perthshire, UK: Clunie.

Mo, P. K., Malik, S. H., & Coulson, N. S. (2009). Gender differences in computer-mediated communication: A systematic literature review of online health-related support groups. *Patient Education and Counseling*, *75*(1), 16–24. doi:10.1016/j.pec.2008.08.029 PMID:19233586

Montigny, F. D., Lacharité, C., & Amyot, É. (2006). The transition to fatherhood: The role of formal and informal support structures during the post-partum period. *Texto & Contexto Enfermagem*, *15*(4), 601–609. doi:10.1590/S0104-07072006000400008

Moorhead, S. A., Hazlett, D. E., Harrison, L., Carroll, J. K., Irwin, A., & Hoving, C. (2013). A new dimension of health care: Systematic review of the uses, benefits, and limitations of social media for health communication. *Journal of Medical Internet Research*, *15*(4), 85–100. doi:10.2196/jmir.1933 PMID:23615206

Morris, M. R. (2014). Social networking site use by mothers of young children. In K. P. O'Hara, M. Massimi, R. Harper, S. Rubens, & J. Morris (Eds.), *Proceedings of the 17th ACM conference on Computer supported cooperative work & social computing* (pp. 1272-1282). ACM. 10.1145/2531602.2531603

Mungham, S., & Lazard, L. (2011). Virtually experts: Exploring constructions of mothers' advice-seeking in online parenting communities. *Radical Psychology*, *9*(2).

Niela-Vilén, H., Axelin, A., Salanterä, S., & Melender, H. L. (2014). Internet-based peer support for parents: A systematic integrative review. *International Journal of Nursing Studies*, *51*(11), 1524–1537. doi:10.1016/j.ijnurstu.2014.06.009 PMID:24998788

Nieuwboer, C. C., Fukkink, R. G., & Hermanns, J. M. (2013). Peer and professional parenting support on the Internet: A systematic review. *Cyberpsychology, Behavior, and Social Networking*, *16*(7), 518–528. doi:10.1089/cyber.2012.0547 PMID:23659725

O'Connor, H., & Madge, C. (2001). Cyber-mothers: Online synchronous interviewing using conferencing software. *Sociological Research Online*, *5*(4). doi:10.5153ro.543

Oakley, A., & Roberts, H. (1981). Interviewing women: A contradiction in terms. In C. Seale (Ed.), *Social Research Methods: A reader* (pp. 261–268). London: Routledge.

Palmén, M., Korpela, M., & Saranto, K. (2012) Identifying health and wellbeing related information management activities and needs in families with young children. *Finnish Journal of eHealth and eWelfare, 4*(3), 165-176.

Parks, M. R. (2011). Social network sites as virtual communities. In Z. Papacharissi (Ed.), *A Networked Self. Identity, community, and culture on social network sites* (pp. 105–123). New York, NY: Routledge.

Plantin, L., & Daneback, K. (2009). Parenthood, information and support on the internet. A literature review of research on parents and professionals online. *BioMed Center Family Practice*, *10*(1), 1–12. PMID:19450251

Qian, H., & Scott, C. R. (2007). Anonymity and self-disclosure on weblogs. *Journal of Computer-Mediated Communication*, *12*(4), 1428–1451. doi:10.1111/j.1083-6101.2007.00380.x

Reichow, B., Halpern, J. I., Steinhoff, T. B., Letsinger, N., Naples, A., & Volkmar, F. R. (2012). Characteristics and quality of autism websites. *Journal of Autism and Developmental Disorders*, *42*(6), 1263–1274. doi:10.100710803-011-1342-6 PMID:21822761

Repetti, R. L., & Wood, J. (1997). Effects of daily stress at work on mothers' interactions with preschoolers. *Journal of Family Psychology*, *11*(1), 90–108. doi:10.1037/0893-3200.11.1.90

Ridgeway, C. L., & Correll, S. J. (2004). Motherhood as a status characteristic. *The Journal of Social Issues*, *60*(4), 683–700. doi:10.1111/j.0022-4537.2004.00380.x

Rogers, E. M. (2003). *Diffusion of innovations* (5th ed.). New York: Free Press.

Saraceno, C. (2003). La conciliazione di responsabilità familiari e attività lavorative in Italia: Paradossi ed equilibri imperfetti. *Polis*, *17*(2), 199–228.

Scaioli, G., Bert, F., Galis, V., Brusaferro, S., De Vito, E., La Torre, G., ... Siliquini, R. (2015). Pregnancy and internet: Sociodemographic and geographic differences in e-health practice. Results from an Italian multicenter study. *Public Health*, *129*(9), 1258–1266. doi:10.1016/j.puhe.2015.06.012 PMID:26210071

Slade, A., Cohen, L. J., Sadler, L. S., & Miller, M. (2009) The psychology and psychopathology of pregnancy. Handbook of infant mental health, 3, 22-39.

Sparks, H., Collins, F. L., & Kearns, R. (2016). Reflecting on the risks and ethical dilemmas of digital research. *Geoforum*, *77*, 40–46. doi:10.1016/j.geoforum.2016.09.019

Spinelli, M., Frigerio, A., Montali, L., Fasolo, M., Spada, M. S., & Mangili, G. (2016). 'I still have difficulties feeling like a mother': The transition to motherhood of preterm infants mothers. *Psychology & Health*, *31*(2), 184–204. doi:10.1080/08870446.2015.1088015 PMID:26359768

Stern, D. N., & Bruschweiler-Stern, N. (1998). *The birth of a mother: How the motherhood experience changes you forever*. Basic Books.

Stuart, J. (2007). Work and motherhood: Preliminary report of a psychoanalytic study. *The Psychoanalytic Quarterly*, *76*(2), 439–485. doi:10.1002/j.2167-4086.2007.tb00264.x PMID:17503624

Suler, J. R. (2002). Identity management in cyberspace. *Journal of Applied Psychoanalytic Studies*, *4*(4), 455–459. doi:10.1023/A:1020392231924

Suler, J. R. (2004). The online disinhibition effect. *Cyberpsychology & Behavior*, *7*(3), 321–326. doi:10.1089/1094931041291295 PMID:15257832

Sundstrom, B. (2016). Mothers "Google It Up:" Extending communication channel behavior in diffusion of innovations theory. *Health Communication*, *31*(1), 91–101. doi:10.1080/10410236.2014.936339 PMID:26075413

Tangherlini, T. R., Roychowdhury, V., Glenn, B., Crespi, C. M., Bandari, R., Wadia, A., … Bastani, R. (2016). "Mommy Blogs" and the Vaccination Exemption Narrative: Results From A Machine-Learning Approach for Story Aggregation on Parenting Social Media Sites. *JMIR public Health and Surveillance, 2*(2).

Thomson, R. (2011). *Making modern mothers*. Policy Press. doi:10.2307/j.ctt1t898c8

Tozzi, A. E., Mingarelli, R., Gonfiantini, M., Pandolfi, E., Carloni, E., Gesualdo, F., & Dallapiccola, B. (2013). The internet user profile of Italian families of patients with rare diseases: A web survey. *Orphanet Journal of Rare Diseases*, *8*(1), 1–8. doi:10.1186/1750-1172-8-76 PMID:23680013

Walther, J. B. (2007). Selective self-presentation in computer-mediated communication: Hyperpersonal dimensions of technology, language, and cognition. *Computers in Human Behavior*, *23*(5), 2538–2557. doi:10.1016/j.chb.2006.05.002

Widarsson, M., Kerstis, B., Sundquist, K., Engström, G., & Sarkadi, A. (2012). Support needs of expectant mothers and fathers: A qualitative study. *Journal of Perinatal Education*, *21*(1), 36–44. doi:10.1891/1058-1243.21.1.36 PMID:23277729

Williams, J. C., & Segal, N. (2003). Beyond the maternal wall: Relief for family caregivers who are discriminated against on the job. *Harvard Women's Law Journal*, *26*, 77–162.

Willson, M. A. (2006). *Technically together: Rethinking community within techno-society*. New York, NY: Peter Lang.

Winnicott, D. W. (1951). Transitional Objects and Transitional Phenomena: A Study of the First Not-Me. *The International Journal of Psycho-Analysis*, *34*(2), 89–97. PMID:13061115

KEY TERMS AND DEFINITIONS

Comparison: The act of consider or estimate the similarities or dissimilarities between two things, ways or people.

Cyber: Relating to or characteristic of computers, computers network, virtual reality and Internet.

E-Group: A number of people that share virtual "place", interests, and experiences.

Motherhood: The state of being a mother; maternity.

Online Support: To help someone emotionally or in a practical way in online contexts, giving encourage, approval, comfort, or reassurance to.

Pregnancy: The state or period of being pregnant.

Tech-Moms: An e-group of mothers and mothers-to-be who use social media and technologies to share their own experiences.

Web Forum: An online meeting "place" in which discussions of issues of public interest can be conducted.

Website: A set of pages on the World Wide Web about a single topic or several closely related topics, usually published by one person or organization.

ENDNOTES

1. In psychoanalysis, the term *transgenerational* refers to the process of the unconscious transmission of inner contents (e.g. the trauma) between generations.
2. These web communities seem to provide an "environment" that is suited to parents' needs, insulating the members from the impact of stress, supporting their emotional expression, putting themselves in the others' place, knowing what they need.

This research was previously published in Global Perspectives on Health Communication in the Age of Social Media edited by Seif Sekalala and Brandon C. Niezgoda; pages 29-58, copyright year 2018 by Medical Information Science Reference (an imprint of IGI Global).

Chapter 5
Teaching Childbirth Support Techniques Using the Prepared Partner and Digital Birth:
The Design and Development of Games for Dads-To-Be

Alexandra Holloway
University of California – Santa Cruz, USA

ABSTRACT

In today's California, a mother's primary social support person in childbirth is her partner, guiding her through a multidimensional experience, helping her make sense of unforgettable emotions and sensations. Preparing the partner is an integral step to making sure that the mother is well-supported in her birth. Because the mother's experience is influenced by the support she receives, and because birth partners need more support than is recognized, we target birth partners with a learning intervention. We investigate video games as a vehicle for knowledge transfer to the birth partner, both as currently available and as a positive learning tool. To address the problem of limited access to childbirth preparation methods, we investigated, designed, and evaluated two games: The Prepared Partner, an online Flash game, and Digital Birth, an iPhone application. Both games allow the user to practice various supportive actions in the realm of childbirth support for a mother in labor. We found that players of The Prepared Partner met learning goals while enjoying the game.

DOI: 10.4018/978-1-7998-2351-3.ch005

INTRODUCTION

Childbirth support – supporting a mother throughout labor and the birth of a child or children – is a complex task, as evidenced by the number of books, websites, and articles available for expectant parents. Most women and their partners receiving prenatal care consider attending childbirth preparation classes, which may include a unit on labor support or comfort measures during labor. Unfortunately, access to printed and online media and in-person childbirth preparation can be limited due to working hours, distance to the classes, economic hardships, and many other reasons.

We present the iterative human-centered, interdisciplinary design and evaluation of two games about childbirth support, The Prepared Partner and Digital Birth, and the surrounding domain research that informed the designs. We applied mixed ethnographic methods of gathering requirements to inform the tools. Our overarching goal was to reach a large number of women and their birth partners, and to increase satisfaction with the birth experience and the feelings of preparedness among first-time parents.

We began by investigating the practice of childbirth preparation by administering an online survey. Participants generally prepared by taking childbirth preparation classes, though not in such large numbers as we expected.

Given our results from the survey, we gathered information about childbirth support from various sources. We developed The Prepared Partner as a pilot or proof-of-concept application, and evaluated it for learning and enjoyment.

This early success led us to continue considering how games might be a good medium for deploying information about childbirth support. Prior to proceeding, we performed a thorough search for childbirth scenes in commercially-available games in order to investigate the landscape surrounding birth in video games.

We conducted further targeted investigation about childbirth support using ethnographic interviews, and observation of childbirth classes. In the interviews, we focused on birth partners' preparation methods, goals and experiences of import when providing childbirth support, and partners' perceived utility as support-providers. For the childbirth education classes, we collected information about the curriculum as it pertained to childbirth support.

Using this information, we developed a second game, Digital Birth, using the feedback from The Prepared Partner together with the interview data. Digital Birth uses the same artificial intelligence engine as The Prepared Partner, but is founded on techniques and user goals from the ethnographic investigations.

CHILDBIRTH PREPARATION

The first stage of our research into a tool to help women have a positive birth experience was to investigate how women and their birth partners prepare for birth. We examine the relationship between the childbirth preparation, feelings of preparedness, learning in childbirth, and overall satisfaction with the birth experience.

Our literature review revealed that childbirth preparation is related to satisfaction regarding childbirth or the choice of childbirth method. However, many of these studies have a limited user base and focus on a few types of childbirth preparation methods.

The Listening to Mothers II survey (LTM) (Declercq, Sakala, Corry, & Applebaum, 2007) summarizes the habits of American women in preparing to conceive, preparing for labor and birth, the birth outcomes and statistics, and postpartum demographics, including breastfeeding incidence and duration. The survey found that the most important source of information about pregnancy and childbirth for first-time mothers (33%, N=146) was books, followed by friends and/or relatives (19%), and the Internet (16%). Childbirth education classes were cited as important only 10% of the time, although most (56%) first-time mothers enrolled and attended such classes.

There has been a significant amount of research about the benefits of childbirth preparation. Lumley and Brown showed that attenders of childbirth education classes did not show increased satisfaction with their birth experience compared to the non-attenders (Lumley & Brown, 1993). Nichols came to the same conclusion: attending childbirth class did not have an effect on childbirth satisfaction (Nichols, 1995). Fabian, et al. found that although there were no statistical differences between attenders and non-attenders of childbirth class in terms of birth experience, those that attended classes were more likely to opt for an epidural during labor (Fabian, Rådestad, & Waldenstro¨ m, 2005).

Goodman, et al. showed childbirth satisfaction was influenced by whether the expectations for labor and delivery were met (Goodman, Mackey, & Tavakoli, 2004). Morgan, et al. described that effective pharmacological pain relief was insufficient for determining maternal satisfaction with labor (Morgan, Bulpitt, Clifton, & Lewis, 1982).

We conducted a survey in May 2010 to attempt to answer the following research questions.

R1: How do expectant parents prepare for childbirth, and how do these choices affect the birth experience they will ultimately attain?
R2: What is lacking in childbirth preparation?
R3: Is "just doing it" really the best preparation?
R4: What preparation methods generate the best results?
R5: How do we measure the "best" outcome of childbirth preparation?

Participants were recruited as part of coursework in an undergraduate human-computer interaction class, open to all majors. Eligible participants had experienced vaginal or Caesarean childbirth, or had assisted their partner in having a child, in the role of main support person. Only one participant per family was eligible to complete the survey. Of the 125 individuals that started the survey, 120 eligible participants completed it in its entirety. Survey responses were collected in the last weeks of May, 2010. The only participants excluded from the study were minors under age 18, and participants that did not fit the eligibility criteria yet still completed the survey. The study received exemption from the Institutional Review Board (IRB) as part of the coursework (HS1308). Data were analyzed using IBM SPSS 18.0.

Most of the participants (70%) were women that gave birth to at least one baby. The remaining 30% replied that their partner or spouse had given birth to at least one baby. This demographic differentiates our survey from surveys specifically for mothers, such as LTM; it differs from those specifically for fathers, such as Chan's (Chan & Paterson-Brown, 2002), Hallgren's (Hallgren, Kilhgren, Forslin, & Norberg, 1999), Odent's (Odent, 1999), Steen's (Steen, Downe, Bamford, & Edozien, 2011) experiences with following fathers; and it differs from work with birth partners, e.g. Somers-Smith's work (Somers-Smith, 1999).

The mean number of births per participant was 2.2, with the mode of 2. The births occurred between 1934 and 2009 (with an average birth year 1990, and mode 1988) in the United States and abroad, including Argentina, Canada, China, France, Philippines, Russia, Singapore, and Taiwan.

The self-reported instrumental delivery rate, deliveries in which forceps or vacuum extraction were used, was 24%. The Caesarean section rate was 45% across all participants, and 39% across all births (i.e., normalized), which included first-time and subsequent births. Twenty percent of first-time mothers had Caesarean sections. The Caesarean section rate in this study was significantly higher than the US average, reported to be 30% of all births (Althabe & Belizan, 2006), and higher than the 32% average rate reported in LTM. It is interesting to note that Caesarean section rates of over 10% are considered detrimental to maternal and infant health (Belizan, Althabe, & Cafferata, 2007). Participants reported that 62% used a pharmacological method of pain relief (e.g., narcotic, epidural, spinal). This is lower than the average reported by LTM (76%), possibly indicating a rise in the use of pharmacological pain relief as most participants in our survey had birthed in the 1980s–1990s; however, without specific geographic data, the effects of geography cannot be discounted. The average birth mass of first babies in our study was 3.33kg.

The remainder of the survey focused on the participants' first birth experience.

Preparing for Childbirth

Experts in the field of childbirth were consulted to compile a list of the most common ways to prepare for childbirth. The experts were childbirth educators, doulas, and doula trainers. The finalized list included talking to a woman who has given birth (e.g., mother, sister, friend); talking to a man whose partner has given birth (e.g., father, brother, friend); taking childbirth preparation classes; reading books, watching videos, and reading Internet sites; talking to a doctor; and talking to another professional (e.g., doula, midwife).

We asked participants four questions about their methods of preparing for childbirth.

1. **Preparation:** How did you prepare for labor and childbirth?
2. **Usefulness:** Which method of preparation did you find to be most helpful?
3. **Repeat Preparation:** If you were to go back in time and have your baby again, how would you learn about the labor and childbirth process?
4. **Recommendation:** If your good friend were going to have a baby, how would you recommend that she learn about the childbirth process?

Multiple answers were allowed only for the preparation, repeat preparation, and recommendation questions. Write-in answers were coded and counted.

One-sample χ^2 tests showed $p < 0.01$ for all items. Figures 1, 2, 3 and 4 summarize the findings described below.

We found that the overwhelming majority of participants (81%) prepared by talking to other women that had given birth, and 26% of participants found this to be the most useful method of preparation, making talking to other women the second most useful method of preparation cited by participants. However, less than half of participants (48%) would recommend preparing by talking to other women. Our results confirmed the LTM results, in which friends were cited as the second most useful method of childbirth preparation by 19% of first-time mothers.

The second-most popular way to prepare for childbirth was through books, videos, and other media (77%) and 20% of participants thought this was the most useful method. Listening to Mothers found 33% of first-time moms found books, and 16% cited the Internet, to be the most important source of information. In our survey, 63% of participants would recommend books and other media to their friends. Not surprisingly, the Internet is gaining popularity, and is ranked among the most influential methods of gaining information about pregnancy and childbirth (Handfield, Turnbull, et al., 2006).

Figure 1. Preparation methods for labor and childbirth

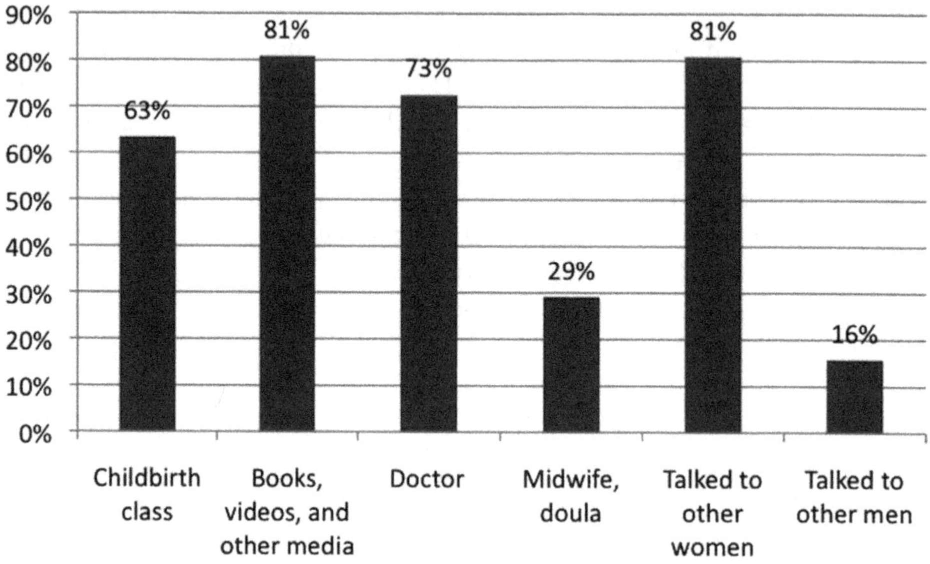

Figure 2. Preparation methods: What was most useful?

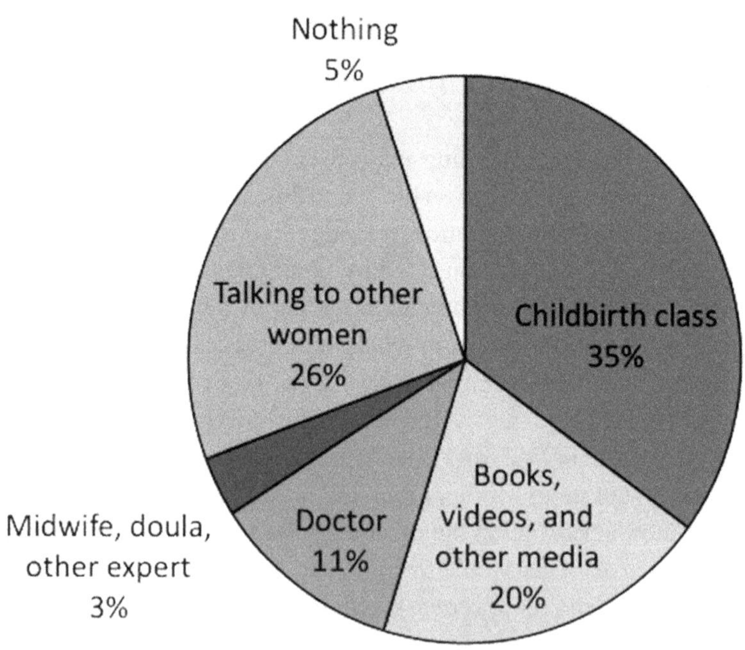

Figure 3. Preparation methods: What would you do again?

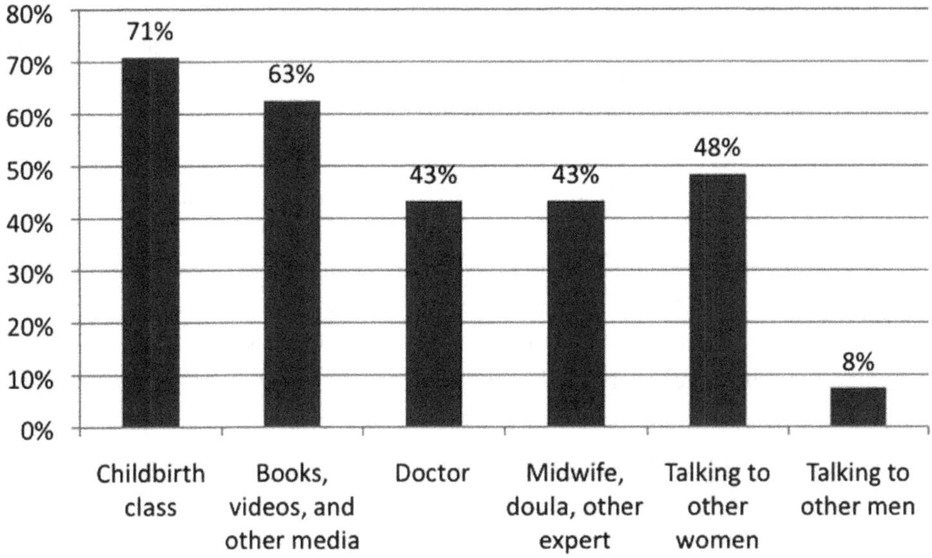

Figure 4. What would you recommend to a friend?

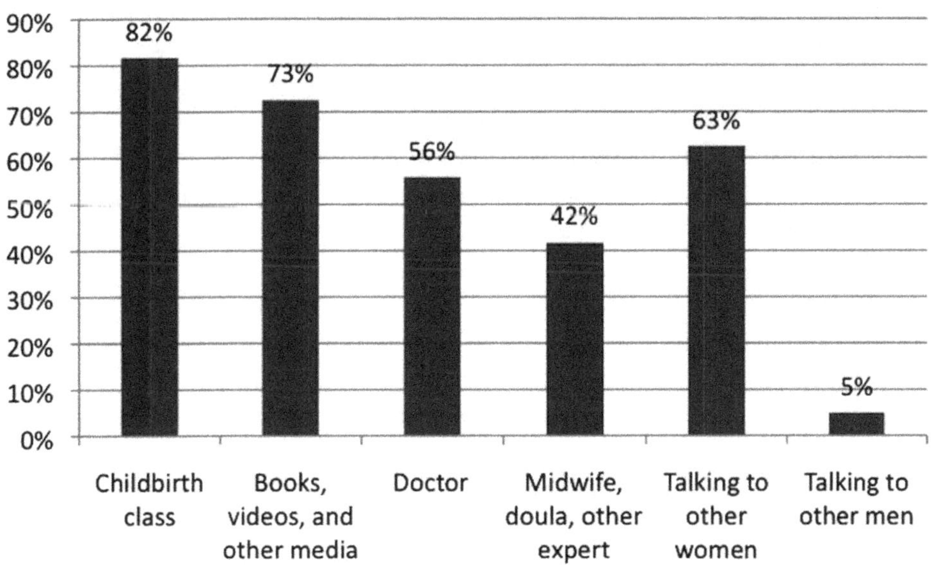

Most (63%) of participants reported preparing for childbirth by taking childbirth preparation classes. Childbirth education classes were seen as the most helpful method of preparation, marked as most useful by 35% of participants. This was a marked difference from the Listening to Mothers survey, in which only 10% of first-time moms found childbirth education classes as the most important source of information about being pregnant and giving birth. In our survey, most participants (71%) would choose to take childbirth classes if they could repeat their preparation, and 82% of participants would recommend childbirth classes to their friends. That is, we found that participants that did not prepare by childbirth class wish they had. Discussing the coming birth with a doctor was a method 56% of participants used to prepare. About a tenth (11%) of participants marked this as the most useful method of preparation. However, only 43% would prepare this way again, indicating that 13% of those that prepared by talking to a doctor would not choose to do this again. More than half (56%) of participants would recommend to a friend to prepare by talking to a doctor. Talking to another professional, such as a doula or midwife, was a method 29% of participants used (although only one participant used a doula in the birth). Only low 3% of participants thought this was the most useful method of preparation, although research suggests that this is the most overall beneficial way to feel supported in childbirth (Van Zandt, Edwards, & Jordan, 2005; Klaus, Kennell, & Klaus, 1993, 2002). Only 10% of participants said that a midwife was present at the birth for continuous labor support, indicating that some participants either spoke with midwives and doulas to prepare, and subsequently chose medical care through family doctors and obstetricians, or some midwives were not present for the entire labor and childbirth process for continuous support. Regardless, 43% would recommend this method of preparation to friends, indicating that new parents recognize the positive influence a midwife or doula can have on a birth experience and birth outcome.

Talking to men whose partner had given birth was not as popular, but present (16%), and few participants said they were likely to prepare by talking to other men again (8%). Not one participant thought this was the most useful method of preparation, and only 5% of participants would recommend talking to men, presumably birth partners, to prepare for birth. We hypothesize that this is a cultural paradigm that is shifting; indeed, men as birth partners in the labor room did not become a norm until the late 1980s (Leavitt, 2009). As of 2003, 93–98% of fathers in the UK attend their partners' births (Kiernan & Smith, 2003), and their presence has tangible benefits to the mothers' birth experience, engagement with the infant, and parental attachment to the baby and to the partner (Fatherhood Institute, 2007).

There was a relationship between preparing by childbirth class with the first child, and choosing to prepare by childbirth class again ($p = 0.006$). There was no similar relationship, however, for any other preparation method.

Support in Childbirth

We asked participants who participated in supporting the mother during childbirth. All answers were significant ($p < 0.001$, one-sample binomial test). The mean number of non-medical personnel present to offer support to the mother was 1.50 ($p < 0.001$, one-sample Kolmogorov-Smirnov test). Most (92%) participants had (or provided) some continuous support during labor (see Figure 5).

Most mothers (78%) had spousal support during labor and childbirth. Some (28%) had parents supporting them. Some were accompanied by a sister or brother (15%), a friend (13%), and/or a midwife (10%). Nine participants (8%) reported having no continuous labor support, aside from the intermittent hospital staff visits from doctors and nurses. Only one participant reported having a doula, or professional childbirth assistant, present at the birth.

We found a significant relationship between the total number of support persons with the participant during labor and childbirth and the total number of different ways the participant prepared for the birth ($p < 0.001$). The more different ways participants prepared for their birth, the more people were present for continuous support during the birth. Participants that had spousal support prepared by reading books ($p = 0.001$), taking childbirth class ($p = 0.001$), and talking to their doctor ($p = 0.001$). As a couple, the woman and her partner were likely to prepare for childbirth

Figure 5. Support during labor: Who was there for continuous labor support?

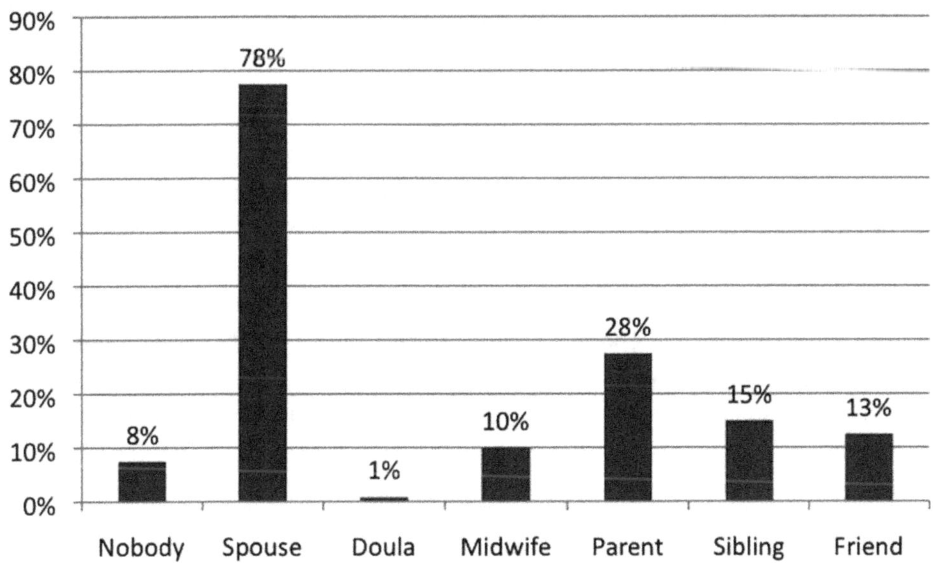

together. Participants that had nobody with them during labor and childbirth for support were likely to prepare for childbirth by reading books ($p < 0.001$); however, there was a negative correlation between having no support person present during the birth and the number of books read.

Pain Relief in Labor

The majority (62%) of participants reported using pharmacological methods of pain relief, such as morphine, Demerol, narcotics, or epidural analgesia during the birth of their first child. Only 22% reported using a non-pharmacological techniques, such as water therapy, aromatherapy, massage, acupuncture, a TENS machine, or another natural method. Further correlations are discussed below.

Satisfaction with Support in Childbirth

DONA International, an organization of birth and postpartum doulas, defines the role of a birth doula as a woman that provides "continuous physical, emotional and informational support to the mother before, during and just after childbirth." We asked participants to rate satisfaction with the different support components during labor, which we defined as emotional support, physical support (e.g., helping the mother move around), cognitive support (i.e., presence and company), and informational support (e.g., telling the mother what is happening). We also asked participants to score their satisfaction with pharmacological pain relief and non-pharmacological, or natural, pain relief. We used a four-point Likert scale (very unsatisfied, unsatisfied, satisfied, very satisfied). The findings are statistically significant ($p < 0.001$, one-sample $\chi 2$) and are summarized in Figure 6.

- **Emotional:** 80% of participants replied they were satisfied with the emotional support received, compared to 15% of participants unsatisfied.
- **Physical:** For physical support (e.g., helping the woman in labor move around) 75% were satisfied with the support received; 18% were unsatisfied.
- **Cognitive:** We define cognitive, or mental, support as presence and company. 76% of participants reported being satisfied with the cognitive support they received in labor, and 18% were unsatisfied with it.
- **Informational:** Informational support, being told what was happening during the stages of labor and during childbirth, was found to be satisfactory by 77% of participants, and unsatisfactory by 19%.
- **Pain Relief Options:** Most (57%) of the participants were satisfied by the pharmacological pain relief (e.g., narcotics or epidural); however, 20% were unsatisfied with it (and 21% answered that this question did not apply to them).

Figure 6. Satisfaction with support in labor

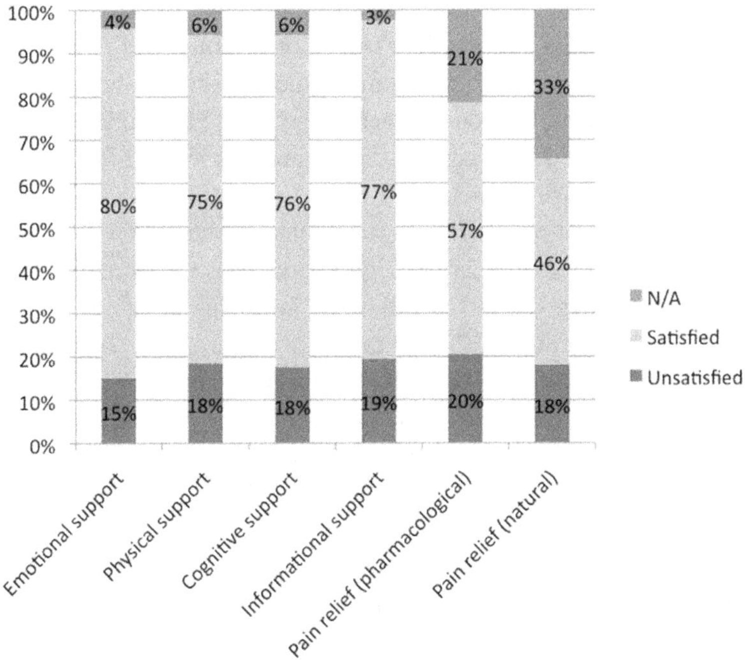

Finally, natural, non-pharmacological pain relief was found to be satisfactory by 46% of participants, and unsatisfactory by 18% (and 33% answered that this question did not apply to them).

Total

We found a significant relationship between the total number of people supporting the mother and the satisfaction rating with respect to emotional support ($\chi 2$, $p < 0.05$), physical support ($p < 0.05$), and cognitive support ($p < 0.05$). The total number of people was also related to the total number of ways the participants prepared for labor and childbirth ($p < 0.01$).

Learning in Labor

Is "just doing it" the best preparation for labor and childbirth? Five percent of participants said there is no best, most useful preparation: "Nothing really prepares you for childbirth except doing it; then you are prepared for the next one." To investigate this phenomenon, we asked participants to rate, on a four-point Likert scale, their feelings about their knowledge level before the birth and after the birth of their first child.

First, we asked: "How much did you know about the labor and childbirth process before your or your partner's first birth?" The options were nothing, a little / I had studied it a long time ago, some / I had studied it recently, and people sought my advice on this. Then, we asked: "How much did you know about the labor and childbirth process after your or your partner's first birth?" The options were nothing, a little / as if I had studied it a long time ago, some / as if I had studied it recently, and people seek my advice on this.

We found that the rating of what participants felt they knew before the labor increased dramatically after the labor. Significance was measured with Wilcoxon Signed Ranks Test, and $p < 0.001$ for all of the following items.

Before the labor, participants' answers were largely split. About half of the participants replied that they knew "some" or a significant amount about the topic. That is, they replied "Some / I had studied it recently" or "people sought my advice on this." These statements were chosen for their concrete, direct interpretations. The other half of participants answered that they knew a little or nothing about the topic, marking "A little / I had studied it a long time ago" or "Nothing" on the survey form.

After the labor, the answers very highly polarized. The majority of participants answered that they had a good or excellent understanding of all items. In particular, very few participants (11% or less) responded that they still knew "nothing" about an aspect of labor and childbirth after the birth. The statistical breakdown is described below:

- **Labor Process (Stages of Labor, etc.):** Participants' responses were an average of 27% higher for the post-birth question than the pre-birth question. After the birth, only 6% of participants replied that they knew only a little or nothing about the labor process. The mode of birth was not a factor — there was no difference between participants that delivered vaginally and participants that delivered by Caesarean section. Figure 7 shows the distribution of answers.
- **Comfort Techniques**: The mean rating for comfort techniques was 19% higher in the post-birth question. However, 20% of participants marked that they still knew a little or nothing about comfort techniques. One possible reason that 20% of participants knew a little or nothing about natural comfort techniques and pain relief options is because of the high first-time Caesarean section rate. There was no correlation between knowledge about comfort techniques and pain relief method or mode of birth (see Figure 7).
- **Non-Pharmacological Pain Relief Options:** Knowledge about non-pharmacological, or natural, pain relief options before the birth was split: nearly half knew "some" or more. After the birth, the number increased by 19%. Unfortunately, a quarter (25%) of participants still knew a little or

nothing about natural pain relief, despite having delivered a baby. As with comfort techniques, one possible reason so few mothers and their partners knew about natural pain relief options is because 20% of these mothers delivered via Caesarean section. Figure 8 shows a summary of this finding.

- **Pharmacological Pain Relief Options:** Twenty-two percent more participants responded that they knew "some" or a significant amount about pharmacological pain relief options after their birth experience than before. However, 16% said they knew a little or nothing (see Figure 8). Because 38% of participants did not use pharmacological pain relief in labor, this number is not surprising.
- **Labor and Birth Positions:** Participants' ratings of their knowledge of labor and birth positions rose by 19% in the post-birth question compared to the pre-birth question. Figure 9 summarizes the participants' answers.
- **Tools and Props for Helping Laboring Women:** Although participants' responses were evenly split before the birth, after the birth, participants' scores for their knowledge of tools and props for helping laboring women rose by 22%. Figure 9 shows a summary graph.
- **Delivery Process:** Twenty-two percent more participants answered that they knew "some" or a significant amount about the delivery process after their birth experience. See Figure 10.
- **Postpartum:** Responses about the early postpartum period on the pre-birth question were split: half of participants said they knew "some" or a significant amount; half said they knew a little or nothing. On the post-birth question, 32% more participants said they knew "some" or a significant amount.

Prepared and Ready

We asked participants if they had felt prepared for labor and childbirth. Answers were provided on a four-point Likert scale (very unprepared, unprepared, prepared, very prepared). In retrospect, most (76%) participants felt some degree of preparation, feeling very prepared (18%) or prepared (58%). The remaining quarter of the participants (24%) felt unprepared (19%) or very unprepared (5%). See Figure 11 for a visual representation of this data. Our survey results are similar to the Listening to Mothers survey, in which 71% of mothers "reported feeling confident as they approached labor" and 24% felt unprepared.

Figure 7. Before and after: how much did you know about the labor process and comfort techniques?

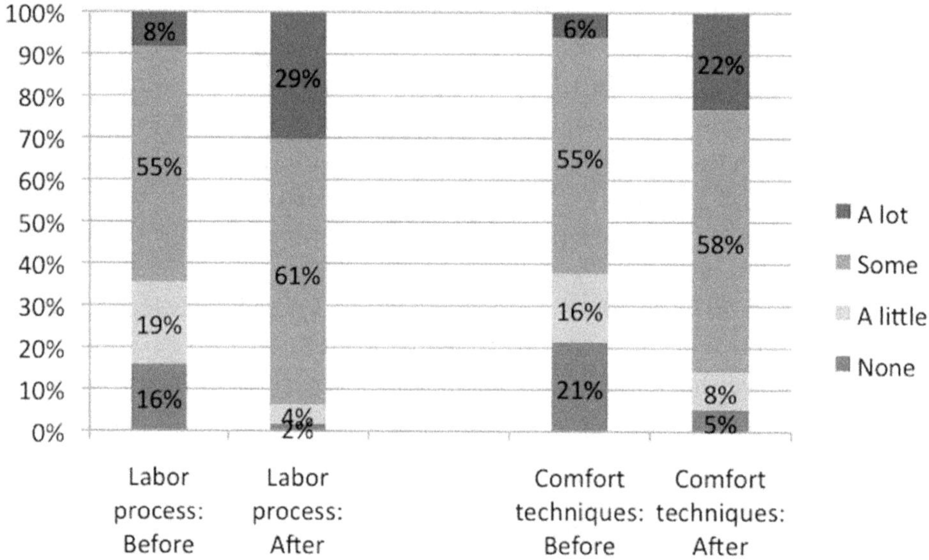

Figure 8. Before and after: how much did you know about pain relief options?

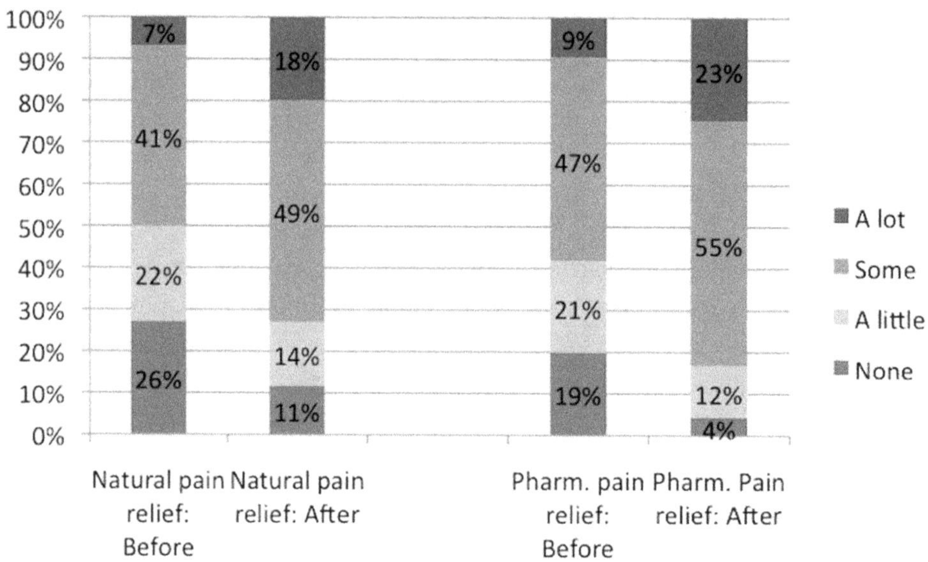

Figure 9. Before and after: how much did you know about labor and birth positions and the tools and props for helping laboring women

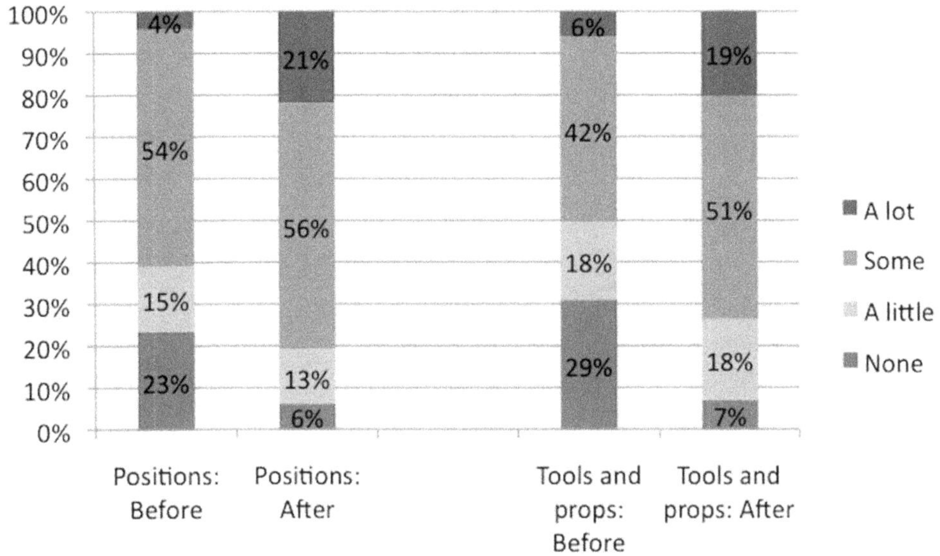

Figure 10. Before and after: how much did you know about the delivery process?

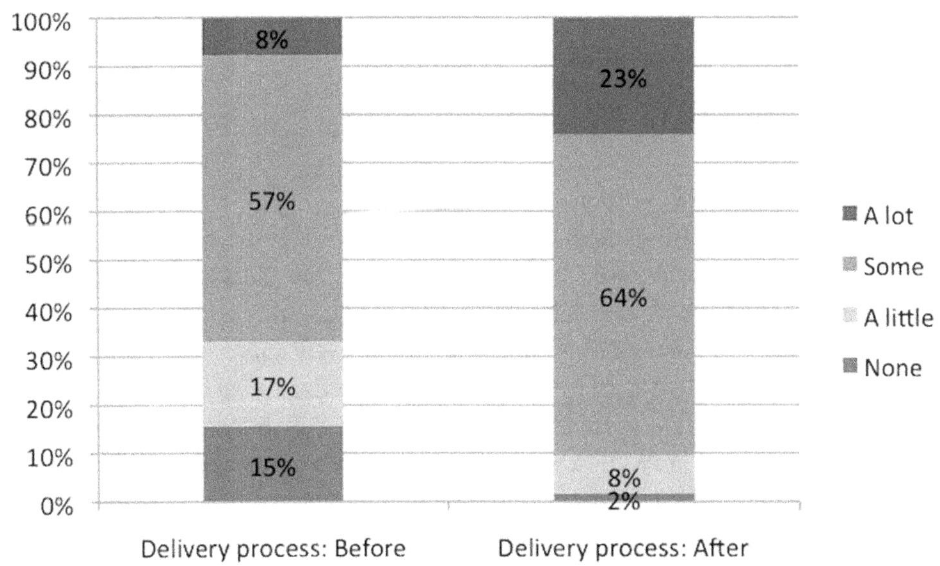

Figure 11. Did you feel prepared for labor and childbirth?

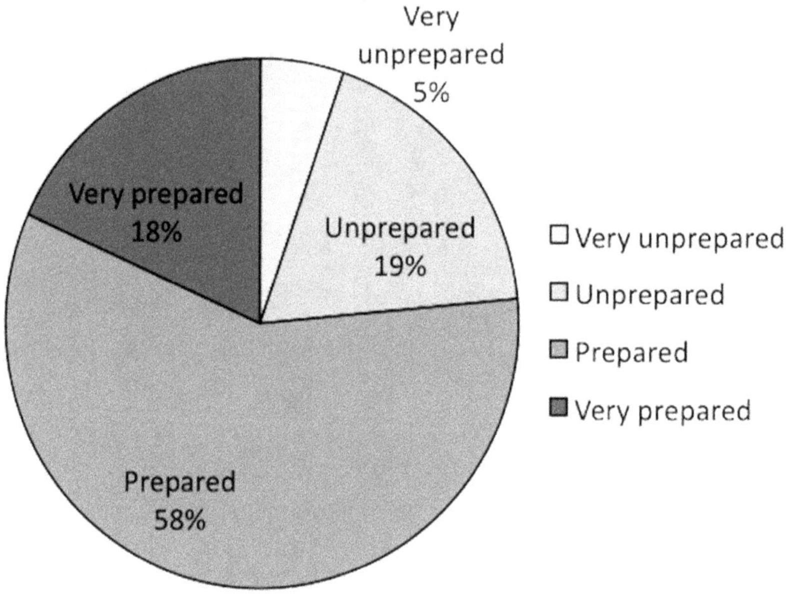

Correlations

Spearman's rho bivariate correlation was used to test non-parametric values. For each correlation table, we note significances at the 0.01 level (2-tailed) with two asterisks (**). Significant correlations at the 0.05 level (2-tailed) are noted with a single asterisk (*):

- **Preparation Methods and Labor Outcome:** We compared the preparation methods participants used and the outcome of the childbirth. Participants that prepared by taking childbirth classes, talking to other men, and talking to professionals (e.g., midwife, doula) were more likely to use non-pharmacological methods of pain management during labor. Using natural techniques was also correlated with the number of books the participants read in preparation. We found that participants that prepared by talking with a doctor (73% of participants said they did this) were also likely to have an instrumental birth (i.e., by forceps or vacuum extraction). These results are summarized in Table 1.
- **Support in Labor and Preparation Methods:** Participants that reported being supported by their spouse were more likely to prepare by taking classes, reading books, and talking to their doctor. However, participants that had no support were unlikely to take classes and read books (see Table 2).

- **Support in Labor and Pain Relief:** Next, we examined support in labor and pain relief options used in labor. Table 3 shows a strong correlation between spousal support and pharmacological methods of pain relief. No such correlation was found for any other support person, including no support. Figure 12 shows that participants supported by a spouse were five times more likely to use pharmacological methods of pain relief than participants without a spouse present (10% vs. 50% — see Figure 12). We also found that participants supported by a midwife were both less likely to use pharmacological methods of pain relief and more likely to use natural pain relief options. Again, no such correlation was found for any other support person.
- **Satisfaction:** Participants that rated highly their satisfaction with any of emotional, physical, cognitive, and informational support during the birth of their first child were likely to rate all of these aspects highly (correlation coefficients all greater than 0.670, $p < 0.01$, two-tailed).

Table 1. Childbirth preparation method versus instrumental birth and whether non-pharmacological methods of pain relief were used in labor

	Instrumental Birth	Used Non-Pharm.
Talking to men	—	.272**
Taking classes	—	.194*
Talking to doctor	.220*	—
Talking to professional	—	.421**
Number of books read	—	.251**

Table 2. Preparation method and support in labor

	Supported by...	
	Spouse	Nobody
Taking classes	.308**	–.204*
Reading books	.335**	–.394**
Talking to doctor	.311**	—
Number of books	.316**	–.302**

Table 3. Support in labor and whether pharmacological or non-pharmacological methods were used

	Used Non-Pharm.	Used Pharm.
Spouse support	—	.206*
Midwife support	.365**	–.303**

Figure 12. Pharmacological methods of pain relief and whether a spouse was present during labor

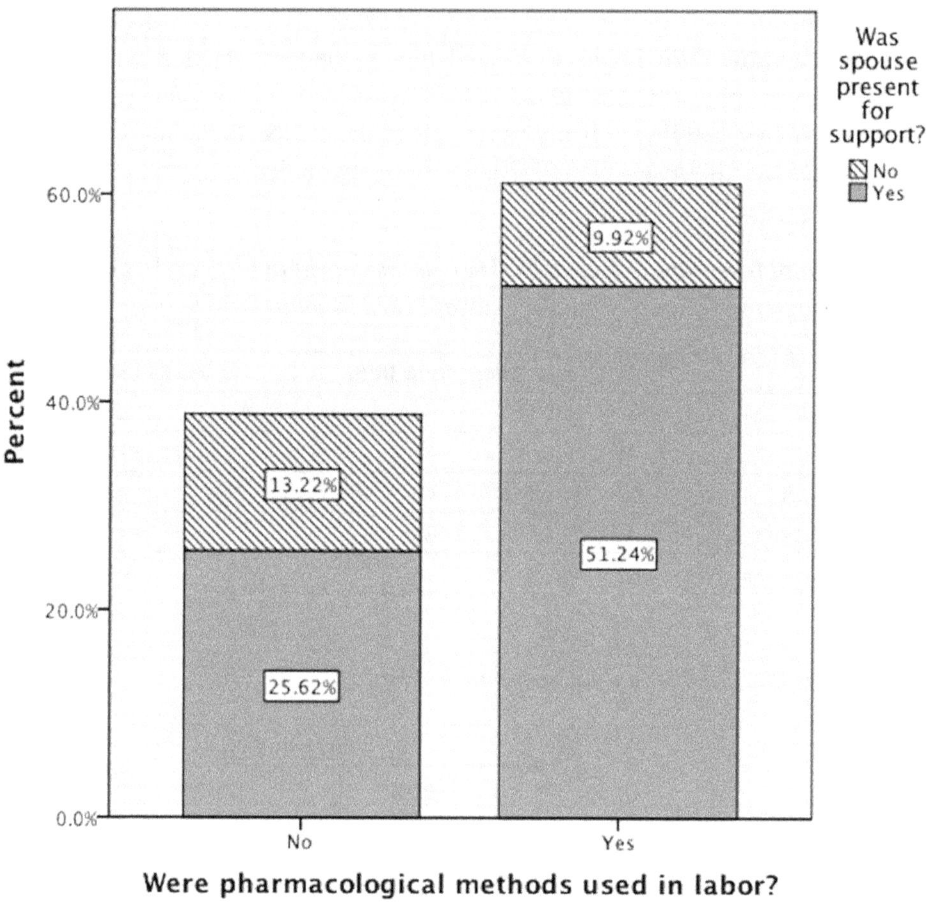

Satisfaction with pharmacological support was also correlated positively with all of the other aspects of labor (correlation coefficients greater than .240, $p < 0.01$, two-tailed). Satisfaction with non-pharmacological support was an exception: it was correlated only with satisfaction with emotional support (correlation coefficient 0.233, $p < 0.05$), and informational support (correlation coefficient 0.231, $p < 0.05$).

There was no correlation between the mode of birth (vaginal or Caesarean section) and satisfaction with the level of support.

- **Satisfaction with Support and Support Person:** We found that both the total number of people supporting the mother during labor and childbirth — spouse, sister, mother, etc. — and the total number of methods used to prepare for childbirth were positively correlated to emotional, physical, and cognitive support satisfaction (see Table 4).

Table 5 shows that we found participants that had no support person(s) with them during their labor were unhappy with the level of emotional, physical, and cognitive support. Although unsurprising, this finding corroborates existing research about the importance of continuous support for a woman throughout her labor and birth. Further, participants with a friend supporting them in labor were more likely to be satisfied with emotional, physical, and cognitive support.

Table 4. Correlation between number of support persons present, the number of preparation methods used, and the satisfaction rating with emotional, physical, and cognitive support in labor

	Satisfaction with...		
	Emotional	**Physical**	**Cognitive**
No. persons	.349**	.278**	.295**
No. of methods	.342**	.358**	.292**

Table 5. Correlation between no support person or having a friend as a support person and satisfaction with emotional, physical, and cognitive support in labor

	Satisfaction with...		
	Emotional	**Physical**	**Cognitive**
Nobody	−.219*	−.227*	−.221*
Friend	—	.192*	.198

- **Satisfaction and Preparation Methods:** We compared participants' satisfaction with the support types in labor with the methods of labor preparation. Table 6 contains the correlation coefficients for these figures.

Talking to a doctor was positively correlated with satisfaction with all but non-pharmacological support. Doctors rarely prepare their patients by discussing natural pain relief options, as a doctor's specialty is with pharmacological methods of relieving pain.

Reading books, one of the most popular methods of preparation (81% of participants marked this option), was positively correlated with satisfaction with emotional, physical, and informational support in labor. me." Another participant wrote: "Class [was most useful to me], because we took it together." However, our results suggest that there was no correlation between taking a childbirth class and feeling supported on a cognitive level through presence and company. Preparing by taking classes was positively correlated only with satisfaction with emotional support and pharmacological pain relief support. That is, participants felt supported emotionally, and were satisfied with the medications they were given (if they chose to use them) to manage labor pain.

Table 6. Preparation methods and satisfaction with support in labor

	Satisfaction with...		
	Emot.	**Phys.**	**Cog.**
Talking to women	—	—	.184*
Talking to men	—	.204*	—
Taking classes	.214*	—	—
Reading books	.276**	.258**	—
No. of books	.287**	.223*	.219*
Talking to doctor	.236**	.291**	.192*
Talking to pro.	.305**	.268**	.282**
	Satisfaction with...		
	Info.	**Pharm.**	**Non-Pharm.**
Talking to men	—	—	.310**
Taking classes	—	.214*	—
Reading books	.238**	—	—
Talking to doctor	.357**	.184*	—
Talking to pro.	.355**	.188*	.277**

Talking to women, the other most popular method of preparation for childbirth (chosen by 81% of participants), was correlated only with satisfaction with cognitive support — that is, the sense of presence and company. However, participants found talking to women to be critical in preparing for childbirth, as one-quarter (26%) of participants cited talking to other women as the single most useful method of preparing for childbirth. One participant explained: "Talking to other mothers [was the most useful method of preparation]. They've been through it and were the most honest about what to expect."

- **Feelings of Preparedness and Support:** Participants that had a midwife or a friend present for support were more likely to respond that they felt prepared for the birth of their first child. No other such correlations were found for any other support person. Participants that used non-pharmacological methods of pain relief were more likely to say they had felt prepared. Feelings of preparedness were positively correlated with attending childbirth class. Table 7 summarizes these findings.

DISCUSSION

In this study, we asked participants to recall their first birth experience. The most common birth year was 1988, and the average was 1990 — most births occurred 22 to 24 years prior to taking this survey. We posit that the memory of the birth does not fade with time. Githens, et al., have found that mothers can remember the details of their births for four to six years (Githens, Glass, Sloan, & Entman, 1993); Tomeo and others saw that this memory can extend much longer: mothers can recall details of their pregnancies and birth weights of their infants 30 years after the birth of their child (Tomeo et al., 1999). Simkin found that women can recall particular details

Table 7. Feelings of preparedness and midwife support, friend support, preparation by childbirth class, and whether non-pharmacological methods were used in labor

	Feelings of Preparedness
Midwife support	.204*
Friend support	.196*
Used non-pharm.	.211*
Childbirth class	.271**

about their birth experience even 20 years later (Simkin, 1992). Because childbirth is a very significant event, we consider the retrospective survey approach a valid way to assess satisfaction with labor support, knowledge, and feelings of preparedness.

Participants were unlikely to prepare for childbirth using just one method. A combination of methods — childbirth class, talking to men, talking to women, and reading a number of books — were positively correlated.

Most (63%) of participants attended organized childbirth preparation classes. This is higher than the Listening to Mothers survey (56% of first-time mothers).

We found that respondents with no labor support also did not prepare for labor and childbirth by other methods, such as taking classes and reading books about childbirth. They were also less likely to have a positive birth experience, with less perceived emotional, physical, and cognitive support in labor than those that had labor support.

We found that participants value the experience of having a child as a method of childbirth preparation. Going through the experience of childbirth was found to be the best way to learn about the subject: participants replied that they knew significantly more about every aspect of childbirth after the fact.

The methods of preparing for childbirth have an effect later, with parents' satisfaction with the labor process. The most popular methods of preparing for childbirth were talking to other women and reading books, watching movies, and browsing the Internet for information. The former was not shown to have a positive correlation with any aspect of the labor and childbirth process other than cognitive support. Talking with other women may contribute to feelings of kinship – feeling a part of a larger whole; feeling connected to all women that have undergone the experience of childbirth (Davis-Floyd, 2004) – and make them feel supported on a mental level by the thought of these women. Participants that prepared with books and other media showed higher scores for emotional, physical, and informational support satisfaction in the birth process. The number of books participants read in preparation for labor was correlated not only with informational satisfaction (that is, how much information the participants received in labor), but also with emotional, physical, and cognitive satisfaction. This indicates that the number of books does not contribute to information alone. Mothers and their partners are preparing on a deeper level with each new book read. They are more likely to imagine a great number of birth outcomes, and prepare both mentally and emotionally for different possibilities. However, because those that prepared with books also prepared with other methods, including talking to other women, taking childbirth classes, and talking to their doctor, and because these same participants were likely to be supported in labor and childbirth by their spouse, it is difficult to draw a conclusion.

Although "just doing it" was found to be the best preparation for childbirth – that is, having a child is the best way to learn about childbirth and prepare for a subsequent birth – parents should have access to preparation methods for their first birth experiences. The most popular method of preparation was talking with other women who had given birth; however, it is an unstructured and anecdotal method. Other most common ways of preparing for a first child were reading books, watching videos, and browsing Internet sites for information. Although taking childbirth classes is the fourth most popular method of preparation, it is seen as the most useful, and is most likely to be recommended to friends – although individual impressions of the utility of childbirth education classes is mixed.

THE PREPARED PARTNER: A PROOF OF CONCEPT

The growing ubiquity of the Internet and other always-on media, such as games, informed our decision to try to incorporate common themes in childbirth education into a game. Because participants considered childbirth education to be important, yet did not necessarily find attending childbirth education classes as a valuable source of information for their own birth experience, we decided to distill the concepts found in childbirth education into a medium that can be easily consumed by a majority of people. We intended to leverage the Internet as a distribution medium, and games as a vehicle for content, in designing and implementing what became The Prepared Partner.

The Prepared Partner was designed to be an educational video game about labor and childbirth. Because literature suggests that fathers and birth partners need more support in labor and childbirth than was previously assumed (Hallgren et al., 1999), the target audience included anyone with an interest in childbirth, including future mothers and birth partners.

We started The Prepared Partner with five main goals for the system. They were as follows (Holloway & Kurniawan, 2010; Holloway, 2010; Holloway & Kurniawan, 2011).

1. To introduce natural coping mechanisms and their effects on labor,
2. To introduce the mechanics of labor and childbirth,
3. To train birth partners to help women in childbirth,
4. To practice interacting with a woman in labor, and
5. To simulate the stages of labor.

We used human-centered design, influenced by the childbirth preparation survey, in designing the game prototype.

Before designing and developing The Prepared Partner, we conducted thorough domain background research – an integral part of usability engineering as research must be completed before prototyping (Holzinger, 2005). We read accounts of childbirth, or birth stories, in popular books suggested to expectant parents, and paid particular attention to information about the stages of labor, relaxation to reduce anxiety, natural techniques to deal with pain and discomfort associated with childbirth, and information about pharmacological options available to mothers in a hospital or birth center (England & Horowitz, 1998; Gaskin, 2003; Goer, 1999; Simkin, 2008). We attended a class for training doulas for their work in continuous support of women throughout labor, birth, and breastfeeding initiation. This class was a thorough introduction to the mechanics of labor, the emotional implications and effects on the woman in labor and her partner, the options available to the parents, and involved hands-on practice of dozens of natural coping mechanisms. We experienced childbirth first-hand and assisted one other woman in the birth of her child, and used these experiences to fuel our research.

The game consisted of a user interface allowing the user to perform supportive actions for Amanda, the mother in labor, and an artificial intelligence unit which reacted to environmental and circumstantial cues (i.e., the progress of labor and the user's interactions with the mother). The game was implemented in Flash. Figure 13 shows a screenshot of the game.

Comfort measures, aggregated from the domain research mentioned above, were converted into a card-game mechanic. In speaking with several doulas, we found that professional childbirth support persons sometimes have a "deck" of support methods written out on index cards and kept in a box as a source of inspiration. The mother and her partner frequently find the "box of tricks" useful, and cite it as an inspiring way to helping them get through a kind of mental block in labor. We adopted this mechanic, creating a deck of about 50 comfort measures that would be randomized at the beginning of the game and then dealt to the player three cards at a time. When all cards had been in play, the deck would be reshuffled and dealt again.

The mother's overall well-being consisted of four traits: energy, emotional support, cognitive support, and the strength of her contractions. The traits were affected by a mathematical formula with a feedback loop, which required player intervention for a successful outcome. The player's selection of comfort measures affected the mother's traits, allowing her to have stronger contractions that would eventually lead to the birth of the child. How each comfort measure affected the mother was determined by her stage in labor, the empirical effectiveness of each comfort measure (Simkin & Bolding, 2004), and a small component of random chance.

Figure 13. Amanda is using chant, mantra, song, or prayer as way to vocalize her experience in active labor. Available actions are affirmation, counter-pressure to her back, and eat a sandwich

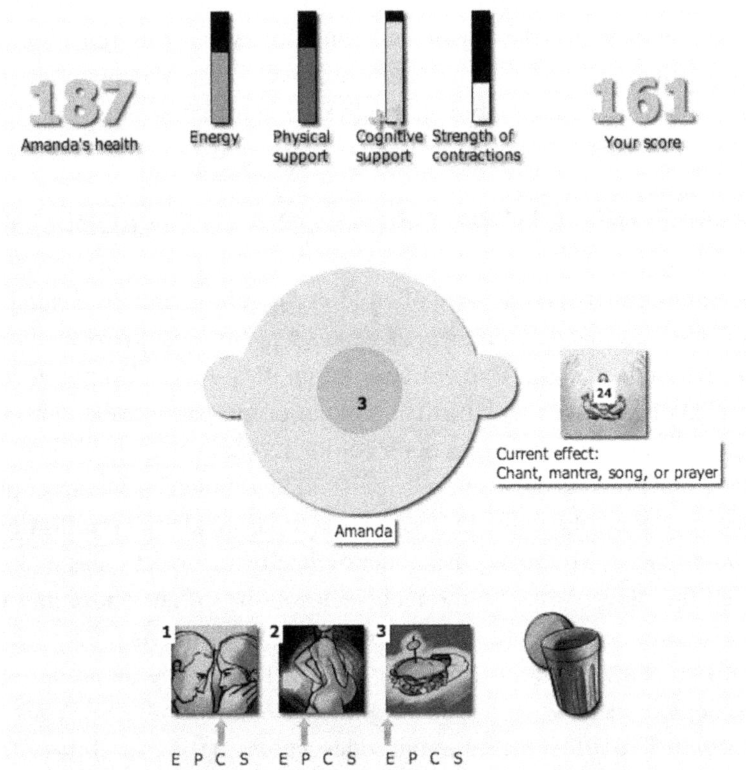

We launched the game as part of a research study using a pre-test, intervention, and post-test (within-subjects) study design. A total of 51 participants completed all portions of the study; about half (47%) had no prior experience with childbirth and most (80%) of the participants were male.

The results of the study (Holloway & Kurniawan, 2011) showed that participants playing The Prepared Partner learned about the mechanics of labor and birth, and answered with more breadth and confidence when asked how to speed up labor naturally. Answers included more concrete actions such as "intimacy," "take a bath," "apply pressure to the lower back," and "acupressure." Before playing The Prepared Partner, the answers were generally more vague and several participants included question marks in their answers, indicating uncertainty. Moreover, participants answered with a broader range of cognitive support methods on the post-test than the pre-test, most of which were presented in the game.

A few months after the study was conducted, one participant contacted the researcher to write that during his recent birth support experience, in the moment, he felt he had forgotten everything except the interactions he saw in The Prepared Partner.

These results indicated that a game was an effective way to transfer knowledge to the birth partner, and prompted further investigation into the nature of childbirth in games, and how to make a more accessible game for knowledge transfer.

VIDEO GAME DEPICTIONS OF LABOR AND CHILDBIRTH

In order to better understand the role of childbirth in commercially-available video games, we first had to determine which games had birth as a part of the story or player interaction. With help from online communities such as Quarter to Three we compiled a list of 34 games with birth as a major or minor game element. It should be noted that childbirth in games is not a common theme.

We found that video games generally paint an incomplete or incorrect picture of the human experience of childbirth from a theoretical standpoint (Holloway, Rubin, & Kurniawan, 2012). Moreover, these incomplete or incorrect ideas expressed by games teach the players these same incorrect notions, often reinforcing negative gender stereotypes, similarly to media effects in other domains.

It is well known that people are negatively influenced by inappropriate, over-sexualized depictions of women in video games (Behm-Morawitz & Mastro, 2009; Downs & Smith, 2010). Hence, though video games do not teach how to have a child, they do suggest the underlying theory of childbirth and childbirth support. Unfortunately, current, commercial video games are lacking in both respects.

Other media depicting childbirth are not without faults. As situational comedies use childbirth for comic relief both in television and in movies (Elson, 1997) the impact of optical media on notions of pregnancy and childbirth are both nontrivial and well documented, affecting perceptions of women's bodies, breastfeeding, and the childbirth process (Morris & McInerney, 2010; Ward, Merriwether, & Caruthers, 2006).

Video games fail to capture the whole gamut of childbirth experiences. There is a wide range of births not captured: women are never shown birthing upright, changing position; they are never shown eating or using comfort techniques in labor. Births are shown as speedy events of pushing out a baby, and only one game half-heartedly models active labor. No game models the third stage of labor (delivery of the placenta), though the mother in one game suggests a few healing spells for herself after the birth. Some games suggest that mothers have to endure some discomfort or pain in the process of birth.

One of the more realistic depictions of the pushing stage of labor, *Assassin's Creed 2* (2009) (Part 1: Birth of the Assassin) shows how Lucy pushes out her baby boy in a semi-sitting position on a table, assisted by two midwives. The midwives coax Lucy to push, and she bears down with all her might in the final pushes necessary to birth the child. In role-playing games such as *Dragon Quest V: Hand of the Heavenly Bride* (2009) and *Harvest Moon DS Cute* (2005) the father waits outside the birthing room, from which pained sounds emanate, and is told in a dialog message that the baby was born in a thematic nod to typical American maternity wards of the 1950s and 1960s.

Having understood the cultural landscape surrounding childbirth in video games, which was largely under-informed and misleading, we investigated the interaction modes. Most games did not allow the player to interact with the birth scene; however, some games allow the player to control the baby's point of view (*Fallout 3* (2008)) or limbs (*Assassin's Creed 2* (2009)) to some extent. In *Sims 3* (2009), the player is allowed to interact with the mother in labor; however, the interaction is limited to involuntary panic, or taking her to the hospital. This form of interaction, in which the player clicks on the mother and selects the only available option through a bubble menu, was fairly intuitive, if lacking in content. *Second Life* (2003) is a simulation game in which the player can purchase a birth package from an online vendor, and participate in the birth of the child. Due to its game-authoring tools, this game has the most diverse representations of birth of any of the games we surveyed. These games are shown in Figure 14.

Figure 14. Representation of childbirth Second Life (2009) and The Sims 3 (2009)

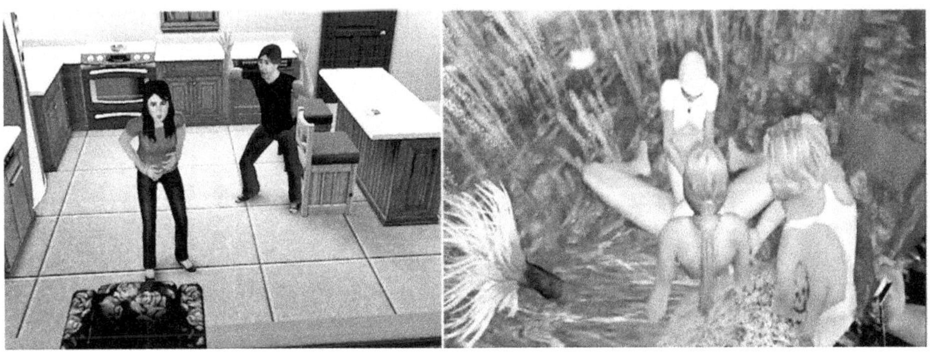

BIRTH PARTNERS' GOALS FOR CHILDBIRTH SUPPORT

We set out to explore the partners experiences of the mothers birth, including attitudes for labor and birth, preparation strategies, labor support goals, birth preferences, and whether the experience unfolded in the way s/he expected. The purpose of the research was to inform a mobile video game about labor and childbirth support as an educational intervention for birth partners.

We wrote an analysis tool that scraped a Website hosting birth stories2. All of these birth stories were authored by women/mothers in the previous year, 2010–2011. In our preliminary analysis, we considered the common themes arising in 100 randomly-selected birth stories. The resulting Wordle is shown in Figure 15. A Wordle is useful for showing graphically common words and themes in a specific body of text. From this image, we determined that it is of high import to model contractions in our system.

Next, we conducted interviews lasting 20 minutes to an hour with 23 birth partners. Some birth partners were recruited before the birth; for them, we asked questions regarding preparation and what they hope to experience in their upcoming role of birth support. For the birth partners that had attended a birth, we asked questions pertaining to their role in the birth support and what they found to be useful (in terms of support strategies) and meaningful (in terms of emotional satisfaction) in the birth experience.

The interviews with birth partners revealed a significant need to feel a connection to the mother and the birth process. Affinity diagrams revealed two main categories of support strategies: emotional support, and physical support.

Figure 15. Wordle, a graphical representation of common topics in 100 random birth stories

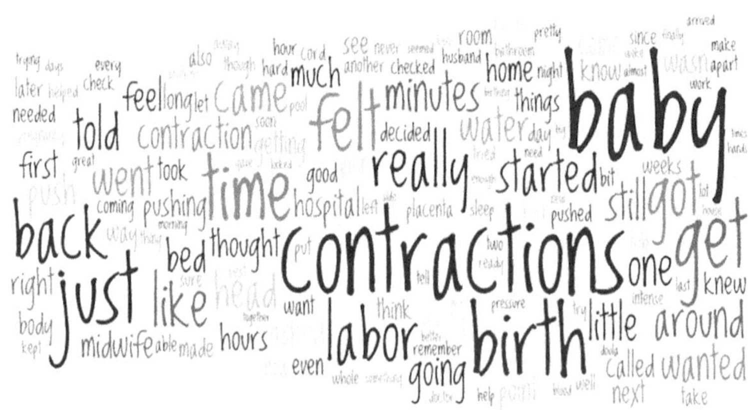

The main goal of emotional support is to calm the mother throughout the discomfort and fear that many mothers experience. Birth partners' stated and implied goals of emotional support were as follows.

- **Physical Presence:** Stay in the room with the mother such that she feels she is never alone.
- **Verbal Care:** Encourage the mother with words and explain that what she is feeling is normal.
- Listen and Respond to the mother's needs promptly and efficiently.
- **Mediate:** Interact with the nursing staff on the mother's behalf, relaying information and normalizing the experience for the mother.
- **Birth Plan Management:** Ensure that a birth plan prepared in advance is followed as closely as possible, and warn and explain to the mother any deviations.

Birth partners placed great import on their role in physical support. While emotional support is different for every person, and is difficult to teach effectively, physical support can be taught in childbirth preparation classes and described in textbooks and other media. The goal of physical support was to make the mothers' bodies more comfortable. The most common types of physical support discussed were rubbing, pushing on, or massaging the mothers back (especially lower back), and holding her hand. Sometimes birth partners would guide and assist the mother in using props such as a birthing (or yoga) ball, or support the mother as she squat, sit, bend over, or stand together to ease labor pain.

Birth partners expressed a desire to know they were needed in the course of the birth. In some cases, mothers become so inwardly focused as the labor progressed that some birth partners felt that they did not receive the feedback they needed. Birth parters felt that physical support gave the best feedback: in supporting a mother physically, they were really doing something, and actively participating in the mother's birth. Emotional support, especially physical presence, was described as a much more passive method of support, and lacking feedback from the mother as she became more inwardly-focused in the course of the birth, and thus more difficult to know how the support was working for the mother.

Our results included that immediate feedback about whether specific action, physical or emotional, was welcome by the mother was key in making birth partners feel necessary and appreciated as support persons.

DIGITAL BIRTH: AN IPHONE SIMULATION OF LABOR

With the knowledge gleaned from our first prototype success, The Prepared Partner; together with the domain knowledge within the fields of childbirth, video games, and user interaction and experience; and added to that the 20+ hours of interview data from expectant and experienced birth partners, prototyped an iPhone game called Digital Birth.

We intended for Digital Birth to be available for free from prenatal clinics and low-cost maternity centers. The game would be distributed at these centers free of charge to any mother or birth partner that wished to obtain a copy of it. Specifically, we built an iPhone game which we targeted for lower-income Latino families from California, who are more likely to surpass whites in their use of data apps from handheld devices such as the iPhone (Smith, 2010).

The mother, Carmen, was the main focus of the game. Carmen was based on our interview data, designed under strict supervision of our anthropology collaborator, and was intended to be age- and race-neutral to appeal to many women or types of women within California. Preliminary inquiries with the target population confirmed that the model of Carmen was acceptable.

Digital Birth is set in a labor and delivery (L&D) room of a hospital-based birth center. The room was designed following visits to L&D wards of California hospitals, including Dominican Hospital of Santa Cruz, University of San Francisco, San Francisco General Hospital, Kaiser Permanente of San Francisco, Redwood City Sequoia Hospital, Good Samaritan Hospital San Jose, Sutter Maternity and Surgery Center of Santa Cruz, and Community Hospital of the Monterey Peninsula. Great import was placed on the use of hydrotherapy (e.g., using the bathtub or shower for pain management) in the visits to the hospitals and from the discussions with the L&D nurses during the tour(s). Thus, we chose to make prominent the large birth tub and the shower in the birth scene in Digital Birth. Other room features include an adjustable hospital bed, large window with window-seat, rocking chair (behind the bed), recessed lighting, hidden compartments for instruments and medical devices, a toilet/shower room with frosted glass, and art on the wall – all designed to create a cozy birthing atmosphere. The room design underwent several iterations, soliciting feedback from our midwifery collaborators until the appropriate level of realism was reached. The game interface can be seen in Figure 16.

Carmen can occupy a variety of positions within the environment, including standing near the bed, sitting up in bed, relaxing in the rocking chair, squatting against the side of the bed, on all fours, slow-dancing with her partner (the player), sitting backwards on a chair, kneeling, lunging, sitting on a birth ball, leaning against the shower wall, walking, sitting on the toilet, and resting against the side of the birth tub while immersed in the tub. Carmen can select one of these positions for herself

Figure 16. Carmen in Digital Birth starts the game by lying on her side in the hospital bed

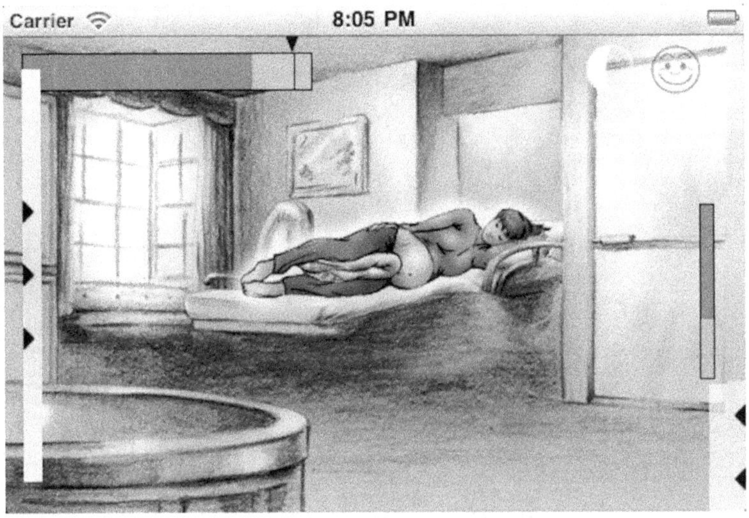

based on her well-being (for example, if she is tired, she will select a lying-down position for herself and will be unable to change to a more vertical position until her energy is replenished), or these positions can be suggested to her by the player. The art used for Carmen's positions is shown in Figure 17.

In any position, Carmen's body glows gold during contractions, and a pull-out contraction monitor can verify the start, end, or peak of a contraction. In our initial interviews, as well as in our birth stories analyses, we found that birth partners typically turn to contraction timing as a supportive activity. Moreover, many of the pregnancy- and birth-related applications we investigated included a contraction timer feature. Thus, we wanted to emphasize the mother's contractions in labor.

The supportive actions available in the game are grouped into six categories: relaxation, breathing, being together (i.e., partner support), position change, and verbal care (e.g., affirmation, tell her how strong she is, etc.). The categories came naturally from affinity diagramming interview responses and comparing them to categories of care in The Birth Partner (Simkin, 2008).

Rather than using "health" or maternal well-being as the main feedback metric about the mother for the player as we did in The Prepared Partner, we decided to use the amount of perceived support a mother feels. From our vast preliminary investigation, it became clear that all mothers are different and all births are different – that is, some mothers want plenty of hands-on support while other mothers just want to feel the presence of their partner. Thus, at the beginning of the game, we auto-generate certain traits for Carmen which we translate into a spectrum of the

Figure 17. Carmen's position art, by Phillip Vaughan, in Digital Birth

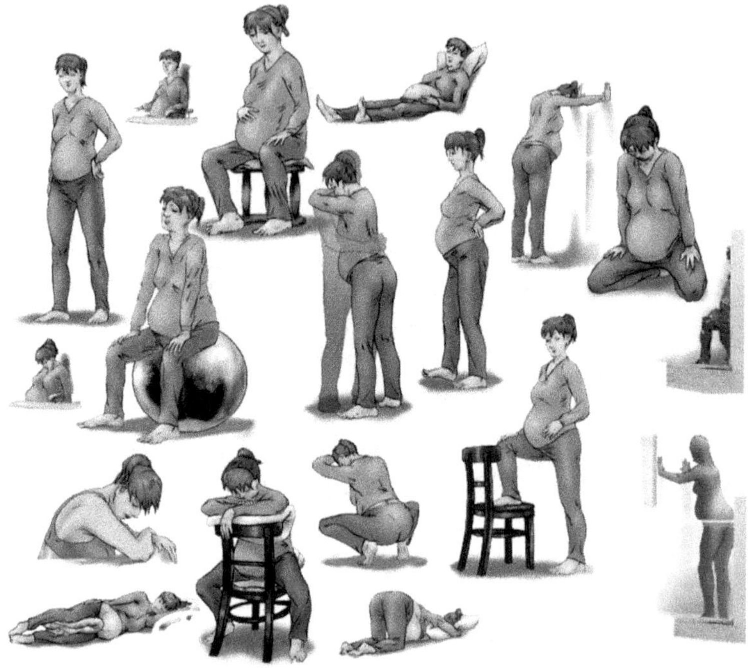

amount of desired support. The player must then stay within a window of that amount by performing actions, or just by being active in the game. If the player is too supportive (i.e., by performing too many actions or suggesting comfort measures too often for Carmen's liking), the results are detrimental to Carmen's labor coping, measured on Simkin's coping scale (Simkin & Bolding, 2004; Simkin, 2011). A visual representation of the spectrum of Carmen's support is shown in Figure 18.

Carmen's overall feelings of support, derived from the amount of support the player provides conflated with her desire for support (and support type aversion multiplier), are translated in realtime into a Simkin-style coping icon (see Figure 19).

We kept the support methods as playing cards metaphor from The Prepared Partner, but instead of dealing three random cards at a time, we decided to make all comfort measures available to the player at all times. In The Prepared Partner, one of our game goals was to show the player as many varied support methods as possible over the course of a play through. For Digital Birth, we wanted to mimic the "tool chest" that doulas describe possessing and accessing during the course of labor support. Thus, all supportive actions were available at all times, when they logistically made sense.

Figure 18. Carmen's desire for support is shown as a green window in this spectrum. The spectrum ranges from a small amount of support (i.e., presence) (A) to a lot of support (i.e., constantly supporting the mother with hands-on actions) (B). The actual amount of support the player is providing is shown as a superscript triangle (C). Carmen's ideal amount of support is shown with the brackets (lower bound D; upper bound E)

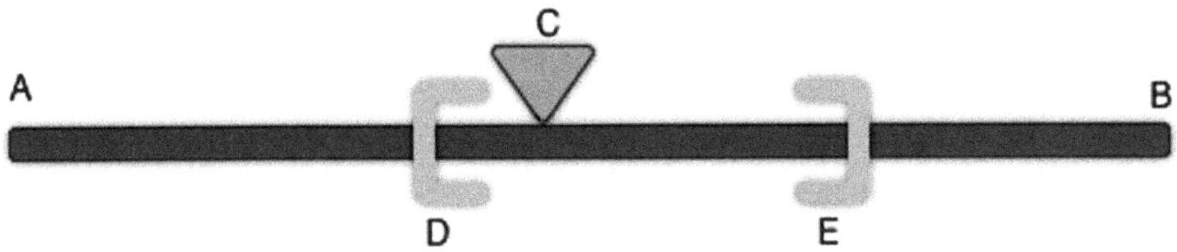

Figure 19. Penny Simkin's pain coping scale for labor and childbirth
Source: Simkin, 2011.

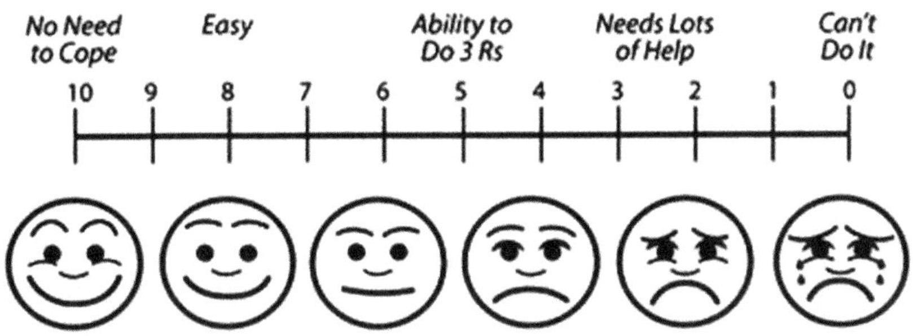

The core component of the way the mother, the non-player character in the game with whom the player interacts, experiences labor is the contraction heartbeat. This is a periodic oscillation that generates uterine contractions in the game, and it is currently implemented with variable contraction durations that correspond to the stages and substages of labor (early labor, active labor, transition, and pushing). The contraction heartbeat is available to the front-end for display via an API call.

The events of the game are not scripted, but are derived from a mathematical formula with a feedback loop that incorporates the stage of labor, the mother's well-being, and the amount of support the player offers the mother. That is, the game elements are procedurally-generated. As in The Prepared Partner, the player's interactions influence Carmen's well-being, and her well-being in turn influences how her labor progresses. At the end of the game, the player is shown a score screen showing a letter-grade corresponding to how well the player supported Carmen – i.e., how well the player stayed within Carmen's desired labor support throughout the birth.

FUTURE WORK

Digital Birth is a prototype game. It is currently undergoing a round of testing with students of nursing-midwifery as a part of their labor support curriculum. We will incorporate the students' feedback into the game. Afterwards, we plan to deploy the game to our intended audience using a within-subjects study design, looking for differences in perceived readiness for childbirth support, understanding of the mechanics of labor and birth and birth support, and childbirth support self-efficacy.

ACKNOWLEDGMENT

The author wishes to thank the following individuals for their contribution to this project at the various stages of work. Rebecca Emrick for her role in Latch Master, a game about teaching breastfeeding; Said Achmiz for his excellent work on the user interface of Digital Birth; Phillip Vaughan for his art design and assets used in Digital Birth; Alaric Holloway for his art used in The Prepared Partner and Digital Birth; Nina Shapiro, Greer Montgomery, and Salvador Contreras for their role in interviewing birth partners; and the author's mentors and advisor, Dr. Megan Moodie, Dr. Jenna Shaw-Battista, and Dr. Sri Kurniawan. The author also wishes to thank the many anonymous individuals that contributed their time to interviews, video game and user interface discussions, and survey data. Specifically, the author acknowledges the participation of the Quarter to Three and Mothering communities.

REFERENCES

Althabe, F., & Belizán, J. (2006). Caesarean section: The paradox. *Lancet*, *368*(9546), 1472–1473. doi:10.1016/S0140-6736(06)69616-5 PMID:17071266

Behm-Morawitz, E., & Mastro, D. (2009). The Effects of the Sexualization of Female Video Game Characters on Gender Stereotyping and Female Self-Concept. *Sex Roles*, *61*(11), 808–823. doi:10.100711199-009-9683-8

Belizán, J., Althabe, F., & Carrerata, M. (2007). Health consequences of the increasing caesarean section rates. *Epidemiology (Cambridge, Mass.)*, *18*(4), 485–486. doi:10.1097/EDE.0b013e318068646a PMID:17568221

Chan, K., & Paterson-Brown, S. (2002). How do fathers feel after accompanying their partners in labour and delivery? *Journal of Obstetrics & Gynaecology*, *22*(1), 11–15. doi:10.1080/01443610120101628 PMID:12521719

Davis-Floyd, R. E. (2004). *Birth as an american rite of passage: With a new preface*. University of California Press. doi:10.1525/california/9780520229327.001.0001

Declercq, E., Sakala, C., Corry, M., & Applebaum, S. (2007). Listening to mothers II: Report of the second national US survey of womens childbearing experiences. *Journal of Perinatal Education, 16*(4), 9–14. doi:10.1624/105812407X244769 PMID:18769512

Downs, E., & Smith, S. (2010). Keeping abreast of hypersexuality: A video game character content analysis. *Sex Roles*, 1–13.

Elson, V. L. (1997). *Childbirth in American movies and television: Patterns of portrayal and audience impact* (Unpublished doctoral dissertation). University of Massachusetts at Amherst.

England, P., & Horowitz, R. (1998). *Birthing From Within: An Extra-Ordinary Guide to Childbirth Preparation*. Albuquerque, NM: Partera Press.

Fabian, H., Rådestad, I., & Waldenström, U. (2005). Childbirth and parenthood education classes in Sweden. Womens opinion and possible outcomes. *Acta Obstetricia et Gynecologica Scandinavica, 84*(5), 436–443. doi:10.1111/j.0001-6349.2005.00732.x PMID:15842207

Fatherhood Institute. (2007). Fathers at the birth and after: Impact on mothers. In *Fatherhood Institute Research Summary: Fathers Attending Births*. Author.

Gaskin, I. (2003). *Ina May's Guide to Childbirth*. Bantam Books.

Githens, P., Glass, C., Sloan, F., & Entman, S. (1993). Maternal recall and medical records: An examination of events during pregnancy, childbirth, and early infancy. *Birth (Berkeley, Calif.), 20*(3), 136–141. doi:10.1111/j.1523-536X.1993.tb00438.x PMID:8240621

Goer, H. (1999). *The Thinking Woman's Guide to a Better Birth*. Perigee.

Goodman, P., Mackey, M., & Tavakoli, A. (2004). Factors related to childbirth satisfaction. *Journal of Advanced Nursing, 46*(2), 212–219. doi:10.1111/j.1365-2648.2003.02981.x PMID:15056335

Hallgren, A., Kilhgren, M., Forslin, L., & Norberg, A. (1999). Swedish fathers involvement in and experiences of childbirth preparation and childbirth. *Midwifery, 15*(1), 6–15. doi:10.1016/S0266-6138(99)90032-3 PMID:10373868

Handfield, B., Turnbull, S., & Bell, R. J. (2006). What do obstetricians think about media influences on their patients? *Australian and New Zealand Journal of Obstetrics and Gynaecology*, *46*(5), 379–383. doi:10.1111/j.1479-828X.2006.00621.x PMID:16953850

Holloway, A. (2010). *System design and evaluation of The Prepared Partner: a labor and childbirth game* (Unpublished master's thesis). University of California, Santa Cruz, CA.

Holloway, A., & Kurniawan, S. (2010). System design evolution of The Prepared Partner: How a labor and childbirth game came to term. In Meaningful play. Academic Press.

Holloway, A., & Kurniawan, S. (2011). The Prepared Partner: Can a video game teach labor and childbirth support techniques? In Information quality in ehealth. Graz, Austria: Academic Press.

Holloway, A., Rubin, Z., & Kurniawan, S. (2012). What video games have to teach us about childbirth and childbirth support. In *Proceedings of the first workshop on design patterns in games* (p. 4). 10.1145/2427116.2427120

Holzinger, A. (2005). Usability engineering methods for software developers. *Communications of the ACM*, *48*(1), 71–74. doi:10.1145/1039539.1039541

Kiernan, K., & Smith, K. (2003). Unmarried parenthood: new insights from the millennium cohort study. *Population Trends - London*, 26–33.

Klaus, M., Kennell, J., & Klaus, P. (1993). *Mothering the Mother: How a Doula Can Help You Have a Shorter*. Perseus Books.

Klaus, M., Kennell, J., & Klaus, P. (2002). *The Doula Book*. Da Capo Press.

Leavitt, J. W. (2009). *How did men end up in the delivery room?* George Mason University's History News Network. Retrieved May 13, 2013, from http://www.hnn.us/articles/116291.html

Lumley, J., & Brown, S. (1993). Attenders and nonattenders at childbirth education classes in Australia: How do they and their births differ? *Birth (Berkeley, Calif.)*, *20*(3), 123–130. doi:10.1111/j.1523-536X.1993.tb00435.x PMID:8240618

Morgan, B., Bulpitt, C., Clifton, P., & Lewis, P. (1982). Analgesia and satisfaction in childbirth (the Queen Charlottes 1000 mother survey). *Lancet*, *320*(8302), 808–810. doi:10.1016/S0140-6736(82)92691-5 PMID:6126674

Morris, T., & McInerney, K. (2010). Media representations of pregnancy and childbirth: An analysis of reality television programs in the United States. *Birth (Berkeley, Calif.)*, *37*(2), 134–140. doi:10.1111/j.1523-536X.2010.00393.x PMID:20557536

Nichols, M. (1995). Adjustment to new parenthood: Attenders versus nonattenders at prenatal education classes. *Birth (Berkeley, Calif.)*, *22*(1), 21–26. doi:10.1111/j.1523-536X.1995.tb00549.x PMID:7741947

Odent, M. (1999). Is the participation of the father at birth dangerous? *Midwifery Today*, (51), 23.

Simkin, P. (1992). Just Another Day in a Womans Life? Part II: Nature and Consistency of Womens Long-Term Memories of Their First Birth Experiences. *Birth (Berkeley, Calif.)*, *19*(2), 64–81. doi:10.1111/j.1523-536X.1992.tb00382.x PMID:1388434

Simkin, P. (2008). The Birth Partner: A Complete Guide To Childbirth For Dads, Doulas, and All Other Labor Companions (3rd ed.). Harvard Common Press.

Simkin, P. (2011, February 28). Part 2: Pain, suffering, and trauma in labor and subsequent post-traumatic stress disorder: Practical suggestions to prevent PTSD after childbirth. *Science & Sensibility*.

Simkin, P., & Bolding, A. (2004). Update on nonpharmacologic approaches to relieve labor pain and prevent suffering. *Journal of Midwifery & Womens Health*, *49*(6), 489–504. doi:10.1016/S1526-9523(04)00355-1 PMID:15544978

Smith, A. (2010). *Mobile Access 2010*. Pew Research Center. Available at http://pewinternet.org/Reports/2010/Mobile-Access-2010/Summary-of-Findings.aspx

Somers-Smith, M. (1999). A place for the partner? Expectations and experiences of support during childbirth. *Midwifery*, *15*(2), 101–108. doi:10.1016/S0266-6138(99)90006-2 PMID:10703413

Steen, M., Downe, S., Bamford, N., & Edozien, L. (2011). Not-patient and and not-visitor: A metasynthesis of fathers' encounters with pregnancy, birth and maternity care. *Midwifery*. PMID:21820778

Tomeo, C., Rich-Edwards, J., Michels, K., Berkey, C., Hunter, D., Frazier, A., ... Buka, S. L. (1999). Reproducibility and validity of maternal recall of pregnancy-related events. *Epidemiology (Cambridge, Mass.)*, *10*(6), 774–777. doi:10.1097/00001648-199911000-00022 PMID:10535796

Van Zandt, S., Edwards, L., & Jordan, E. (2005). Lower epidural anesthesia use associated with labor support by student nurse doulas: Implications for intrapartal nursing practice. *Complementary Therapies in Clinical Practice*, *11*(3), 153–160. doi:10.1016/j.ctcp.2005.02.003 PMID:16005832

Ward, L., Merriwether, A., & Caruthers, A. (2006). Breasts are for men: Media, masculinity ideologies, and men's beliefs about women's bodies. *Sex Roles*, *55*(9), 703–714.

This research was previously published in Transforming Gaming and Computer Simulation Technologies across Industries edited by Brock Dubbels; pages 154-182, copyright year 2017 by Information Science Reference (an imprint of IGI Global).

Chapter 6
MotherCare App for Expectant Mothers in Interior Parts of Pakistan

Muhammad Abdul Tawab Khalil
City University of Science and Information Technology, Pakistan

Saifullah Jan
IQRA National University, Pakistan

Wajid Ali
IQRA National University, Pakistan

Adnan Khan
IQRA National University, Pakistan

ABSTRACT

Pregnancy, as a matter of fact, is always physically and emotionally challenging for women. Rapid physical changes with baby's growth in the womb exposes the mother to severe mood swings from short spell of merriment to long spells of anxiety and depression about upcoming child's health, its wellbeing, and so on. Most of the third world countries with their struggling economies have patriarchal social fabric, a fact that makes it worse for women of these societies to healthily tackle or seek help during gestation. The main goal of the proposed application, MothersCare, is to help the expecting mothers when they need it most. It will help them choose the right physician and request appointments from the comfort of homes, barring cumbersome wait for turn in long queues in rush hours for appointments with doctors at hospitals. This app is absolutely user-friendly in terms of simplicity of use and wide spectrum of maternal healthcare services it offers.

DOI: 10.4018/978-1-7998-2351-3.ch006

INTRODUCTION

With the fast development of mobile technology, mobile devices are becoming ever more importantly ubiquitous. With the recent improvement on mobile devices, their humanitarian utility has become multifaceted. Their multipurpose service not only includes facilitation of one-on-one or one-on-group interaction but education, personal security, healthcare, etc. A number of software packages, embedded or downloadable in one's mobile, offer a range of services—a fact that has easified day to day affairs of mobile users.

MotherCare is one such app through which we seek to assist an expecting mother in maintaining her own health as well as that of the baby during pregnancy. Meant for Pakistani women, specifically the women of District Swat in Khyberpakhtunkhwah, the app intends to save moms-to-be the labor of queuing up for allotment of appointment number and then waiting for the turn to see a doctor. It facilitates female patients to locate doctors and set appointments easily. This app also provides weekly information illustrated with images to the patients regarding their pregnancy. Hence, our app aims to provide consultancy and tips to the expecting mothers with the help of mobile phones by making maternity care service more interactive and accessible.

BACKGROUND

Pakistan, which is fifth most populous country of the world with a population of over 209,970,000 people (Stimson & Haynes 2012), has a 60.78% rural population (Trading Economics, 2018). The economic façade of the country has changed rapidly in recent years from a dominantly agricultural to an evolving industrial economy. Many settled areas in less known parts of the country have already put on an urban or at least suburban array such as Kohaat, Nooriabad, Nowshera, Mirpur Khas, etc. Residents of these areas enjoy access to basic amenities of life. All the same, there are certain interior parts of Pakistan where development has been slow to make its mark. These areas are physically and temperamentally rustic. Unavailability of smooth tarmacked roads to travel long distances and absence of basic medical facilities are the regular nuance to the residents, for instance, underdeveloped parts of Haala and Tharparkar Districts in Sindh, and Charsadda District in Khyberpakhtunkhwa.

Female residents especially suffer greater due to unavailability of basic healthcare facilities near their homes. They suffer worse because, being a patriarchal society to the core, male members of the family feel shy to allow the ailing women of their families to travel long distances and get themselves checked by proper physicians or specialists in cities for prenatal care. Men's attitude becomes more rigid towards women who are in the family way. Instead of letting their women visit a maternity care centre or such a department in a hospital, they prefer to engage an obstetrician with or without certified training for baby's birth at home. This augments hazards to expectant mother's health, as well as that of her to-be-born baby's.

According to official records, one in 89 women loses her life due to gestational or/and child-birth related complications (Rau, 2015). In Ashrita Rau's words: "Rural women are less likely to have access to a hospital. The rate of maternal mortality is consequently higher in rural areas than urban areas—23 percent in rural areas rather than 14 percent in urban areas. One major reason for comparatively high maternal mortality rate in rural areas is the home births that are extremely common. A total of 74 percent of women in rural areas give birth at home, compared to 43 percent of women in urban areas", (Rau, 2015)

Since in Pakistani society, women as daughters, wives and sisters are generally regarded an economic liability on the male members of the family, any expense on their medical care is frowned upon and evaded to the best. So goes for the pregnant lady in the family.

In addition, the shortage of doctors, nurses, and beds at government hospitals also imperceptibly discourages general public, especially expectant women, to take all the trouble of travelling to a hospital, lining up for allotment of appointment time, and finally waiting for hours for the turn to see a gynecologist. Worse still, a good number of regular staff in a gynecological department of a hospital are postgraduate trainees who lack knowledge and skill to handle gestational complications (Rau, 2015).

Lack of general education and ignorance about the significance of prenatal or antenatal care for an expectant lady's and her evolving baby's health are additional factors that discourage a majority of Pakistani women to seek a healthcare service. Ashrita Rau, a writer for the Borgen Project, observes that 96% percent of educated women go for prenatal care. However, the figure tapers down to just 50% in case of uneducated prenatal or antenatal care seekers. "One third of pregnant women in Pakistan do not get prenatal care at all, due to the feeling (or misperception that) it is unnecessary or that it costs too much money. Prenatal care can help prevent complications and decrease the maternal mortality rate. While prenatal care visits have increased, as of 2007, only 28 percent of Pakistani women went to the recommended four prenatal care visits," Ashrita Rau comments (Rau, 2015).

Since education ratio is much higher in foreign countries, the women and their families are well aware of the significance of antenatal care and ways to prevent complications that involve pregnancy induced depression, insomnia, anxiety, exhaustion, dietary issues and so on. According to a report on Google, 22,000 women search for the tips and planning regarding their pregnancy per day. Besides searches on symptoms like nausea, heartburn and constipation, food carving is another common search amongst pregnant women across the world. The trend is on the increase in Pakistan, too, amongst the educated women.

Keeping in view the ground issues that face the expectant women in Pakistan, as well as the significance of their accessibility to antenatal counseling and care, through MotherCare app, we have tried to offer a handy solution. It has been designed to provide week by week guidelines on the development of pregnancy and baby, health tips and exercises to suit every key stage of gestation, facility to set an appointment with a nearby gynecologist, and a record of these appointments. Any woman with some smatterings of English language, ability to read English language and the know-how of using an android mobile phone can highly benefit from the key features of the app, and save herself cumbersomely long travels and wait at hospitals/maternity care centers.

MOTHERSCARE AND RIVAL APPS

A number of apps already exist in order to guide and assist expectant women about their antenatal and postnatal health. These help the women schedule appointments with doctors and seek guidance on healthcare. They are easy to download in mobile phones with android or iOS support. These include:

My Pregnancy Day by Day

Claimed to be a complete app on pregnancy related issues, cautions and guidelines, My Pregnancy Day by Day app has been offered and developed by iBoo Mobiles. It is helpful to a pregnant mom in many ways. It helps them keep important pregnancy notes, consult nutrition guide, find out about right exercises for each key stage of pregnancy, follow a to do list before and after childbirth, search list of easy-to-access hospitals, seek tips on handling labor, get amazing cards to notify birth to friends and family, and choose appropriate name for the baby from a list of 1000+ names (iBoo, 2017). These features are illustrated in Figures 1, 2 and 3 below:

This app can be easily downloaded in any android mobile phone. However, all the key features on this app are only available to use after payment of around $2. No payment, no service!

Pregnancy Week by Week

This app shares information/guidelines on exercises suited to each important stage of pregnancy including kegel exercises. It also features information, as well as health advice on week by week development of pregnancy and the baby's evolving size, pregnancy calendar, regular checks on one's weight during pregnancy through a weight tracker, kick counter to keep a track of baby kicks, a vigilance for false and real

Figure 1. List to choose your baby's name (iBoo, 2017)

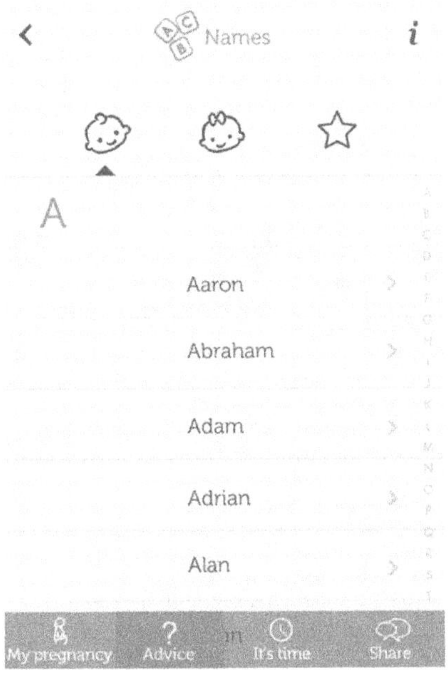

Figure 2. Information on week-wise development of pregnancy and the baby (iBoo, 2017)

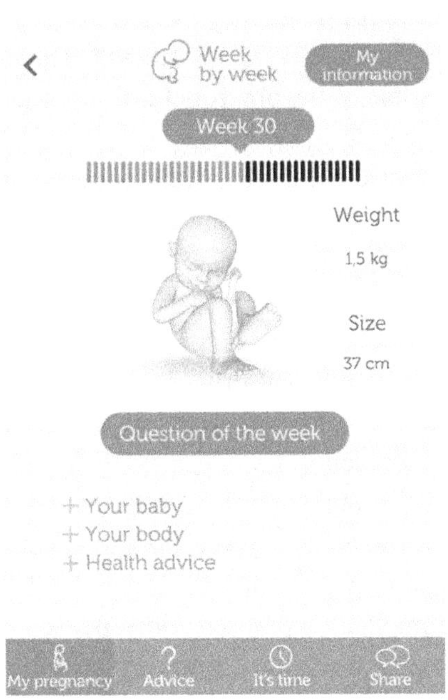

Figure 3. Illustrated tips on exercises at key stages of pregnancy (iBoo, 2017)

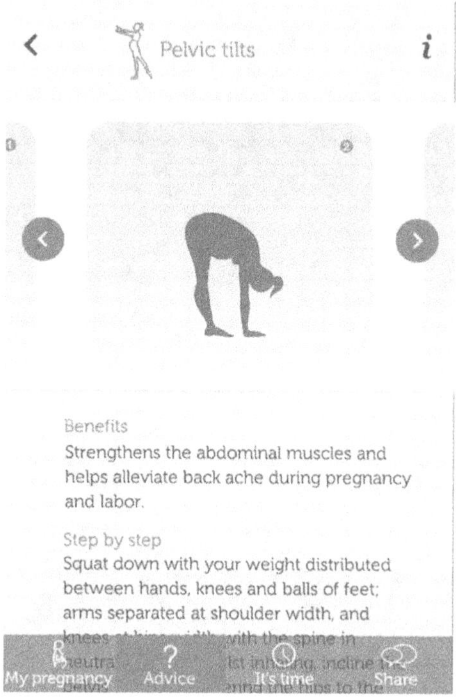
Pelvic tilts
Benefits
Strengthens the abdominal muscles and helps alleviate back ache during pregnancy and labor.
Step by step
Squat down with your weight distributed between hands, knees and balls of feet; arms separated at shoulder width, and
My pregnancy
Advice
It's time
Share

contractions, and note keeper of pregnancy symptoms such as sickness, pregnancy induced physical changes and doctor appointments. This app is downloadable in android mobile phones. Some of the app functions are illustrated below in Figures 4 and 5 (Amila, 2018).

Though the app provides useful tips on gestational issues, it is sans any mechanism for searching nearby gynecologists and setting appointments with them.

I'm Expecting

The key features of this app are that it provides weekly updates on body changes and baby development. It also offers videos on week-based pregnancy, as well as baby development. It lets women in the family way keep track of their pregnancy symptoms and compare with other moms-to-be. The app also facilitates a check on weight throughout the pregnancy stages. The expectant mom-cum-app user can compare the baby's weekly growth with images in fetal development videos developed by concerned medical experts. Besides being a due date calculator, the app, like Pregnancy Week by Week app, offers a platform to expecting mothers to engage in a supportive interaction with a community of moms, registered on this

Figure 4. Track baby kicks (Amila, 2018)

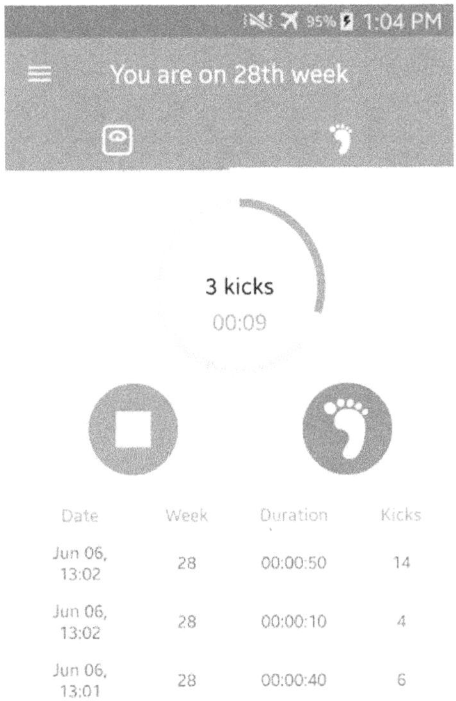

app as users, by sharing pregnancy related questions and answers. There are also articles to tip off expectant moms about pregnancy, childbirth and postnatal care.

The app also, in a detailed way, informs the users of symptoms of weekly pregnancy development along with a to-do list and health tips (StayWell, 2018). One of the app services is illustrated below in Figure 6.

MOTHERCARE APP

In contrast, our designed application, MotherCare app is intended to assist expectant moms, situated anywhere in the Swat District of Khyberpakhtunkhwa, Pakistan, to access guidelines for handling pregnancy related complications, and set appointments with nearby gynecologist all from the cozy comfort of their home. A search bar helps navigate for the nearest gynecologist, and set consultancy time with them by SMS or call. The ability of the MotherCare App to facilitate the expecting moms-cum-users to schedule a check-up session with nearby gynies gives the app an edge over its competitors. Besides, it has user-friendly interface.

Figure 5. Weight tracker chart (Amila, 2018)

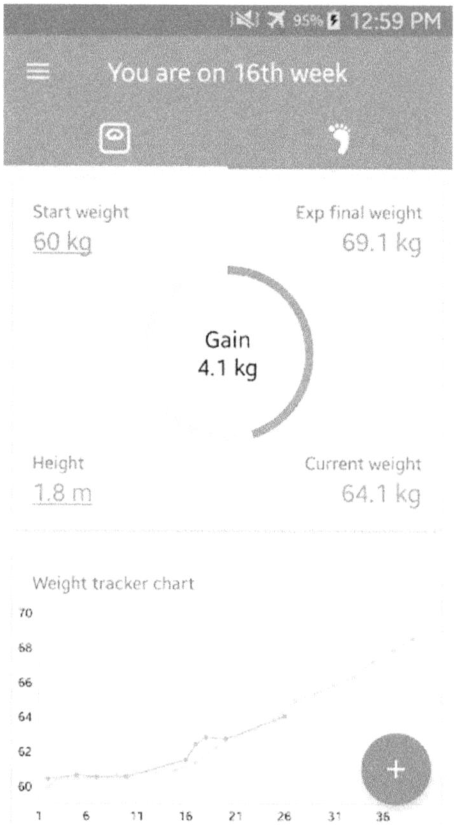

WHY USE MOTHERSCARE APP

In addition to its serviceability to the expectant moms, our proposed application, MotherCare app, has certain technical features that enhance its user-friendliness. These not only include its design and interface, but security of personal data. Details are given as follows:

1. An application should have an interface that is convenient and engaging for users to interact with. A user friendly application must be simple and easy to use; otherwise it loses its charm for the user before long. The overall design and interface of MotherCare app take care of these significant facts.
2. Android happens to be the world's most commonly used smart phone platform and is used by many different phone manufacturers. On the contrary, iOS, another contemporary operating system is only used on Apple devices, such as the iPhone

Figure 6. Tip off on baby's weekly size (StayWell, 2018)

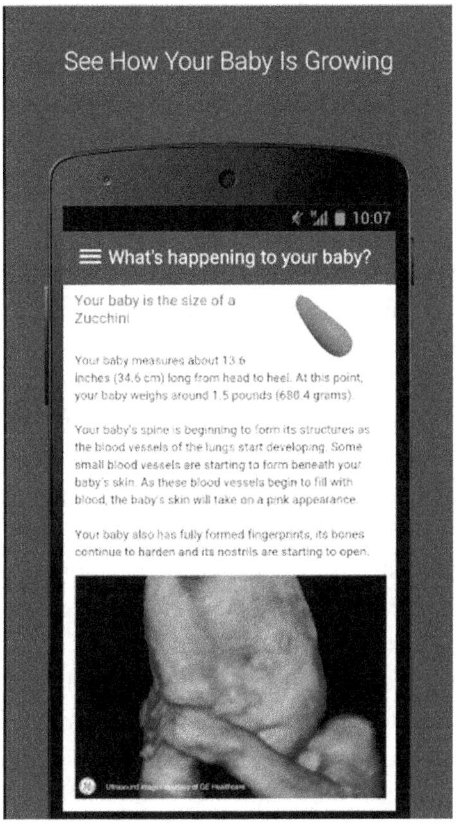

(Diffen, 2017). Therefore, the compatibility of MotherCare app with android adds to its accessibility to the general public, especially expecting mothers.

3. MotherCare app has been designed to make right yet prompt response to user's activity, consuming system resources modestly. This feature adds to the efficiency of the app and its subsequent user-friendliness.
4. MotherCare app has extensibility enough to maintain it by further improvement or adjustment of features.
5. User privacy has been assured by restricting its use to registered users.
6. This app works reliably and robustly. It has been proofed against any tendency to crash.
7. The code of this app has been carefully tested to make it bug-proof.
8. This is a professional software app with clear and readable source code. It is based on open standards, allowing for further improvement on its performance in order to enhance its efficiency.

9. The app has been developed in line with Data Protection Act (DPA) of the UK, as well as the Computer Misuse Act in order to secure user privacy. This app cannot access a user's system, and modify or delete their files without authorization.

DEVELOPMENT AND USE OF MOTHERSCARE APP

We have developed MotherCare app in conformation with the framework of an application development life cycle in order to ensure its accuracy and usability. An illustration is given in Figure 7 below:

MotherCare app is easy to download in an android mobile phone or smartphone from Google App Store. After installation, the user is required to register themselves by entering their name, address, cell phone number and email ID in order to fully utilize the app. As they open the app, illustrated in Figure 8, the first button they come across is Week by Week. A tap on this opens another screen where the user can select a week from a list of 40 weeks for information on pregnancy and baby's development. After the selection of a week, relevant information opens up detailing out the gestational progress with clear illustrations.

Next key button on home screen of the app is General Tips. A thumb touch leads the user to a list of weeks for tips on care during pregnancy in a given week. The user selects the week of their choice to access precautionary guidelines related to that week. This information is particularly useful to help the expectant mother to maintain her own health, as well the health of her growing baby.

Figure 7. MothersCare Development Life Cycle

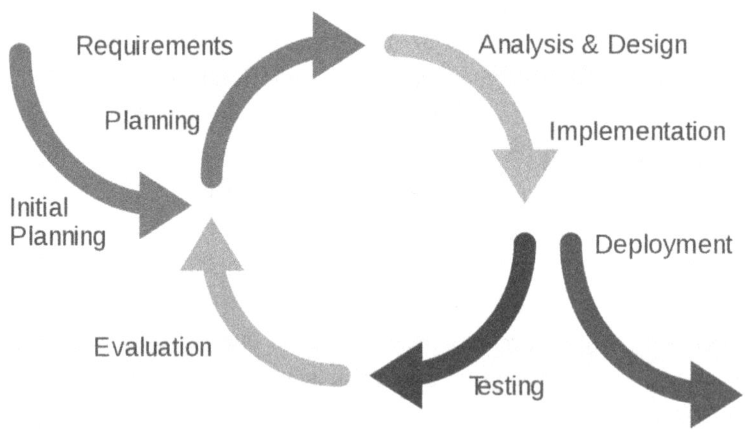

Figure 8. Use Case Diagram of MothersCare App

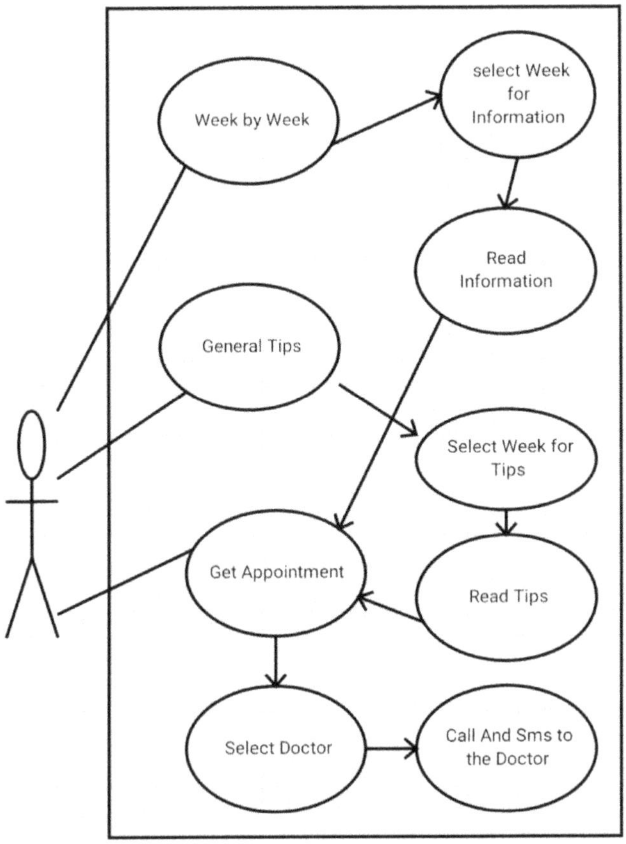

Third key button on the homepage of the app is Get Appointment. A click on this opens a list of gynecologists under the title Select Doctor. After selecting a doctor from the list, next window offers two choices to contact the doctor by call and/or SMS. Homepage of the app is illustrated in Figure 9 below:

On Thumb Press of Week by Week Button

A tap on this very first button opens a whole list of 40 weeks. An expectant mother can here select the week to search information on pregnancy development and physical changes during that week. The information is also illustrated with images of the shape and size of the evolving baby during entire gestation right from Week 1 to the Week 40. The illustrations are given in Figures 10 and 11 below:

Figure 9. Homepage of MothersCare App

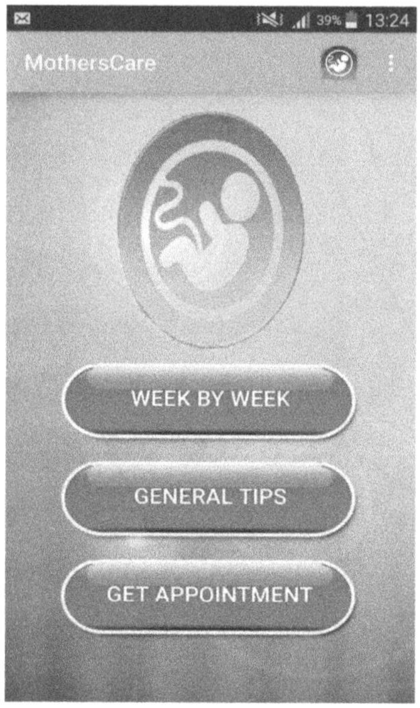

Figure 10. Weeks listed according to gestational progress

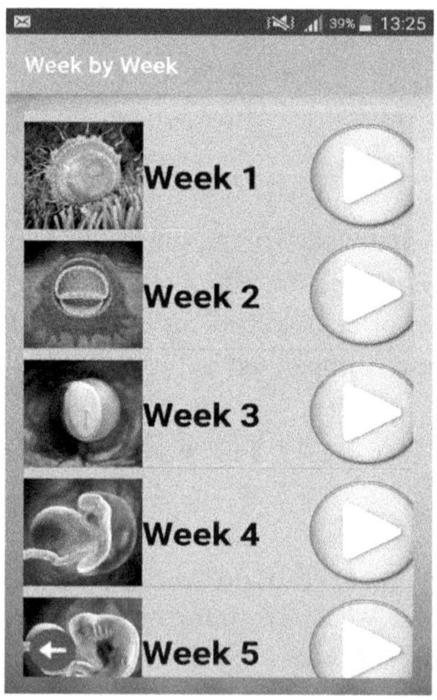

Figure 11. An illustration of week-wise information on pregnancy progress

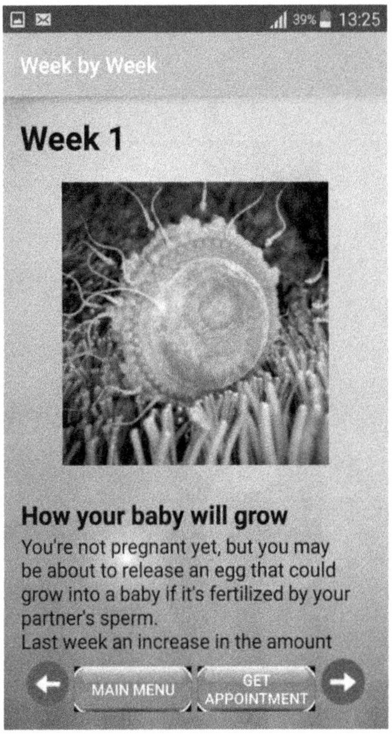
13:25
Week by Week
Week 1
How your baby will grow
You're not pregnant yet, but you may be about to release an egg that could grow into a baby if it's fertilized by your partner's sperm.
Last week an increase in the amount
MAIN MENU
GET APPOINTMENT

On Thumb Press of General Tips Button

With a click on this button, another list of 40 weeks, which make up the general time span of a mother's pregnancy, opens up. This is illustrated in Figure 12 below:

A thumb press on the rightward thick arrow of a week leads the user to the pregnancy-related health tips and cautions. This also prepares the to-be-moms about their physical and emotional constitution during the given week so that she can handle it effectively. This is illustrated in Figure 13 below:

On Thumb Press of Get Appointment Button

A click on the Get Appointment button opens a list of gynecologists located in nearby area(s) of the user. They have choice to pick doctors that are comparatively easy to access. This facility is illustrated in Figure 14 below:

Figure 12. Week-wise general tips on pregnancy

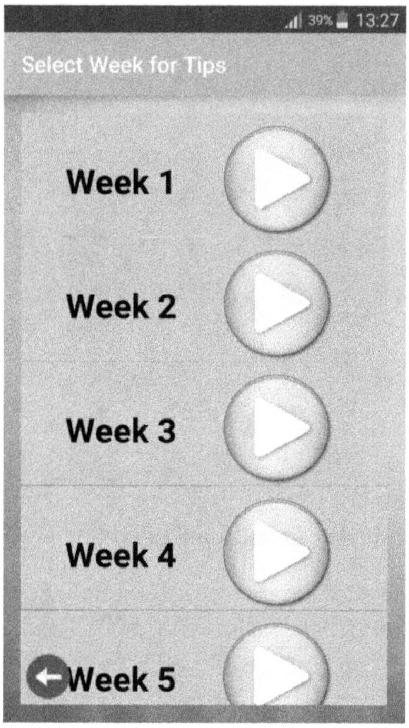

Figure 13. Pregnancy-related general tips for to-be-moms

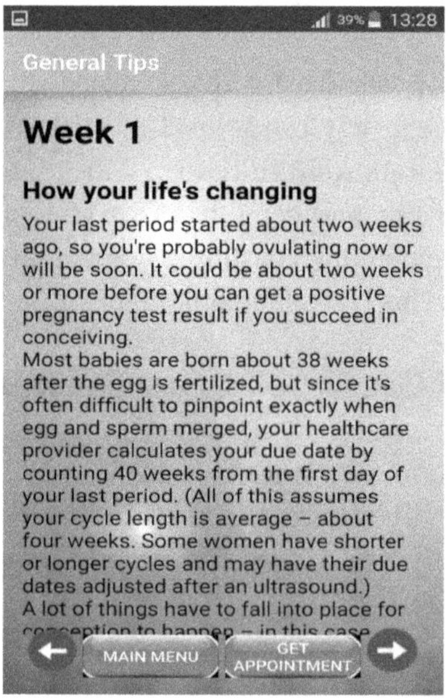

Figure 14. List of nearby doctors/gynecologists

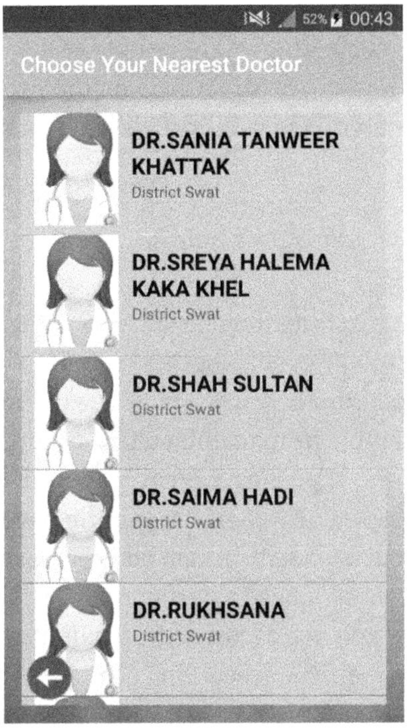

Figure 15. An illustration of a doctor's profile

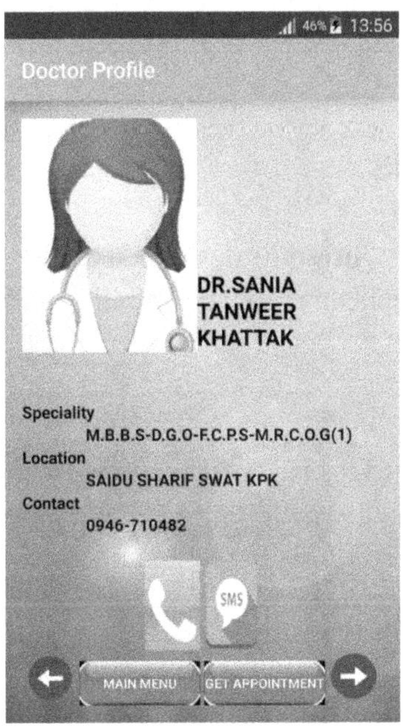

After the user clicks on the name of a doctor, their full profile flashes across the screen, next. The profile consists of name, location and description about their field of specialty. There are two green buttons at the bottom of a doctor's profile for making a call and/or sending SMS to get expert advice on the overall health of pregnancy and/or fix the appointment with the doctor. This is illustrated in Figure 15 below:

CONCLUSION

In a county like Pakistan, travelling long distances and then waiting in long queues for securing appointments with gynecologist(s) is quite a painful labor next to the labor pains for an expectant mother. In view of the difficulties expectant women from rural areas or areas far off from mainland face, we have tried to come up with an application that saves the expecting patient many troubles in accessing timely healthcare services. Our proposed MotherCare app is intended to assist the gestational mothers with timely approach to medical care and necessary health tips to maintain their baby's, as well as their own health during pregnancy. In order to optimize its user-friendliness, we have built in it a feature that facilitates making a call to a doctor and/or sending an SMS to them for scheduling an appointment. Besides, like other competitor pregnancy-related apps, this app provides detailed health guidelines to expecting mothers on the progress of their pregnancy, subsequent physical and emotional changes, tips to handle these changes, and weekly updates on baby's growth within a mom's womb. Moreover, the app has a user-friendly design and interface, making it an efficient support for expectant mothers.

FUTURE DIRECTIONS

MotherCare app has been currently developed for the women of Swat Valley in Khyberpakhtukhwah, Pakistan. Its accessibility and user-friendliness can be improved by:

1. Adding Video call.
2. Adding multiple languages like Urdu and regional languages of Pakistan.
3. Spreading it city wise.
4. Distributing the gynecologists city-wise and providing a search bar to search gynecologists in a specific city.

REFERENCES

Amila. (2018). *Pregnancy Week By Week*. Retrieved on March 24, 2018 from https://play.google.com/store/apps/details?id=com.easymobs.pregnancy&hl=en

Diffen. (2017). *Android vs. iOS*. Retrieved on March 25, 2018 from https://www.diffen.com/difference/Android_vs_iOS

iBoo. (2017). *My Pregnancy Day by Day*. Retrieved on March 24, 2018 from https://play.google.com/store/apps/details?id=com.iboomobile.heroembarazointer

Rau, A. (2015). *Maternal Mortality in Pakistan*. Retrieved on March 20, 2018 from https://borgenproject.org/maternal-mortality-pakistan/

StayWell. (2018). *I'm Expecting*. Retrieved on March 25, 2018 from https://play.google.com/store/apps/details?id=org.medhelp.iamexpecting&hl=en

Stimson, R., & Haynes, K. E. (2012). *Studies in Applied Geography and Spatial Analysis: Addressing Real World Issues*. Edward Elgar Publishing. doi:10.4337/9781781007969

Trading Economics. (2018). *Pakistan - Rural population*. Retrieved on March 23, 2018 from https://tradingeconomics.com/pakistan/rural-population-percent-of-total-population-wb-data.html

ADDITIONAL READING

BabyCenter. (2015). Expert Info for Pregnancy & Parenting. Retrieved on March 20, 2015 from https://www.babycenter.com/

Barron, P., Peter, J., LeFevre, A. E., Sebidi, J., Bekker, M., Allen, R., ... & Pillay, Y. (2018). Mobile health messaging service and helpdesk for South African mothers (MomConnect): history, successes and challenges. BMJ global health, 3(Suppl 2), e000559.

Bhargava, H. K., & Tanghetti, J. (2016). Mobile health technologies. In The UCLA Anderson Business and Information Technologies (BIT) Project: A Global Study of Technology and Business Practice (2016) (pp. 167-185). doi:10.1142/9789814733564_0009

Chang, C. W., Hsu, Y. Y., Kuo, S. E., & Hou, T. W. (2018). *Maternal body weight and diet management system*. Contemporary Clinical Trials Communications.

Coleman, J. C. (2004). The Construction and Experience of 'Risk' in Pregnancy and Childbirth in Australia (Doctoral dissertation, University of Michigan).

Dahl, A. A., Dunn, C. G., Boutté, A. K., Crimarco, A., & Turner-McGrievy, G. (2018). Mobilizing mHealth for Moms: A Review of Mobile Apps for Tracking Gestational Weight Gain. *Journal of Technology in Behavioral Science*, *3*(1), 32–40. doi:10.100741347-017-0030-6

Deparkes, (2015). How to Use Firefox SQLite Manager. Retrieved on May 30, 2015 from https://deparkes.co.uk/2016/03/04/use-firefox-sqlite-manager/

Dolan, B. (2013). Report finds pregnancy apps more popular than fitness apps. Mobi Health News, 14.

Frazer, C., Hussey, L., Bosch, E., & Squire, M. (2015). Pregnancy apps: A closer look at the implications for childbirth educators.

Golden, A., & Krauskopf, P. (2016). Eponyms and MommyMeds. *The Journal for Nurse Practitioners*, *12*(3), e133–e134. doi:10.1016/j.nurpra.2015.12.005

Gourevitch, R. A., Mehrotra, A., Galvin, G., Karp, M., Plough, A., & Shah, N. T. (2017). How do pregnant women use quality measures when choosing their obstetric provider? *Birth (Berkeley, Calif.)*, *44*(2), 120–127. doi:10.1111/birt.12273 PMID:28124390

Gunter, J. Practice Extender, App Corner Sprout Pregnancy Essentials An app to help your patient track her pregnancy September 2012· Vol. 2

Haelle, T. (2018). Pregnancy Apps: Your Patients Use Them—Are You Up to Speed?.

Hussain, A., Mkpojiogu, E. O., Fadzil, N., Hassan, N., & Zaaba, Z. F. (2018). A Mobile Usability Evaluation of a Pregnancy App. Journal of Telecommunication, Electronic and Computer Engineering (JTEC), 10(1-11), 13-18.

Javapoint, (2015). Android Tutorial. Retrieved on June1, 2017 from https://www.javatpoint.com/android-tutorial

Larsen, H., Nielsen, G. L., Schønheyder, H. C., Olesen, C., & Sørensen, H. T. (2001). Birth outcome following maternal use of fluoroquinolones. *International Journal of Antimicrobial Agents*, *18*(3), 259–262. doi:10.1016/S0924-8579(01)00390-9 PMID:11673039

Latchem, C. (2018). Health care, Childcare, Safe Water, Sanitation and Hygiene. In *Open and Distance Non-formal Education in Developing Countries* (pp. 121–130). Singapore: Springer. doi:10.1007/978-981-10-6741-9_12

Lau, Y., Cheng, L. J., Chi, C., Tsai, C., Ong, K. W., Ho-Lim, S. S. T., ... Tan, K. L. (2018). Development of a Healthy Lifestyle Mobile App for Overweight Pregnant Women: Qualitative Study. *JMIR mHealth and uHealth*, *6*(4), e91. doi:10.2196/mhealth.9718 PMID:29685868

Leaver, T. (2017). Born digital? Presence, privacy, and intimate surveillance.

Lupton, D., & Pedersen, S. (2016). An Australian survey of women's use of pregnancy and parenting apps. *Women and Birth; Journal of the Australian College of Midwives*, *29*(4), 368–375. doi:10.1016/j.wombi.2016.01.008 PMID:26874938

Lupton, D., & Thomas, G. M. (2015). Playing pregnancy: the ludification and gamification of expectant motherhood in smartphone apps. M/C Journal, 18(5).

Material Design, (2015). Understanding Layout. Retrieved on August 3, 2015 from https://material.io/design/components/buttons.html#implementation

Mendez, I., Holt, T., McKinney, V., & Keays-White, D. Smart Technology. In Congress on Circumpolar Health.

Murkoff, H. (2016). *What to expect when you're expecting*. Workman Publishing.

Osman, N. F., & Mohamed, H. H. (2016, October). Islamic pregnancy mobile learning application. In e-Learning, e-Management and e-Services (IC3e), 2016 IEEE Conference on (pp. 150-155). IEEE. 10.1109/IC3e.2016.8009057

Paradis, M., Atkinson, K. M., Hui, C., Ponka, D., Manuel, D. G., Day, P., ... Wilson, K. (2018). Immunization and technology among newcomers: A needs assessment survey for a vaccine-tracking app. *Human Vaccines & Immunotherapeutics*, 1–5. doi:10.1080/21645515.2018.1445449 PMID:29482427

ProgrammingKnowledge. (2015). Android SQLite Database Tutorial 1 + 2. Retrieved on May 15, 2015 from http://programmingknowledgeblog.blogspot.com/2015/04/android-sqlite-database-tutorial-1.html

Radin, J. M., Steinhubl, S. R., Su, A. I., Bhargava, H., Greenberg, B., Bot, B. M., ... Topol, E. J. (2018). The Healthy Pregnancy Research Program: Transforming Pregnancy Research Through a ResearchKit App. *bioRxiv*.

Rodger, D., Skuse, A., Wilmore, M., Humphreys, S., Dalton, J., Flabouris, M., & Clifton, V. L. (2013). Pregnant women's use of information and communications technologies to access pregnancy-related health information in South Australia. *Australian Journal of Primary Health*, *19*(4), 308–312. doi:10.1071/PY13029 PMID:24004661

Sinthanayothin, C., Bholsithi, W., Wongwaen, N., & Xuto, P. (2014, July). ZBaby: Android application for pregnancy due date, fetus development simulation and weight gain during pregnancy. In Computer Science and Engineering Conference (ICSEC), 2014 International (pp. 62-66). IEEE.

Stackoverflow, (2012). How do I get my solution in Visual Studio back online in TFS. Retrieved on June 30, 2015 from https://stackoverflow.com/questions/.../how-do-i-get-my-solution-in-visual-studio-bac.com/questions/26346727/android-material-design-button-styles

Thomas, G. M., & Lupton, D. (2016). Threats and thrills: Pregnancy apps, risk and consumption. *Health Risk & Society*, *17*(7-8), 495–509. doi:10.1080/13698575.2015.1127333

West, D. M. (2015, March). Using mobile technology to improve maternal health and fight Ebola: A case study of mobile innovation in Nigeria. In Center for Technological Innovation at Brookings. The Institute for Peace and Security Studies (IPSS) gathered a group of experts for a workshop on AfSol from (Vol. 26, pp. 26-27).

Wu, C. T., Tzeng, Y. F., Ho, T. W., Chen, S. W., Gau, B. S., Lai, F., & Chiu, H. Y. (2016, August). A smart phone application in improving healthy lifestyles and health outcomes for school-age children with asthma. In Advances in Social Networks Analysis and Mining (ASONAM), 2016 IEEE/ACM International Conference on (pp. 1034-1037). IEEE. 10.1109/ASONAM.2016.7752368

KEY TERMS AND DEFINITIONS

Accessibility: A facility that is easy to reach or use.

Antenatal Care: Healthcare given to an expectant mother before birth; prenatal.

App: A downloadable application that has been developed to serve certain purpose.

Appointment: A session scheduled for consultancy between a doctor and a patient.

Complications: Issues. In context of the chapter, this means health issues facing a pregnant woman.

Expectant Mother: An adult female animal or human pregnant with a baby.

Gestation: The time period during which an infant animal or human develops inside its mother's womb until its birth.

Gestational: Related to a woman's pregnancy.

Gynecologist: A physician specializing in women's health issues related to reproductive system.

Maternity Care Centre: A care center for health issues of women.

Moms-to-Be: A woman in the family way (i.e., expecting, or pregnant with a child).

Prenatal Care: Healthcare given to an expecting woman before the birth of a baby. This is also called antenatal care. Its antonym is postnatal care which relates to healthcare after birth of a baby.

This research was previously published in Mobile Devices and Smart Gadgets in Human Rights edited by Sajid Umair and Muhammad Yousaf Shah; pages 132-152, copyright year 2019 by Information Science Reference (an imprint of IGI Global).

Section 2
Complications and Risks

Chapter 7
The Decision-Making Processes of Pregnant Women at High Risk

Marta Ferraz
Entidade Reguladora da Saúde, Portugal

Ana Margarida Pisco Almeida
Universidade de Aveiro, Portugal

Alexandra Matias
Universidade do Porto, Portugal

INTRODUCTION

Under the context of the new health communication paradigms, this chapter explores the implications and challenges that the current online search and open publication practices may have on the decision-making process of pregnant women with an associated maternal pathology.

Acknowledging the importance of the concepts of autonomy and mediation in understanding the strategies and mechanisms of e-health information searching, this chapter presents the results of a study which main purpose was understanding how the decision-making process of pregnant women is influenced by the search for information provided by institutional and/or commercial website; moreover we intended to understand whether the nature, quantity and quality of information is taken into account when choosing a source of information and whether the participation

DOI: 10.4018/978-1-7998-2351-3.ch007

of pregnant women in social networks increases the ability of decision-making and if the views and stories shared by other pregnant women influence their decisions; finally our study aimed at comprehend if the decision-making process is supported by the opinions expressed by health professionals or by self-guided web search.

Background

A survey conducted in the United States revealed that over 75% of pregnant women stated they had searched information on pregnancy and labour in digital networks (Declercq, Sakala, Corry, & Applebaum, 2007). Nevertheless, the literature revision points out the lack of reliability and up-to-date of some of the available medical information (Eysenbach & Kohler, 2002; Kunst, Groot, Latthe, Latthe, & Khan, 2002; Weiss & Moore, 2003), as well as the lack of quality (Eysenbach & Kohler, 2002). Indeed, the information available online fails by the absence of regulation, which makes it difficult for the average citizen to distinguish reliable sources from not credible ones (Bernhardt & Felter, 2004; Dhillon, Albersheim, Alsaad, Pargass, & Zupancic, 2003). Some authors even mention the potentially hazardous and damaging nature of the information acquired by the citizen, without the necessary monitoring (Skinner et al., 2003). Many pregnant women have declared to have felt more anxious and confused after reading specific information on the internet (De Santis et al., 2010).

In Japan the decision-making process of pregnant women with a risk pregnancy was analysed. As a result, Usui et al. (Usui, Kamiyama, Tani, Kanagawa, & Fukuzawa, 2011) clarified the main problems of using online medical information during pregnancy in patients of a single Japanese health institution who had been diagnosed with foetal malformation. The authors drew on a survey, via anonymous questionnaire, directed at 155 pregnant women in the aforementioned conditions, during the period between 2005 and 2009. Participants were asked about the diagnosis regarding their foetal complication, the gestational age at which it had been detected, whether they had searched it on the Internet and what type of information they had found, as well as their impression regarding their level of reliability and if they had established a comparison between the online information and that provided by their physician. They were also asked whether they would use the searched information and which particular information they would like to obtain if they lived the situation once again. .In terms of results, 57.3% of the respondents resorted to online information during pregnancy. In 60% of the cases, the impression was different concerning the information gathered from the web and the one provided by the health professional. In the first case, 60% of those inquired considered online information more frightening and negative than the one provided by the physician. The authors concluded that the number of pregnant patients who search the Internet has increased significantly in recent years, being these the ones who have experienced feelings of greater anxiety and pessimism, regarding the seriousness of the illness suffered by their babies.

The internet produced a shift in pregnancy policies and it is in this context that the study of Cohen & Raymond emerges (Cohen & Raymond, 2011), analysing the culture of three public online forums in which pregnant women share experiences. According to these authors, pregnancy is a borderline state between health and illness, since the woman can suffer from some pathology derived by her state of pregnancy. In addition, the burden of uncertainty regarding the possibility of spontaneous miscarriages, foetal harm or their own death is carried by the majority of pregnant women. It is in this context that online forums for pregnant women emerge, contributing for their empowerment.

A study conducted in 2012 in China, aiming to understand how Chinese pregnant women use the internet as a tool of information (Gao, Larsson, & Luo, 2012) analysed dimensions such as: the frequency in which health information was searched by pregnant women; the type of searched information; the way it was assessed; the degree of reliability of that information; and whether it was shared with the health professional. Regarding the reliability's level assessment of the information, the interviewed pregnant women elected the matching between the reported facts on other sources as the first reliability factor (64%). The supply of references (42%) and the expert revision (34%) were the second and third factors. It is relevant that 80% of the participants held a university degree and mainly all belonged to the middle class, which might have somehow contributed to the abovementioned findings. Taking into account the interaction with their health professional, 75.1% of the respondents revealed they had not talked to their ob regarding their web search. 32% mentioned to have sought additional information regarding issues which were debated with the childbirth educator.

In "Internet Use in Pregnancy Informs Women's Decision Making: A *Web*-Based Survey", Lagan *et al.* (Lagan, Sinclair, & Kernohan, 2010), present the results of an online questionnaire filled in by 613 women among 24 countries during 12 weeks. Search engines (mainly Google) were used by 97% of the interviewed to identify web pages with pregnancy related information (1), to find support groups (2) and to do online shopping (3). Moreover, about 94% of the sample stated to have resorted to the web to complement the information that had been previously given by their health physician, while 83% declared that the research was carried out with the intention to aid in the decision-making process, especially since about half the interviewed mentioned the lack of time and the little information provided by the health professional as reasons to encourage the online search.

Methods

Aiming to better understand the decision-making process of Portuguese pregnant women, we have conducted an exploratory survey applied to 178 Portuguese pregnant and post-partum women in 2013. Of the 178 overall respondents, 49 answered the section devoted to gestational problems, 32 to maternal pathology and 17 to the foetal pathology. From the 136 respondents who were identified as being frequent users of the web, 37 answered the gestational problems section: 27 regarding maternal problems and 10 regarding foetal problems. From the 34 respondents identified as medium frequency users, 7 answered to that section: 3 regarding maternal problems and 4 regarding foetal problems. From the three respondents who were considered non users: 1 answered to the maternal pathologies and 2 to the foetal ones.

Our paper-based questionnaire was divided in five sections: 1. background demographic and socio-economic information on the individuals; 2. pregnancy separated in two groups, one to be responded by pregnant women and another by post-partum women; 3. the influence of the web on the decision-making processes, includes 11 questions; 4. the relation established with the health professional; 4. pathologies related to gestation.

Survey Results

Web Search

Considering the respondents with associated maternal pathology (AR - 32), 23 stated they had conducted an online search in the context of their condition, 7 claimed the contrary and 2 didn't answer. From the Frequent web users group (FWU - 27), 21 searched in the same context, 4 didn't and 2 didn't answer. In what concerns Medium frequency users (MFU - 3), 2 searched in this context, one did not.

To perform that search, 8 of the 32 AR chose the search engines "often" and 10 "always". 4 selected "sometimes" and 1 "never". FWU: 8 selected "often" to search engines and 9 "always"; 3 selected "sometimes" and 0 "never"; 6 didn't answer. In the MFU group, 1 used search engines "always" using the and one other "sometimes"; The third did not answer (See Table 1).

It is clear that the distinction between institutional/governmental and commercial websites is relevant in any dimension related to health, moreover if an illness is diagnosed. Indeed, 4 of AR "always" used governmental websites. The "often" was chosen by 6, relating to the governmental websites and by 3 relating to the commercial ones. On the FWU group, 4 chose "always" for governmental and 0 for the commercial. The MFU respondents had the following results: 1 selected "hardly ever" for both types of websites and 2 did not answer. Concerning "never", 4 of AR

Table 1. AR' search engine use

		Always	Often	Sometimes	Hardly Ever	Never
Yes	**22**	10	8	4		
No	2	-	-	-	1	1
N/A	8	-	-	-		-

marked it for the governmental websites, however 8 did it for the commercial ones. The same scale was observed for the FWU: 3 for the governmental and 7 for the commercial ones. Hence, the majority of respondents with a maternal pathology diagnosis preferred to search their doubts in governmental websites, over commercial (See Table 2).

One of the main goals of this investigation is to evaluate if the peer social support stemming from online communities influences the decision-making process of the pregnant woman. In the context of pathology, this assessment becomes even more relevant, given the understandable state of vulnerability and anxiety. Considering the main AR group, 1 respondent selected "always" for the discussion forums, but not for the online support communities. As for "often", 8 respondents selected it for both spaces. These values match with those of the FWU. "Sometimes" was marked by 6 AR, regarding communities and for 9 regarding the forums. FWU: 5 selected "sometimes" for communities and 7 for forums. MFU: 1 selected "sometimes" for communities and 2 for forums. As for "never", 5 AR selected it for communities and 4 for forums. FWU: 4 selected "never" for communities and 3 for forums.

In what concerns social networks and blogs, our results show that participants did not so frequently use them. 3 of AR selected "often" for social networks and 5 for blogs. "Sometimes" was selected by 3 AR for social networks and by 4 for blogs. In the FWU group 3 respondents selected "often" in both options. 1 MFU also selected it for blogs. "Never" was the most chosen option: 11 AR selected it for social networks and 8 for blogs. 9 of the FWU did the same for social networks and 7 for blogs. One MFU also chose "never" for social networks (See Table 3).

Table 2. AR's governmental and commercial websites use

	Always	Often	Sometimes	Hardly Ever	Never	N/A
Governmental	4	6	4	4	4	10
Commercial	0	3	6	4	8	11

Table 3. AR's forums, online communities, social networks and blogs use

	Always	Often	Sometimes	Hardly Ever	Never	N/A
Forums	1	8	9	1	4	9
Online communities	0	8	6	3	5	10
Social networks	0	3	3	5	11	10
Blogs	0	5	4	5	8	10

Purpose of the Search

The following question of our questionnaire intended to assess the purpose of the performed search. The result was clear: 18 from AR agreed with the option "to gather additional information" and 7 "fully agreed". In the FWU group, 16 agreed with this statement and 7 fully agreed. Concerning MFU, 2 agreed and the NU did not answer. Likewise, 16 of AR agreed with the options "check the existence of similar cases" and "have access to similar case reports". 3 of these "fully agreed" with both hypotheses. With the FWU the same results were obtained, as 15 agreed with both the checking of identical cases as theirs existence as with the access to the reports and 3 "fully agreed". In the MFU group, 1 agreed with both hypotheses. The NU didn't answer.

It is curious that, despite willing to know or recognise identical cases, AR seem not to be not interested in contacting those individuals: 11 of them wished "to contact other individuals with the same situation", while 7 disagreed and 3 "fully disagreed". Yet 6 of these didn't answer. Peculiarly, the FWU group demonstrated more interest in this contact with peers in an identical situation, possibly due to that same condition. Thus, 11 of them agreed with the statement while only 5 disagreed and 3 "fully disagreed". The 1 MFU who opted to answer this question, disagreed. The NU did not answer.

The option "confirm the information provided by the health professional" was selected by 13 of AR, who agreed, and by 3, who "fully agreed". Nevertheless, 6 disagreed and 5 "fully disagreed". Similar were the figures associated to the FWU: 11 agreed and 2 "fully agreed". However, 6 disagreed and 4 "fully disagreed". One of the MFU agreed with this option, while the other 2 did not answer. The NU "fully agreed" with "confirm the information provided by the health professional".

There is a diffuse attitude concerning the hypothesis of searching the web to validate the information provided by the physician. Combining the "agree" and "fully agree" and contrasting them with "disagree" and "disagree fully", the result is that agreement is superior; nonetheless, the difference is not striking. The answer to this question deals greatly with each of the respondents' sensibility, as well as their previously established correlation with their health professional. Most likely, those who had had a greater proximity with the doctor won't admit the search for validation. Concerning the option "finding contacts of other health professionals", although 7 of AR agreed, 6 disagreed and 7 "fully disagreed". Similarly, 6 of FWU agreed with this search for alternative contacts, but 4 disagreed and 10 "fully disagreed". In the MFU group, 1 "fully agreed", 1 disagreed and the last did not answer, as well as the NU. This last hypothesis was not popular, even because it could be perceived as the will to change doctors and not simply to have a second opinion. The majority of pregnant women with associated maternal pathology wish to have all the available information regarding their case, confirming what had been said by their health professional. Moreover, they also wish to be able to access similar cases, which may provide a greater feeling of comfort and lessen the anxiety. (See Table 4).

Level of Confidence

When questioned about the level of confidence provided by the information found in the internet, 11 of the AR claimed to have felt "reasonably more confident"; 12 felt "slightly more confident"; only 2 felt "much more confident" after having read web information concerning their pathology; 5 considered it "indifferent". In the FWU group, 11 respondents felt "reasonably more confident" after reading digital information and 10 "slightly more confident"; just 1 felt "much more confident". The level of indifference reached 4 of these users. Considering MFU, 1 felt "slightly more confident" and another "much more confident". The searched digital information increased the level of confidence of pregnant women with associated maternal pathology (See Table 5).

Table 4. AR 'purpose of the maternal pathology searches

	Fully Agree	Agree	Disagree	Indifferent	Fully Disagree	N/A
Gather additional info	7	18	1	1	1	4
Check similar cases	3	16	3	3	2	5
Access similar cases reports	3	16	3	3	2	5
Contact others with same situation	0	11	7	5	3	6
Confirm info provided by HP	3	13	6	1	5	5
Find contacts of other HP	0	7	6	4	10	5

Table 5. AR' level of confidence in the context of a maternal pathology

Much More	Reasonably	Slightly	Indifferent	N/A
2	11	12	5	2

Influence of Web Search and Online Contact

17 of AR felt influenced by the Internet search and 3 were "fully influenced"; 16 of the FWU felt influenced by this search and 3 "fully influenced". Considering the MFU opinions differed: 1 felt "influenced", other "little influenced" and the last "nothing". The NU didn't answer. The FWU had the most expansive mood regarding the digital search influence in the context of their maternal pathology diagnosis.

Online contact was not very influencing. Communication with the physician: 14 AR, the selected "nothing" and 7 selected "little influence"; the remaining 4 selected "indifferent" and only 1 selected "influence". FWU: 11 selected "nothing"; 7 selected "little influence"; 4 selected "indifferent" and just 1 felt "influenced". Two thirds of the MFU selected "nothing". The NU did not answer.

As for the role of the nurse, only the MFU were influenced by this health professional, which cannot be seen as noteworthy. AR: 3 selected "indifferent"; 11 selected "little influence" and 12 selected "nothing". 10 of the WF selected "little influence" and "nothing", whereas 3 selected "indifferent". As mentioned, 1 MFU felt influenced and one other "fully influenced". The NU did not answer.

Other pregnant women were also not very influencing. AR: 2 felt influenced and 1 even felt "fully influenced", however 3 selected "indifferent" and 4 selected "little influence". On the other hand, 17 selected "nothing". The same was observed with the FWU: 1 was "fully influenced" and 2 were influenced. Nevertheless, besides 2 others who selected "indifferent", 4 selected "little influence" and 15 "nothing". Two thirds of the MFU equally selected "nothing" and the NU did not to answer.

It is noteworthy that family and friends were slightly more relevant for the expectant mothers than their peers. Therefore, 2 of AR were even "fully influenced" and 4 were influenced. However, 5 felt "little influence" and 10 selected "nothing". MFU and NU weren't influenced. In fact, pregnant women with a maternal pathology not only intended to find identical cases on the web, as they also seemed to feel better by communicating online with their most inner circle.

Concerning the chemist and doula, the outlook remained steady throughout the whole result presentation. The diagnosis of a maternal pathology did not alter its lack of influence regarding the pregnant and postpartum women. Generally, there was no influence of the chemist in any of the analysis groups. 18 of AR selected "nothing"; 7 selected "little influence"; one selected "indifferent" and 6 did not answer. 15 of

Table 6. Influence of web search and online contact in AR in the event of a maternal pathology diagnosis

	Fully Influenced	Influenced	Little Influenced	Nothing Influenced	Indifferent	N/A
Internet search	3	17	5	2	3	2
Contact with physician	0	1	7	14	4	6
Contact with nurse	0	1	11	12	3	6
Contact with other pregnant women	1	2	4	17	3	5
Contact with family/ friends	2	4	5	13	2	6
Contact with chemist	0	0	7	18	1	6
Contact with doula	0	1	4	22	0	5

the FWU selected "nothing"; 7 selected "little influence", 1 selected "indifferent" and 4 did not answer. 2 MFU selected "nothing" and 1 did not answer as the NU. Regarding the doula, 22 AR selected "nothing" and 4 selected "little influence", but 1 felt "influenced" and 5 did not answer. Also 20 FWU selected "nothing"; 3 felt "little influenced" and 3 did not answer. Still, 1 felt influenced by this labour coach. 3 MFU selected "never" and 1 did not answer (See Table 6).

Influence of Face-to-Face Contact

This kind of contact has different results. The doctor is fully influential for 18 AR and influential of 9; only 2 selected "never". The FWU were substantially influenced by the presence of their doctor: 15 were "fully influenced" and 8 were influenced. These findings are extremely relevant since they show that even skilled web users appreciate face-to-face contact, especially with the health professional and in the context of a maternal pathology. MFU were also influenced and 2 were "fully influenced". The NU was also "fully" influenced.

In second place is the face-to-face contact with a nurse. 13 AR felt "fully influenced" and 6 were influenced, only 2 selected "nothing". 12 FWU were also "fully influenced" and 5 were influenced; having just 2 selected "nothing at all". MFU: 1 was "fully influenced" by the nurse, one other was influenced and the last did not to answer, like the NU. The expectant mother feels closer to the health professional following their advice and clearing her doubts. In the event of a maternal problem, the pregnant women, even searching information on the internet, do not do without the face-to-face contact with the doctor and the nurse.

Table 7. Influence of the face-to-face contact in AR in the case of a maternal pathology diagnosis

	Fully Influenced	Influenced	Little Influenced	Nothing Influenced	Indifferent	N/A
Contact with physician	18	9	0	2	1	2
Contact with nurse	13	6	4	2	3	4
Contact with other pregnant women	1	9	6	11	1	4
Contact with family/friends	1	9	5	10	2	5
Contact with chemist	0	0	8	15	3	6
Contact with doula	0	0	5	21	1	5

As far as peers and family/friends are concerned, 1 AR felt "fully influenced" by peers and 9 were influenced, whereas 11 selected "nothing". Similarly, 1 WFU felt "fully influenced, 8 influenced and 9 "nothing". Only 1 MFU was influenced by their counterparts, having the other 2 selected "nothing". The NU did not answer.

Family and friends results' were similar, with exception to the MFU who were not influenced by these agents. Thus, 1 AR was "fully influenced" and 9 were influenced, while 8 selected "never". The NU didn't answer.

The chemist and the doula are left to the end again, due to their complete lack of influence. 21 AR selected "nothing" and "little influence" for the doula. The same is true for 19 FWU who selected "nothing" and 5 selected "little influence" for this professional. 2 MFU selected "nothing" and 1 did not answer, like the NU. This also happened with the chemist, even if with less enthusiastic figures: 15 AR selected "never" and 8 selected "little influence"; 14 FWU also selected "nothing" and 7 selected "little influence". 1 MFU selected "nothing", other "little influence" and the last did not answer, like the NU (See Table 7).

Influence of Media and Scientific Literature

Regarding the last two agents, it can be stated that the media only influenced 2 and 14 AR selected "nothing", 6 selected "little influence" and 5 selected "indifferent". In the FWU group, only 2 felt influenced by the media, whereas 12 were not influenced; 6 were "little influenced" and 4 selected "indifferent". However, 2 MFU were influenced, the other didn't answer, like the NU.

Scientific literature, not having influenced 7 AR, influenced 10 and "fully influenced" 6. Concerning FWU, 8 and 6 felt, both, influenced and "fully influenced", having 6 others selected "nothing". It is worth reminding that 46.6% of the respondents to the survey had a university degree, which surely had an impact on these results.

FUTURE RESEARCH DIRECTIONS

Since the questionnaire was distributed throughout the year of 2013, it is important to conduct follow-up analysis, addressing the issue of the influence of online communities and social networks in the pregnant woman decision-making process, since these platforms are, currently, extremely used. Indeed, the results of the survey identify several interesting future research directions, and allowed an already conducted case study of an online community "Rede Mãe". The results of this analysis as well as in-depth interviews conducted will help to build upon the results obtained in the survey and hence characterize more deeply the studied scenario.

CONCLUSION

Pregnant women with associated pathology are influenced by online searches considering their status. However, it is the doctor that still is the most influent agent.

The web search influences pregnant women with associated pathology decisions in several dimensions, but mainly concerning the differences between institutional/governmental and commercial websites as the former seems to be more influential than the latter. Despite some influence, online communities and social networks are promptly overtaken by the contact with relatives and friends and mainly through the face-to-face communication with the physician, whose influence still prevails. Mediation and patients' autonomy are core-concepts when analysing new media influence on health decisions.

REFERENCES

Bernhardt, J. M., & Felter, E. M. (2004). Online pediatric information seeking among mothers of young children: Results from a qualitative study using focus groups. [Evaluation Studies]. *Journal of Medical Internet Research*, *6*(1), e7. doi:10.2196/jmir.6.1.e7 PMID:15111273

Cohen, J. H., & Raymond, J. M. (2011). How the internet is giving birth (to) a new social order. *Information Communication and Society*, *14*(6), 937–957. doi:10.1080/1369118X.2011.582132

De Santis, M., De Luca, C., Quattrocchi, T., Visconti, D., Cesari, E., Mappa, I., ... Caruso, A. (2010). Use of the Internet by women seeking information about potentially teratogenic agents. *European Journal of Obstetrics, Gynecology, and Reproductive Biology*, *151*(2), 154–157. doi:10.1016/j.ejogrb.2010.04.018 PMID:20478650

Declercq, E. R., Sakala, C., Corry, M. P., & Applebaum, S. (2007). Listening to Mothers II: Report of the Second National U.S. Survey of Women's Childbearing Experiences: Conducted January-February 2006 for Childbirth Connection by Harris Interactive(R) in partnership with Lamaze International. *Journal of Perinatal Education, 16*(4), 9–14. doi:10.1624/105812407X244769 PMID:18769512

Dhillon, A. S., Albersheim, S. G., Alsaad, S., Pargass, N. S., & Zupancic, J. A. (2003). Internet use and perceptions of information reliability by parents in a neonatal intensive care unit. [Comparative Study]. *Journal of Perinatology, 23*(5), 420–424. doi:10.1038j.jp.7210945 PMID:12847540

Eysenbach, G., & Kohler, C. (2002). How do consumers search for and appraise health information on the world wide web? Qualitative study using focus groups, usability tests, and in-depth interviews. *British Medical Journal, 324*(7337), 573–577. doi:10.1136/bmj.324.7337.573 PMID:11884321

Gao, L. L., Larsson, M., & Luo, S. Y. (2012). Internet use by Chinese women seeking pregnancy-related information. *Midwifery*. doi:10.1016/j.midw.2012.07.003 PMID:22958935

Kunst, H., Groot, D., Latthe, P. M., Latthe, M., & Khan, K. S. (2002). Accuracy of information on apparently credible websites: Survey of five common health topics. *BMJ (Clinical Research Ed.), 324*(7337), 581–582. doi:10.1136/bmj.324.7337.581 PMID:11884323

Lagan, B. M., Sinclair, M., & Kernohan, W. G. (2010). Internet Use in Pregnancy Informs Women's Decision Making: A Web-Based Survey. *Birth-Issues in Perinatal Care, 37*(2), 106–115. doi:10.1111/j.1523-536X.2010.00390.x PMID:20557533

Skinner, T. C., Howells, L., Greene, S., Edgar, K., McEvilly, A., & Johansson, A. (2003). Development, reliability and validity of the Diabetes Illness Representations Questionnaire: Four studies with adolescents. *Diabetic Medicine, 20*(4), 283–289. doi:10.1046/j.1464-5491.2003.00923.x PMID:12675641

Usui, N., Kamiyama, M., Tani, G., Kanagawa, T., & Fukuzawa, M. (2011). Use of the medical information on the internet by pregnant patients with a prenatal diagnosis of neonatal disease requiring surgery. *Pediatric Surgery International, 27*(12), 1289–1293. doi:10.100700383-011-2965-6 PMID:21833721

Weiss, E., & Moore, K. (2003). An assessment of the quality of information available on the Internet about the IUD and the potential impact on contraceptive choices. *Contraception*, *68*(5), 359–364. doi:10.1016/j.contraception.2003.07.001 PMID:14636940

This research was previously published in the Encyclopedia of E-Health and Telemedicine edited by Maria Manuela Cruz-Cunha, Isabel Maria Miranda, Ricardo Martinho, and Rui Rijo; pages 901-909, copyright year 2016 by Medical Information Science Reference (an imprint of IGI Global).

Chapter 8
County Socioeconomic Deprivation and Preterm Birth Risk Between White and Black Mothers in Georgia, USA

Wei Tu
Georgia Southern University, USA

ABSTRACT

Past studies have reported the association between living in a socioeconomically deprived neighborhood and elevated preterm births (PtB) risk after adjusting certain individual level confounders. This article examined the association between county-level deprivation and PtB risk of three stratified racial groups, white, black, and the others. The author built two level random intercept logistic regression models using 112,589 single live births retrieved from vital statistics record in Georgia, USA in 2010. Although county level deprivation was found to be insignificant for PtB risk for the entire study population, it had a significant yet modest effect on magnifying the PtB risk of black women (The odds ratio (OR) = 1.063,95% CI = 1.02, 1.12). In addition, the Median Odds Ratio (MOR) (1.229) indicated a weak neighborhood effect on PtB risk and the Interval Odds Ratio (IOR)-80% (0.68-1.49) suggested large unaccounted county-level heterogeneity. Future research will include more confounders at both levels in analysis as well as addressing the uncertain geographic context problem (UGCoP).

DOI: 10.4018/978-1-7998-2351-3.ch008

INTRODUCTION

Preterm births (PtB) are births occurring earlier than the 37th week gestation. As a significant health issue, PtB is closely associated with infant mortality, infant morbidity, and numerous childhood developmental disabilities (Callaghan, MacDorman, Rasmussen, Qin, & Lackritz, 2006; Goldenberg, Culhane, Iams, & Romero, 2008; Shapiro-Mendoza & Lackritz, 2012). Many previous studies have shown that pregnant women, particularly black women, living in more socioeconomically deprived neighborhoods had been at an elevated risk of adverse birth outcomes including PtB, after adjusting for individual socioeconomic status (SES) (Ma et al., 2015; Messer et al., 2006; Tu, Tu, & Tedders, 2014). However, the reported relationship between neighborhood deprivation and PtB risk among racial and/or ethnic groups has not always been consistent. Some studies found little difference among ethnic groups (Elo et al., 2009) while some reported a stronger effect on the non-Hispanic white group (Cubbin et al., 2008; O'Campo et al., 2008). Further, other studies found the greatest magnitude of an association among Hispanic Caribbean women (Janevic et al., 2010).

Although past research has rather consistently shown that neighborhood SES has a moderate-weak but statistically significant effect on health outcomes (Pickett & Pearl, 2001; Robert, 1999; Subramanian, Kim, & Kawachi, 2002), important challenges such as the definition of neighborhoods and identification of relevant neighborhood characteristics are also acknowledged (A.V. Diez Roux, 2001; Kwan, 2012a). Overall, scholars agree that risk factors at the individual and the neighborhood level may jointly influence specific health outcomes (Marmot, 1998). Thus, knowledge about the association between health risks and the neighborhood SES may provide valuable insights to formulate innovative approaches for community level interventions. In some instances, neighborhood SES may be viewed as an upstream effect in the causal pathway influencing health outcomes (Adler & Newman, 2002; Bharmal, Derose, Felician, & Weden, 2015). The biological and behavioral characteristics of downstream individuals may then be affected by neighborhood level SES, consequently influencing health outcomes such as PtB. For instance, pregnant women residing in neighborhoods with high SES are more likely to have better access to higher quality prenatal care services, lower exposure to stress and environmental pollution, and more pleasant built environment, thereby resulting in a decreased risk of PtB (Meng, Thompson, & Hall, 2013).

In the State of Georgia, the raw PtB rates in 2015 for white, black, and all other racial groups were 9.3% (total case = 7003), 13.7% (total case = 6165), and 8.8% (total case = 954), respectively (Georgia Department of Public Health, 2016a). While the PtB rates of the white group and the others group have met or exceeded the Healthy People 2020 goal of 11.4% and even a more ambitious target rate of 9.6% set by the March of Dimes (2016), the rate of black group has not. So, there was an obvious disparity in PtB rate between black and the other two racial groups.

Figure 1a illustrates county-level unadjusted PtB rates for all births in Georgia in 2015. The high rates were observed mostly in central counties while low rates were observed mostly in suburban Atlanta metropolitan area and southern and southeastern region of the state. Figure 1b illustrates the demographic clusters of Georgia at the census tract level based on 25 selected 2010 census variables (Georgia Department of Public Health, 2016b). All the census tracts were divided into four classes (A, B, C, and D) with A representing the highest SES and D the lowest. Across the state, the downtown areas of large cities (particularly Atlanta) and rural areas tended to be more socioeconomically deprived while the suburban areas of large cities overall enjoyed a much higher SES. When visually comparing Figures 1a and 1b, it appeared that higher PtB prevalence tended to occur in lower SES level areas.

Figure 1. Raw PtB rates in Georgia 2015 and demographic clusters in Georgia 2010

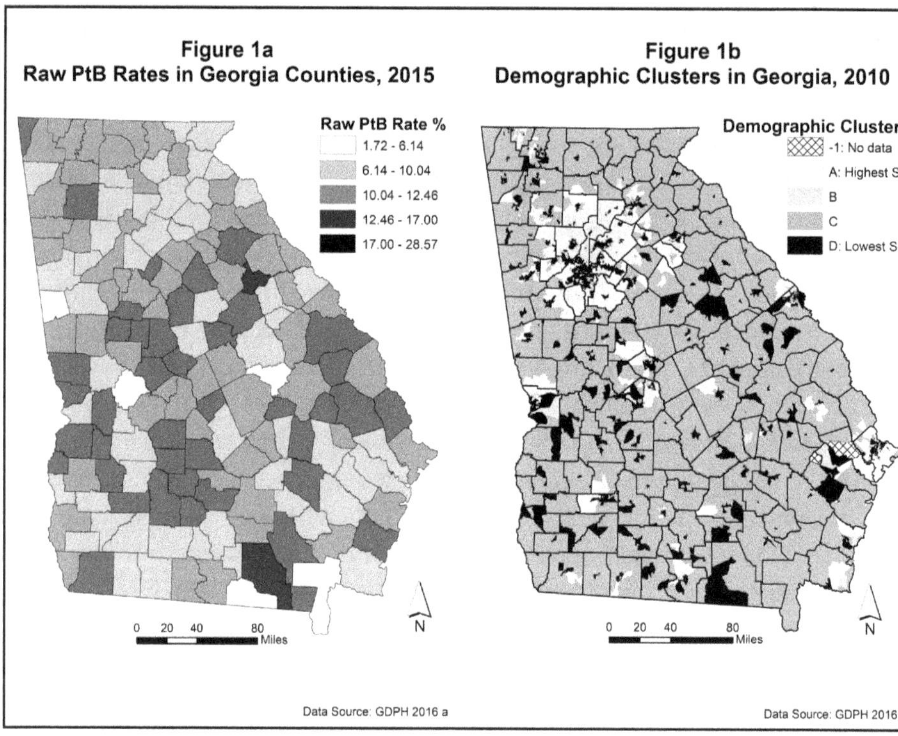

This study sought to examine the association between neighborhood deprivation and PtB risk using 2010 Georgia birth data. Births were stratified into three racial groups, the white group, the black group, and the others group. Using multilevel regression (MLR) models, we partitioned the outcome (PtB or not PtB) variation between the individual and neighborhood level risk factors and compared how and to what extent neighborhood deprivation affected the PtB risks among the three racial groups. We were particularly interested in understanding how the deprivation effect might impact the white and the black group differently. A neighborhood deprivation index (NDI) was constructed to synthesize the multidimensional neighborhood deprivation measures to allow for easier interpretation and comparison to other studies with similar design (Messer et al., 2006). In addition, the Median Odds Ratio (MOR) and the Interval Odds Ratio (IOR) were calculated to facilitate the quantification and interpretation of the neighborhood effects produced from MLR models. Findings from this study may shed light on effective community-based prevention and intervention strategies, as well as how to make neighborhood SES as a possible mediator of PtB risk among high risk populations.

DATA AND METHODS

Individual-Level Data

The birth data in year 2010 were obtained from the Georgia Department of Public Health (Georgia Department of Public Health, 2016c). Only live and singleton births with complete information on the six individual-level variables were used in our analyses. These variables were race (black, white, others), sex (male or female), age (mother's age in years), marital status (married or unmarried), education (mother received less than nine years of education, yes or no), and tobacco use during pregnancy (yes or no).

Neighborhood-Level Data

We chose to use counties (N = 159) to approximate neighborhoods in this study. Counties were much less used than census tracts as a proxy of neighborhood among studies using U.S. census boundaries as analytical units (Janevic et al., 2010; Krieger, Chen, Waterman, Rehkopf, & Subramanian, 2003; O'Campo et al., 2008; O'Campo, Xue, Wang, & Caughy, 1997; Tu, Tu, & Tedders, 2015). However, counties do have several often overlooked advantages over census tracts. As the smallest political, legal, and geographical entities in most of the U.S. states, counties are responsible for providing a variety of socioeconomic and health care services. They also have more stable sociopolitical and geographic boundaries that will allow for consistent data collection and comparison. From a management perspective, counties are more practical units for organizing and implementing healthcare policies and interventions programs (Warren, 1978). In addition, results from county based studies may be compared with those from census tracts to help understand how modeling results would respond to the change in analytical units. Finally, counties have been treated as a proxy of neighborhoods and/or communities in previous health studies (Arcaya, Brewster, Zigler, & Subramanian, 2012; Chaix, Merlo, & Chauvin, 2005; DeFranco, Lian, Muglia, & Schootman, 2008).

Messer et al. (2006) constructed a NDI using eight socioeconomic variables that had been selected from 20 U.S. census variables after a thorough literature review. The authors then tested the index using birth datasets collected from 19 cities in four U.S. states. The index was later adopted by other studies on the neighborhood effect on birth outcomes in the U.S. (Janevic et al., 2010; O'Campo et al., 2008). Since U.S. census variables are easily accessible, this index can be easily replicable to allow a consistent comparison among studies conducted in other regions with similar design, especially the ones using U.S. data. In this study, we modified the index slightly to make it better suit the situation in Georgia. Our index was made by nine census variables including poverty, female household head, household income less than $25,000, occupation in management sectors, unemployment, percent population receiving public assistance, average household size, vehicle ownership, and population receiving less than high school education. The county level census data were collected from the American Community Survey 5-year (2008-2012) estimates (American Community Survey, 2016).

Principle Component Analysis (PCA) without rotation was performed on the nine county level census variables to reduce the data dimensionality. The eigenvalues of the top three principal components (Factor 1, Factor 2, and Factor 3) were respectively 4.11, 1.24, and 1.10, explaining 45.7%, 13.7%, and 12.2% of the total variance in the 2010 data, respectively. Factor 1 had high positive loadings on household income less than $25,000, percentage of population living under the poverty line, and lack the access to vehicles and a high negative loading on working population in management and professional occupations. Factor 2 had high positive loadings on household size, unemployment rate, and public assistance receiving rate and high negative loading on working population in management and professional occupations. Factor 3 had high positive loadings on percentage of female headed households and working population in management and professional occupations.

Factor 1 is clearly a county poverty measure. High Factor 1 values indicate high level of poverty or low SES. The meanings of Factors 2 and 3 are less straightforward and both explained much less total variance than Factor 1. Thus, only Factor 1 was retained, standardized (with a mean of 0 and a standard deviation of 1) and used in the regression models as the NDI measure (Jolliffe, 2002). Factor 1 was linked to the individual variables using the geocoded self-reported mailing addresses of mothers.

Statistical Analysis

Compared with ordinary least square (OLS) regression, MLR can partition the variance between individual and neighborhood levels to determine the respective contribution of the predicting variables from different levels to the total variance of the outcome variable (Goldstein, Browne, & Rasbash, 2002). In this study, individuals (mothers, level 1) were nested within neighborhoods (counties, level 2) and the outcome variable was dichotomous (1s for a PtBs and 0s for non PtBs). We assumed that the PtB risk had varied across counties and the coefficients of the individual predicting variables had been constant, so random intercept logistic regression models were built to analyze the association between neighborhood deprivation and PtB risk after adjusting six individual level predicting variables.

Predicting variables were selected based on the established individual risk factors in the literature as well as the theoretical association of PtB with neighborhood deprivation (Behrman & Butler, 2007; Messer et al., 2006; O'Campo et al., 2008). We first fit a null single level regression model (M00) and a null MLR model (M0) as benchmark models. We then fit a single level regression model with all the predicting variables from both levels (M1). Next, we fit a MLR model (M2) with only individual predicting variables. We finally updated M2 by adding the NDI and an interaction term between the NDI and race (M3). Thus, M3 was considered the full model in this study.

M3 can be described conceptually as: PtB (yes or no) = newborn's sex + mother's age-25 + mother's race (white, black and others) + mother's marital status (Married or unmarried) + mother's tobacco use during pregnancy (Yes or no) + county-level deprivation (Factor 1) + county-level deprivation (Factor 1) x mother's race + random effects. The description of the formal statistical notations and model specifications for MLR models is beyond the scope of this paper but can be found elsewhere (Gelman & Hill, 2007; Snijders & Bosker, 2012). The random part (level 1 and 2 variances) and the fixed part (regression coefficients) of the models were estimated using maximum likelihood with the Laplace approximation. All the statistical analyses were conducted using R v. 3.2.3 (R Core Team, 2016).

Variance Partition and the Interpretation of Neighborhood Effects

For MLR models with continuous outcome variables, Intraclass Correlation Coefficient (ICC) is a common measure for calculating the proportion of variation attributable to the neighborhood level variation. The range of ICC is between 0 and 1. Larger the ICC value, more outcome variance can be explained by the difference in the neighborhood characteristics. Furthermore, variance at the individual and the neighborhood level is at the same measurement scale in MLR models with continuous outcome variables. However, in MLR models with dichotomous outcome variables, the individual level variance is on the probability scale while the neighborhood level variance is on the logistic scale, making it difficult to compute and interpret ICC (Merlo et al., 2006).

To overcome this problem, we introduce MOR and IOR, two alternative statistic that are both at the Odds Ratio (OR) scale to measure the neighborhood heterogeneity (Larsen & Merlo, 2005; Sanagou, Wolfe, Forbes, & Reid, 2012). MOR can be computed with the following equation:

$$\mathrm{MOR} = \exp\left[\sqrt{2\times\tau^2}\times 0.6745\right] \approx \exp\left(0.95\tau\right) \qquad (1)$$

where, τ^2 is the neighborhood level variance. 0.6745 is the 75th centile of the cumulative distribution function of the standard normal distribution (mean = 0 and variance = 1). MOR should be equal to or greater than 1. If the MOR is equal to 1, then there is no neighborhood heterogeneity. That would mean, in this study, that individuals having the same individual level characteristics but residing in different neighborhoods would have the same PtB risk. The larger the MOR, more variation in the outcome variable (e.g., probability of having a PtB) can be explained by the neighborhood-level characteristics (Merlo et al., 2006).

To quantify the neighborhood effect on the individual outcome variable, it is necessary to compare individuals residing in different neighborhoods. However, the common OR measure for the single level logistic regression model cannot be used to interpret the neighborhood effect in MLR because individuals residing in the same neighborhood would have the same neighborhood characteristics (e.g., NDI). The IOR accounts for the fixed effect as well as the random residual variation at the neighborhood level. More specifically, IOR-80 is an interval of OR between two individuals with identical individual-level characteristics but differing in the neighborhood-level measure by 1, so it covers the middle 80% of the OR. IOR-80 can be computed using the following equation:

$$IOR-80\%_{\frac{lower}{upper}} = \exp(\beta \pm 1.2816\sqrt{2 \times \tau^2}) \approx \exp(\beta \pm 1.81\tau) \quad (2)$$

where, β is the regression coefficient of the neighborhood-level predicting variable, τ^2 is the neighborhood-level variance, and -1.2816 and +1.2816 are respectively the 10th and the 90th centiles of the standard normal distribution (mean = 0 and variance = 1). IOR-80 is calculated using a two-step approach. The first step is to calculate the OR of all pairs of individuals with identical individual level characteristics from two neighborhoods differing in the neighborhood-level measure by 1; the second step is to retrieve an interval that contains 80% of the OR values according to the distribution of all the calculated OR from the first step. A small between-neighborhood variation (τ^2) will result in a narrow IOR-80 while a large between-neighborhood variation (τ^2) will result in a wide IOR-80. Moreover, if IOR-80 contains 1, then the un-modeled neighborhood level variation is larger than the modeled neighborhood level effect (Merlo et al., 2006).

RESULTS

Descriptive Statistics

There were 133,668 total births in the State of Georgia in 2010, among which 128,356 (or 96.0% of all the births) were live and singleton births. After excluding records with missing individual predicting variables, a total of 112,589 (or 84.2% of all the births) were used in the following analyses. Table 1 provides the summary descriptive statistics of both individual and county level variables. At the individual level, The percentage of PtB, male newborn babies, white mothers, married mothers, and mothers who used tobacco products during pregnancy were 11.15%, 50.40%, 62.46%, 62.55%, and 8.33%, respectively. The mean value of mothers' age was 26.48.

At the county level, 21.36% of the population was below the federal poverty line, 33.10% of the households had income less than $25,000, 10.24% of the households with dependent children were female headed, and 1.76% of the households received public assistance. In addition, 28.00% of the working population was in management and professional occupations, the average household size was 2.66 persons, the unemployment rate was 10.97%, 21.17% of the population did not complete high school, and 7.44% of the households did not have vehicles (either owned or rental). Further, the standard deviation measures indicated sizable variation in several variables. For example, the SD of household income was 9.17%.

Table 1. Summary statistics of the level 1 and 2 variables

Variable	Method of Computation/Unit	Categorical variables: % the samples with the value of 1 Continuous variables: Mean ± SD
Level 1 (N = 112,589)		
Gestation Weeks	<37 weeks = 1; >=37 weeks = 0	11.15%
Mothers' Race	White =1; Black =2; Others =3	62.46%
Children's sex	Male =1; Female =0	50.40%
Mothers' age		26.48 ± 6.13
Mothers' marital status	Married = 0; Unmarried = 1	37.45%
Mothers' use of tobacco During Pregnancy	Yes =1; No =0	8.33%
Level 2 (N = 159)		
Poverty	% living below federal poverty	21.36±6.80
Household income	% households with income less than $25,000	33.10±9.17
Female household head	% female headed households with dependent children	10.43±2.99
Public Assistance	% households receiving public assistance	1.76±1.02
Occupation	% in management	28.00±5.95
Household size	Average household size	2.66±0.20
Unemployment	% unemployed population	10.97±3.21
Education	% no high school education	21.17±6.19
Vehicle ownership	% households with no vehicle	7.44±3.53

Results of the Regression Models

Table 2 presents the ORs and 95% CIs for the individual and county level effects of three (M1, M2 and M3) out of the five regression models that were fit. M00 and M0 were respectively null single level logistic regression model and null logistic MLR model. M1, an single level logistic regression model with all the predicting variables at both levels; M2, a logistic MLR model adjusting only individual level predicting variables; and M3, an update of M2 by adding the NDI and an interaction between the NDI and the race at the individual level. Examining the individual level ORs in M3, race was the strongest predicting factor (Race: black, OR: 1.442, 95% CI: 1.381-1.506), mothers older than the average age (26.48) had a slightly higher risk (OR: 1.022, 95% CI: 0.946-1.104), and the effects of marital status (OR: 1.282, 95% CI: 1.229-1.337) and tobacco use (OR: 1.226, 95% CI: 1.148-1.309) were in similar magnitude.

Table 2. Partial results from the regression models

	M1		M2		M3	
Level 1	OR	95% Cl	OR	95% Cl	OR	95% Cl
N=112,589						
Sex (Female)	0.972	(0.940,1.006)	0.973	(0.941,1.007)	0.973	(0.941,1.007)
Race (Black)	1.406	(1.351,1.464)	1.454	(1.393,1.518)	1.442	(1.381,1.506)
Race (Other)	1.009	(0.936,1.088)	1.019	(0.948,1.096)	1.022	(0.946,1.104)
Age (centered)	1.018	(1.015,1.021)	1.019	(1.016,1.022)	1.019	(1.016,1.022)
Marriage (No)	1.279	(1.226,1.334)	1.287	(1.234,1.342)	1.282	(1.229,1.337)
Smoking(Yes)	1.245	(1.167,1.328)	1.220	(1.142,1.302)	1.226	(1.148,1.309)
Level 2						
N = 159						
Factor1	1.050	(1.025,1.077)			1.004	(0.959,1.052)
Factor1: Race(Black):	1.028	(0.992,1.066)			1.063	(1.021,1.106)
Factor1: Race(Other):	1.033	(0.9551.116)			1.034	(0.954,1.120)
Random effect						
U_{0j}				0.048		0.047
MOR				1.231		1.229
IOR-80						(0.678,1.488)
Model Fit						
AIC	90006		89456		89267	

Comparing the results of M1 and M3, the NDI was significant in M1 (OR: 1.050, 95% CI: 1.025-1.077) but not in M3 (OR = 1.004, 95% CI: 0.959-1.052). However, the interaction between the NDI and race (black) was significant (OR: 1.063, 95% CI: 1.021-1.06) in M3 but not in M1. This result could be interpreted as living in a more deprived county would amplify the PtB risk of the black mothers after controlling for individual level predictors. In addition, the 95% CIs of the NDI in M3 (0.959-1.052) was wider than that in the M1 (1.025-1.077), indicating that MLR model took into account between county heterogeneity.

MOR was 1.229 in M3. This could be interpreted as, if a mother moves to another county with a higher propensity of having PtB, the median increase in the odds of having a PtB would be 1.229-fold. This effect was comparable with the magnitude of the tobacco use at the individual level and also much higher than the fixed the county level effect (OR: 1.004, 95% CI: 0.959-1.052).

The IOR-80% was 0.68 to 1.49. This interval could be interpreted as, when comparing two randomly chosen mothers with identical individual level predicting variables and residing in counties with NDI differing by 1, the OR for the comparison would, with an 80% probability, lie between 0.68 and 1.49. The interval was relatively wide and containing the OR value of 1, indicating considerable uncertainty in the county deprivation effect on mothers' PtB risk. In other words, there was substantial between county residual that could not be explained by the NDI alone.

Multilevel Model Adequacy and Selection

We chose the likelihood ratio test to compare the difference and determine the statistical significance between models (Raudenbush & Bryk, 2002). The chi-square values between M0 and M00 and between M3 and M1 were 324.4 and 196.3, respectively. Both numbers were significantly higher than 3.84, the 5% point of distribution on 1 degree of freedom. These numbers justified the use of MLR models over single-level models and a MLR model controlling both level predicting variables over the one controlling only individual level predicting variables. In addition, the Akaike Information Criterion (AIC) values were 89456, 89267, and 89262 for M1, M2, and M3, respectively (Akaike, 1974). M3 had the lowest AIC value among the three models, indicating that it was a better modeling choice among the three.

DISCUSSIONS

Past studies have suggested that epidemiologic studies considering a broader socioeconomic context would help establish the association adverse birth outcomes and their risk factors. The primary rationale behind broadening the socioeconomic context is due to the fact that the individual characteristics alone could not fully explained the variation in outcome variables. In this study, we used MLR models to examine the effect of county socioeconomic deprivation on PtB risk, particularly on how and to what extent this effect might impact the white and the black group differently using the data from Georgia, USA. We adopted and modified a NDI based on a well cited approach in a previous pregnancy risk study (Messer et al., 2006; O'Campo et al., 2008). In addition to the ORs, we calculated MOR and IOR-80% to help interpret the neighborhood effect as well as the between-neighborhood heterogeneity in MLR models.

Our MLR model results showed that the association between county level deprivation and PtB risk for the entire study population was insignificant. However, living in a more deprived neighborhood would increase the PtB risk of the black mothers. Thus, our main findings were overall consistent with the past studies using a similar design, there was significant but moderate-weak association between neighborhood deprivation and neighborhood deprivation might operate by different mechanisms among different racial groups (Janevic et al., 2010; O'Campo et al., 2008; Tu et al., 2014). Substantial un-modeled between county heterogeneity warrants further investigation of other significant neighborhood level factors.

We should note the limitations of this study. The nature of the U.S. vital record data determines that the quality and the breadth of the individual level confounders are far from ideal. For instance, as self-reported data, certain variables such as smoking tended to be under reported. Drinking during pregnancy, another known risk factor of PtB was not controlled in our models because the variable was missing in approximately 20% of our birth records. However, our results as well as those reported from previous studies showed that the changes in crude ORs were unlikely to be large by adjusting for more individual-level confounders (Luo et al., 2004; O'Campo et al., 2008). Further, vital records also lacked information about the length of residence of women in the neighborhood where the mailing addresses were located. The possibility that some women might move to another neighborhood during their pregnancy presents challenges to the analysis. As such, it is impossible to measure the actual exposure of neighborhood deprivation, and we were unable to assess the impact of this problem on our findings. Moreover, racial groups were only crudely categorized in this study as our major research objective was to understand the disparity between black and white mothers. This limitation prevented us from analyzing the association between the neighborhood deprivation and smaller minority racial groups as well as recent immigrants.

We admit that county is a crude proxy of neighborhood at best. Our choice of county was based largely on the advantages of that they are more stable boundaries, they allow more complete and consistent data collection, and they are more operational sociopolitical units for organizing and implementing community-based prevention and intervention policies. Although the main findings in this study were overall consistent with another Georgia study using census tract as unit of analysis (Tu et al., 2015), it is unclear how and to what extent artificial administrative boundaries such as U.S. census geographic units is able to capture factors such as social and cultural customs, values, and perceptions that are critical to delineating true neighborhoods. Defining appropriate neighborhood itself is indeed a complicated, yet fundamental research frontier in spatial epidemiology and health geography that has great potential (A. V. Diez Roux, 2007; Kwan, 2012b).

MLR models have provided a promising methodology framework to quantify the neighborhood effect on adverse birth outcomes. They are, however, vulnerable to the modifiable areal unit problem (MAUP) (Gehlke & Biehl, 1934; Openshaw, 1983). Firstly, measures of variation are dependent upon how neighborhoods are defined. Secondly, neighborhoods have been treated in most of the existing MLR analysis as spatially independent units so that potential spatial autocorrelation might be neglected in the analyses. In other words, variation measure of most MLR models considered correlation only among individuals within neighborhoods but not between neighborhood units. These technical issues of MLR could lead to incorrect model calibration, unreliable results, and inferential errors (Briant, Combes, & Lafourcade, 2010; Chaix et al., 2005; Swift, Liu, & Uber, 2008).

We will seek to mitigate the impacts of the MAUP on MLR models in our future projects. We plan to construct MLR models using neighborhoods definition other than census units. For instance, Mu and Wang (2008) has proposed a modified scale-space clustering method (MSSC) that would create neighborhoods with both attribute homogeneity and spatial contiguity (Mu & Wang, 2008; Mu, Wang, & McLafferty, 2010). We also plan to run spatial mixed models that will take account into the potential spatial autocorrelation among neighborhood units across the study area (Chaix et al., 2005; Kleinschmidt, Sharp, Clarke, Curtis, & Fraser, 2001; R Core Team, 2016). Moreover, there are several other well-developed NDI other than the one that was adopted in this study that may be tested and compared (Health Innovation Program, 2014; Krieger et al., 2003).

Previous studies have shown that neighborhood SES may influence birth outcomes by shaping maternal behavioral risks. Our findings further suggest that the interaction effect between contextual and compositional factors may be different across racial groups. Future studies should also examine more direct measures of neighborhood stress, such as perceived neighborhood disorder, and evaluate alternative mechanisms by which neighborhood factors influence individual behaviors (e.g., social norms and access to goods and services) (Schempf, Strobino, & O'Campo, 2009).

This study is not designed to provide any concrete measures to directly lower PtB risk. This study would however advance the modeling strategies so that neighborhood effects could be more precisely qualified and quantified. Better models would then provide useful information to help design and implement community- and/or population-based prevention and intervention programs. These programs have the great potential to impact multiple health outcomes for a large number of individuals at a time. So this study is indirectly relevant to the process of health policy-making.

CONCLUSION

We constructed two-level random intercept logistic regression models to investigate the impact of county socioeconomic deprivation on PtB risk among white and black women using birth data from Georgia, USA in 2010. We calculated a NDI based on nine county level census SES variables. In addition to traditional ORs, we computed two statistics, MOR and IOR-80%, to better interpret the neighborhood effect from the MLR models in addition to the regular OR measures. Overall, findings from our analysis are consistent with past studies using similar research designs. Our results suggest that living in deprived neighborhood would increase the PtB risk for black women and there was large unexplained between county heterogeneity. For future research, efforts should be made to include more relevant individual as well as neighborhood level variables in analysis and to seek innovative approaches to address the MAUP and the Uncertain Geographic Context Problem (UGCoP) (Kwan, 2012a).

REFERENCES

Adler, N. E., & Newman, K. (2002). Socioeconomic Disparities in Health: Pathways and Policies. *Health Affairs*, *21*(2), 60–76. doi:10.1377/hlthaff.21.2.60 PMID:11900187

Akaike, H. (1974). A new look at the statistical model identification. *IEEE Transactions on Automatic Control*, *19*(6), 716–723. doi:10.1109/TAC.1974.1100705

American Community Survey. (2016). Summary file data. Retrieved from http://www.census.gov/programs-surveys/acs/

Arcaya, M., Brewster, M., Zigler, C. M., & Subramanian, S. V. (2012). Area variations in health: A spatial multilevel modeling approach. *Health & Place*, *18*(4), 824–831. doi:10.1016/j.healthplace.2012.03.010 PMID:22522099

Behrman, R. E., & Butler, A. S. (2007). *Preterm Birth: Causes, Consequences, and Prevention. Washington, D.C.: Institute of Medicine of the National Academies*. Washington, D.C.: National Academies Press.

Bharmal, N., Derose, K. P., Felician, M., & Weden, M. (2015). Understanding the upstream social determinants of health (Working Paper No. WR-1096-RC). Retrieved from https://www.rand.org/content/dam/rand/pubs/working_papers/WR1000/WR1096/RAND_WR1096.pdf

Briant, A., Combes, P., & Lafourcade, M. (2010). Dots to boxes: Do the size and shape of spatial units jeopardize economic geography estimations? *Journal of Urban Economics*, *67*(3), 287–302. doi:10.1016/j.jue.2009.09.014

Callaghan, W. M., MacDorman, M. F., Rasmussen, S. A., Qin, C., & Lackritz, E. M. (2006). The contribution of preterm birth to infant mortality rates in the United States. *Pediatrics*, *118*(4), 1566–1573. doi:10.1542/peds.2006-0860 PMID:17015548

Chaix, B., Merlo, J., & Chauvin, P. (2005). Comparison of a spatial approach with the multilevel approach for investigating place effects on health: The example of healthcare utilisation in France. *Journal of Epidemiology and Community Health*, *59*(6), 517–526. doi:10.1136/jech.2004.025478 PMID:15911650

Cubbin, C., Marchi, K., Lin, M., Bell, T., Marshall, H., Miller, C., & Braveman, P. (2008). Is neighborhood deprivation independently associated with maternal and infant health? Evidence from Florida and Washington. *Maternal and Child Health Journal*, *12*(1), 61–74. doi:10.100710995-007-0225-0 PMID:17562150

DeFranco, E. A., Lian, M., Muglia, L. A., & Schootman, M. (2008). Area-level poverty and preterm birth risk: A population-based multilevel analysis. *BMC Public Health*, *8*(1), 316. doi:10.1186/1471-2458-8-316 PMID:18793437

Diez Roux, A. V. (2001). Investigating Neighborhood and Area Effects on Health. *American Journal of Public Health*, *91*(11), 1783–1789. doi:10.2105/AJPH.91.11.1783 PMID:11684601

Diez Roux, A. V. (2007). Neighborhoods and health: Where are we and were do we go from here? *Revue d'Epidemiologie et de Sante Publique*, *55*(1), 13–21. doi:10.1016/j.respe.2006.12.003 PMID:17320330

Elo, I., Culhane, J., Kohler, I., O'Campo, P., Burke, J., Messer, L., ... Holzman, C. (2009). Neighbourhood deprivation and small-for-gestational-age term births in the United States. *Paediatric and Perinatal Epidemiology*, *23*(1), 87–96. doi:10.1111/j.1365-3016.2008.00991.x PMID:19228318

Gehlke, C. E., & Biehl, K. (1934). Certain Effects of Grouping upon the Size of the Correlation Coefficient in Census Tract Material. *Journal of the American Statistical Association*, *29*(185A), 169–170.

Gelman, A., & Hill, J. (2007). *Data Analysis Using Regression and Multilevel/Hierarchical Models*. Cambridge, New York: Cambridge University Press.

Georgia Department of Public Health. (2016a). OASIS Web Query - Maternal Child Health (MCH) Statistics. Retrieved from https://oasis.state.ga.us/oasis/oasis/qryMCH.aspx

Georgia Department of Public Health. (2016b). Demographic clusters in Georgia 2011. *retrieved from* https://oasis.state.ga.us/gis/demographiccluster/DemoClusters2011.htm

Georgia Department of Public Health. (2016c). Health Data and Statistics. *retrieved from* https://dph.georgia.gov/health-data-and-statistics

Goldenberg, R. L., Culhane, J. F., Iams, J. D., & Romero, R. (2008). Epidemiology and causes of preterm birth. *Lancet*, *371*(9606), 75–84. doi:10.1016/S0140-6736(08)60074-4 PMID:18177778

Goldstein, H., Browne, W., & Rasbash, J. (2002). Partitioning Variation in Multilevel Models. *Understanding Statistics*, *1*(4), 223–231. doi:10.1207/S15328031US0104_02

Health Innovation Program. (2014). *Retrieved from* https://www.hipxchange.org/ADI

Janevic, T., Stein, C. R., Savitz, D. A., Kaufman, J. S., Mason, S. M., & Herring, A. H. (2010). Neighborhood deprivation and adverse birth outcomes among diverse ethnic groups. *Annals of Epidemiology*, *20*(6), 445–451. doi:10.1016/j.annepidem.2010.02.010 PMID:20470971

Jolliffe, I. T. (2002). *Principal Component Analysis* (2nd ed.). New York: Springer-Verlag New York.

Kleinschmidt, I., Sharp, B. L., Clarke, G. P., Curtis, B., & Fraser, C. (2001). Use of generalized linear mixed models in the spatial analysis of small-area malaria incidence rates in Kwazulu Natal, South Africa. *American Journal of Epidemiology*, *153*(12), 1213–1221. doi:10.1093/aje/153.12.1213 PMID:11415957

Krieger, N., Chen, J. T., Waterman, P. D., Rehkopf, D. H., & Subramanian, S. V. (2003). Race/ethnicity, gender, and monitoring socioeconomic gradients in health: A comparison of area-based socioeconomic measures--the public health disparities geocoding project. *American Journal of Public Health*, *93*(10), 1655–1671. doi:10.2105/AJPH.93.10.1655 PMID:14534218

Kwan, M. P. (2012a). The uncertain geographic context problem. *Annals of the Association of American Geographers*, *102*(5), 958–968. doi:10.1080/00045608.2012.687349

Kwan, M. P. (2012b). How GIS can help address the uncertain geographic context problem in social science research. *Annals of GIS*, *18*(4), 245–255. doi:10.1080/19475683.2012.727867

Larsen, K., & Merlo, J. (2005). Appropriate assessment of neighborhood effects on individual health: Integrating random and fixed effects in multilevel logistic regression. *American Journal of Epidemiology*. PMID:15615918

Luo, Z. C., Kierans, W. J., Wilkins, R., Liston, R. M., Mohamed, J., & Kramer, M. S. (2004). Disparities in birth outcomes by neighborhood income: Temporal trends in rural and urban areas, british columbia. *Epidemiology (Cambridge, Mass.)*, *15*(6), 679–686. doi:10.1097/01.ede.0000142149.34095.88 PMID:15475716

Ma, X., Fleischer, N. L., Liu, J., Hardin, J. W., Zhao, G., & Liese, A. D. (2015). Neighborhood deprivation and preterm birth: An application of propensity score matching. *Annals of Epidemiology, 25*(2), 120–125. doi:10.1016/j.annepidem.2014.11.021 PMID:25523896

March of dimes. (2016). US preterm birth rate hits healthy people 2020 goal seven years early. Retrieved from http://www.marchofdimes.org/news/us-preterm-birth-rate-hits-healthy-people-2020-goal-seven-years-early.aspx

Marmot, M. G. (1998). Improvement of social environment to improve health. *Lancet, 351*(9095), 57–60. doi:10.1016/S0140-6736(97)08084-7 PMID:9433438

Meng, G., Thompson, M. E., & Hall, G. B. (2013). Pathways of neighbourhood-level socio-economic determinants of adverse birth outcomes. *International Journal of Health Geographics, 12*(1), 32. doi:10.1186/1476-072X-12-32 PMID:23786633

Merlo, J., Chaix, B., Ohlsson, H., Beckman, A., Johnell, K., Hjerpe, P., & .... (2006). A brief conceptual tutorial of multilevel analysis in social epidemiology: Using measures of clustering in multilevel logistic regression to investigate contextual phenomena. *Journal of Epidemiology and Community Health, 60*(4), 290–297. doi:10.1136/jech.2004.029454 PMID:16537344

Messer, L. C., Laraia, B. A., Kaufman, J. S., Eyster, J., Holzman, C., Culhane, J., ... O'Campo, P. (2006). The development of a standardized neighborhood deprivation index. *Journal of Urban Health, 83*(6), 1041–1062. doi:10.100711524-006-9094-x PMID:17031568

Mu, L., & Wang, F. (2008). A Scale-Space Clustering Method: Mitigating the Effect of Scale in the Analysis of Zone-Based Data. *Annals of the Association of American Geographers, 98*(1), 85–101. doi:10.1080/00045600701734224

Mu, L., Wang, F., & McLafferty, S. (2010). *Analyzing Spatial Patterns of Late-Stage Breast Cancer in Chicago Region: A Modified Scale-Space Clustering Approach.* Springer Netherlands.

O'Campo, P., Burke, J. G., Culhane, J., Elo, I. T., Eyster, J., Holzman, C., & ... . (2008). Neighborhood Deprivation and Preterm Birth among Non-Hispanic Black and White Women in Eight Geographic Areas in the United States. *American Journal of Epidemiology*. PMID:17989062

O'Campo, P., Xue, X., Wang, M. C., & Caughy, M. (1997). Neighborhood risk factors for low birthweight in Baltimore: A multilevel analysis. *American Journal of Public Health, 87*(7), 1113–1118. doi:10.2105/AJPH.87.7.1113 PMID:9240099

Openshaw, S. (1983). *The modifiable areal unit problem*: Norwick: Geo Books.

Pickett, K. E., & Pearl, M. (2001). Multilevel analyses of neighbourhood socioeconomic context and health outcomes: A critical review. *Journal of Epidemiology and Community Health, 55*(2), 111–122. doi:10.1136/jech.55.2.111 PMID:11154250

R Core Team. (2016). *R: A language and environment for statistical computing*. Vienna, Austria: R Foundation for Statistical Computing.

Raudenbush, S. W., & Bryk, A. S. (2002). *Hierarchical Linear Models: Applications and Data Analysis Methods*. SAGE Publications.

Robert, S. A. (1999). Socioeconomic position and health: The independent contribution of community socioeconomic context. *Annual Review of Sociology, 25*(1), 489–516. doi:10.1146/annurev.soc.25.1.489

Sanagou, M., Wolfe, R., Forbes, A., & Reid, C. M. (2012). Hospital-level associations with 30-day patient mortality after cardiac surgery: A tutorial on the application and interpretation of marginal and multilevel logistic regression. *BMC Medical Research Methodology, 12*(1), 28. doi:10.1186/1471-2288-12-28 PMID:22409732

Schempf, A., Strobino, D., & O'Campo, P. (2009). Neighborhood Effects on Birthweight: An Exploration of Psychosocial and Behavioral Pathways in Baltimore, 1995–1996. *Social science & medicine (1982), 68*(1), 100-110.

Shapiro-Mendoza, C. K., & Lackritz, E. M. (2012). Epidemiology of late and moderate preterm birth. *Seminars in Fetal & Neonatal Medicine, 17*(3), 120–125. doi:10.1016/j.siny.2012.01.007 PMID:22264582

Snijders, T. A. B., & Bosker, R. J. (2012). Multilevel analysis: An introduction to basic and advanced multilevel modeling (2nd ed.). Los Angeles: London: SAGE.

Subramanian, S. V., Kim, D. J., & Kawachi, I. (2002). Social trust and self-rated health in US communities: A multilevel analysis. *Journal of Urban Health, 79*(4 Suppl. 1), S21–S34. doi:10.1093/jurban/79.suppl_1.S21 PMID:12473696

Swift, A., Liu, L., & Uber, J. (2008). Reducing MAUP bias of correlation statistics between water quality and GI illness. *Computers, Environment and Urban Systems, 32*(2), 134–148. doi:10.1016/j.compenvurbsys.2008.01.002

Tu, W., Tu, J., & Tedders, S. (2014). Estimating Neighborhood-level Socio-Economic Effect on Preterm Births Using a Multilevel Approach: A Case Study of Georgia, USA. *Annals of GIS, 20*(3), 181–191. doi:10.1080/19475683.2014.945483

Tu, W., Tu, J., & Tedders, S. (2015). A Multilevel Analysis of Neighborhood Socioeconomic Effect on Preterm Births in Georgia, USA. *AIMS Public Health, 2*(4), 638–654.

Warren, R. (1978). *The community in America*. Boston: Houghton Mifflin.

This research was previously published in the International Journal of Applied Geospatial Research (IJAGR), 9(3); edited by Donald Patrick Albert and Samuel Adu-Prah; pages 18-30, copyright year 2018 by IGI Publishing (an imprint of IGI Global).

Chapter 9
A Predictive Analytic Model for Maternal Morbidity

Edgardo Palza
École de technologie supérieure, Canada

Jorge Sanchez
Universidad Peruana Unión, Peru

Guillermo Mamani
Universidad Peruana Unión, Peru

Percy Pacora
Hospital Nacional Docente Madre Niño "San Bartolomé", Peru

Alain Abran
École de Technologie Supérieure, Canada

Jane Moon
University of Melbourne, Australia

ABSTRACT

This chapter presents a predictive analytic model for preventing neonatal morbidity through the analysis of patterns of risky behavior regarding morbidity in newborns. The chapter presents the design and implementation of a forecasting model of Neonatal morbidity. The model developed is based on artificial intelligence using Bayesian Networks, Influence Diagrams and principles of traditional statistics. The model research is based on a repository of 10,000 medical records at a hospital in Peru. The model aims to identify the factors that are causes of morbidity in newborns, is based on data mining techniques and developed using the CRISP-DM methodology.

DOI: 10.4018/978-1-7998-2351-3.ch009

INTRODUCTION

The World Health Organization (WHO) defines maternal morbidity as "Maternal death is the death of a woman while pregnant or within 42 days of termination of pregnancy, irrespective of the duration and site of the pregnancy, from any cause related to or aggravated by the pregnancy or its management but not from accidental or incidental causes" (OMS, UNICEF, UNFPA, & Banco Mundial, 2005).

Morbidity in the pregnancy period is one of the leading causes of death in women: WHO mentions that around 800 women die every day from complications related to pregnancy or childbirth. For instance, 287 000 women died in 2010 before, during and after the pregnancy and childbirth (OMS, 2014).

A key problem encountered in maternity consultations or emergencies, is the complexity of identifying risk factors of morbidity in order to minimize or eliminate them through a timely and accurate diagnosis (Say L, Pattinson RC, & Am G., 2004). Therefore, hospitals and clinics require adequate processes starting with collecting necessary data to create assertive knowledge about the patient and therefore offer an adequate treatment.

Our research aimed to create knowledge related to medical diagnosis. To analyze data from this database Influence Diagrams and Bayesian probabilities will be used to create a model for the detection of morbidity patterns and risk factors in the pregnant mothers during consultations or in intensive care units (ICU).

This research work was carried out with the collaboration of the National Teaching-Hospital Mother-Child "San Bartolomé" (HNDSB) in Lima (Peru) whose most important activities are maternal education, monitoring of pregnant women, delivery care and care of the newborns.

This chapter presents the empirical context and the project phases for the development of the predictive analytic model with examples of diagnosis scenarios developed using this predictive model and the knowledge repository available for research purposes.

RELATED STUDIES

Bulegon *et al.* (Bulegon, Bortoleto, & Roman, 2009) discuss the creation of data models in the context of health. They propose an entity-relationship model that includes cardiovascular risks, tests, exams, risks and other considerations that allow monitoring of the patient's conditions and they suggest some specific data mining techniques to explore the data.

Flores *et al.* (Flores C, Barros P, & S, 2013) present criteria for creating and modeling of Bayesian networks and propose a multi-agent software that simulates clinical cases for learning within an academic environment. Their knowledge database was created by experts in the domain and their system uses influence diagrams to organize a teaching strategy.

Fernandes *et al.* (Fernanez J, Martínez-Selles M, & Arredondeo MT, 2004) present a model for decision support systems based on Bayesian networks and influence diagrams. Their model attempts to provide a solution to determine the best treatment for patients suffering systolic heart failure disease. Their model also offers a probability of a patient's developing systolic heart failure. In terms of prediction, their model uses the signs, symptoms, risk factors, previous heart problems and test results; in addition, this model reports the most appropriate corrective treatment.

Kayaalp (Kayaalp M, 2012) reports on a study to predict, with some degree of accuracy, the mortality of a patient in an intensive care unit (ICU). Variables used in the study include physiological measurements of the patient in the first 48 hours. The Bayesian model proposed predicts the result with a posterior probability.

THE EMPIRICAL CONTEXT AND THE DEVELOPMENT PHASES FOR THE PREDICTIVE ANALYTIC MODEL

Empirical Context

The HNDSB has a Perinatal Information System (PIS) which records the basic history of the mother and child, including all tests and controls that have been undertaken from the beginning of pregnancy until the time of delivery. PIS was one of the most important sources of data for the Analytic Model, while others were social reports. The population available in the PIS database consisted of about 65,000 medical records of pregnant patients collected between 2000 and 2010.

Research Objectives for the Analytic Model

For understanding and developing a consensus for the model's predictive functionality in the context of a perinatal unit, various meetings were held with both medical residents and staff physicians. The following research objectives were identified:

- Prediction of birthweight less than 500g, 1000g, 2500g, 3000/4000g, or greater.
- Prediction of whether the child will be born sick, die within the first seven days or born healthy.

- Prediction of birth before 37 weeks.
- What is the risk of neonatal death in multiparous women with at least one child.
- What are the risks of death in women older than 34 years old
- What is the relationship between weight and morbidity in infants?
- The extent of the mother's difficulty factor in pregnancy.
- Analysis of the newborn "Apgar Score" at 1 minute and 5 ("In the Belly of the Medical Machine," 2007).
- Epidemiological study of maternal anemia and its effect on newborns.
- Quantify the amount of vaginal bleeding during childbirth
- Establish causes of other maternal morbidity during a caesarean
- Identify the fetus with growth restriction.
- Epidemiological study of fetal deaths including the effects of social, nutritional and metabolic factors and maternal obesity.
- Epidemiology of preterm birth.

This paper does not address all of these objectives individually, but proposes a generic approach to develop an analytic model which can then be used to develop a predictive diagnosis scenario for each one.

To create an analytic model, particular considerations were established:

1. Inclusion criteria: patients who completed the whole process of pregnancy, birth and postpartum.
2. Exclusion criteria: mothers who already had some disease or complications just before the pregnancy.
3. Elimination criteria: medical records with incomplete data in the medical record.

Figure 1. presents the phases and steps to build the analytic model. It starts by establishing, with the assistance of clinical experts, the objectives of an influence diagram and an assessment of the variables in the medical records.

The influence diagram represents a cause-effect map that allows selection and extraction of data from medical records (Almond, Mislevy, Steinberg, Yan, & Williamson, 2015; Mazur, 2015). To validate the hypothesis embedded within the influence diagram, a statistical analysis is applied to the cause-effect data extracted. Upon the completion of this analysis, a revised influence diagram is validated based on relationships. Next, the "a priori" and "a posteriori" probabilities are calculated, determined according to the number of variables in the influence diagram. Finally, tests have to be performed to verify the accuracy of the diagnosis model, creating past events using simulations with the model, and the whole procedure is documented.

The six main phases of this research methodology are presented next in more detail – see Figure 1.

Phase 1: The Proposal of an Influence Diagram

The objective in this phase is to create an influence diagram capable of establishing a probabilistic diagnosis of a disease for a pregnant mother. The diagram should be based on a set of factors that influence the pregnancy process, from its beginning till childbirth (Bain, 2003).

The Maternal Morbidity Working Group (MMWG), (Cross S, Bell J, & W., 2010) has defined a framework in order to identify principles about maternal morbidity:

(i) Identification and measurement of the selected maternal conditions should be feasible and evidence-based;
(ii) Maternal morbidity should not be viewed as consisting only of the conditions themselves, but also their complications; and
(iii) Morbidity conditions should be prioritized on the basis of their frequency and impact.

Considering the analysis provided by WHO, the following values were selected for the "maternal morbidity" variable (Denison et al., 2015; Rocha Filho et al., 2015):

- Value 1: Healthy (when the mother has no complications).
- Value 2: Pathological (when the mother develops pathology or complications after pregnancy).
- Value 3: Death (when the mother died in childbirth or after 42 hours).

Phase 2: Definition of Variables

In phase 2, the definitions and values for each variable are identified and are presented next.

Variable "Genesic Interval"

This variable specifies the period that the mother rests between two pregnancies (Mironov, 2001). This variable may take the following three values:

- Value 1: Short (less than 12 months).
- Value 2: Long (greater than 60 months).
- Value 3: Normal (greater than 12 months and less than 60 months).

Figure 1. Phases for the Development of the Predictive Analytic Model

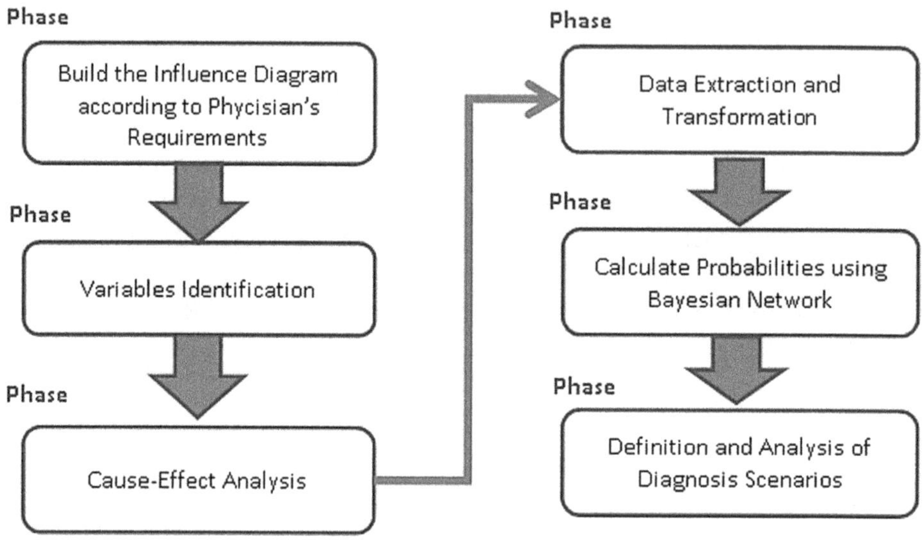

Variable: "Preterm Birth"

This variable refers to the childbirth that occurs after 20 weeks and before 37 weeks; it may take two values:

- Value 1: Yes (if it exists)
- Value 2: No (if it does not exist)

Similarly we proceeded to define constraints for all the variables involved in the influence diagram; they are illustrated in the diagrams presented in this chapter.

Phase 3: Cause-Effect Analysis in the Influence Diagram

Twenty four (24) variables were identified as directly and indirectly influencing maternal morbidity. Figure 2 represents them in the influence diagram, including target variables and their related influence factors.

At this stage the directional arrows are hypotheses raised by experts which must be validated through statistical analysis of historical data from the medical records.

Phase 4: Data Transformation and Statistical Approaches

Initial Data Collection

As a first step, data were exported from the Perinatal Information System (PIP) (which contains the history of the patient) to spreadsheets. The data contain general references about the patients, such as age, marital status, education level, as well as examinations and tests such as blood tests (diabetes, anemia, HIV, etc.), measurement of the fetus, and other medical requirements such as muscle mass, diseases, family and personal history, etc. For this research two years of patient's records were considered.

Data Preparation

In this step the quality of the data was verified: for instance verifying zero contents, duplicates, inconsistencies. The format of the data was also reviewed, that is scalar, nominal, ordinal values. Where appropriate, conversions were performed according to the requirements of the analysis. In the case of transformation of nominal values, we used SQL Queries and Stores Procedures (Bain, 2003).

After converting data into standard or linear records, data were reanalyzed via SQL queries to create specific cases or scenarios requested by physicians and related to maternal morbidity. This allowed the identification of candidate attributes that may have greater impact on the conditions of the mother.

Statistical Approach

The first version of a Prediction Model design was tested statistically before involving physicians. Test was prepared using the Chi Square technique with some variables identified. In this first version of a scenario each relationship between variables was distributed in a model and historical data were used to validate the model using the Chi Square technique. The Chi Square technique was repeated 6 times, to eliminate variables that do not show strong relationship. The most important variables identified are depicted in figure 2.

Phase 5: Probabilities - a Priori and a Posteriori

Figure 3 shows the influence diagram in its initial state. The diagram shows nodes without parents: this means that they do not have any a priori conditions. It should be noted that nodes with parents that have conditional probabilities and are called a posteriori. In order to calculate the a priori and a posteriori probabilities we used Bayes theorem (Smith, 2011).

Figure 2. Causal diagram of maternal morbidity

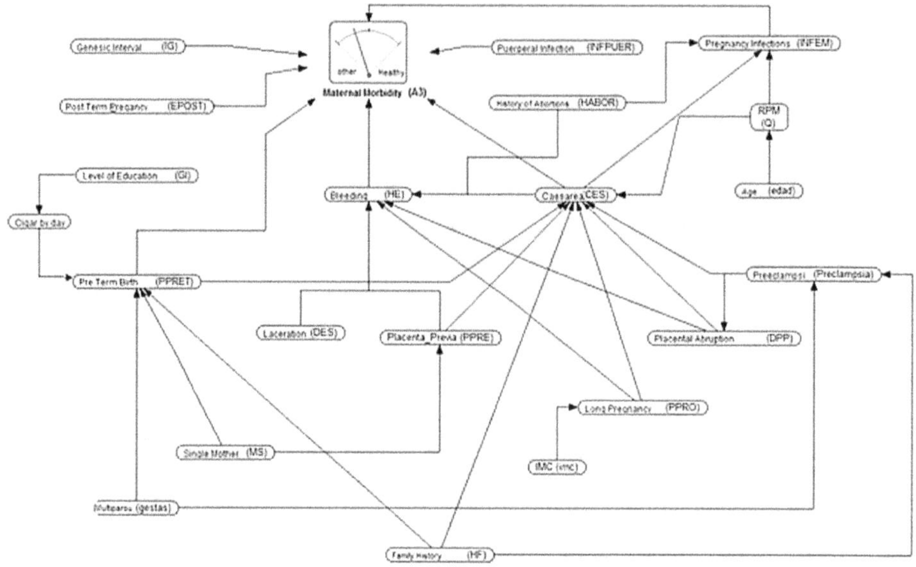

Figure 3 presents the initial state of the generic influence diagram with twenty four (24) variables. It is composed of 24 nodes or variables, and each variable is represented by a probability of occurrence. From the probabilities presented in Figure 3, there are eight factors significantly and directly influencing maternal morbidity: genesic range, pregnancy post-term, degree of education, pre-delivery term hemorrhage, caesarean, history of abortion, puerperal infection

Generalized Bayes theorem is the conditional probability distribution of a random variable A given B [$\Pr(A_i|B)$] in terms of the conditional probability distribution of the variable B given A [$\Pr(B|A_i)$] and marginal probability distribution of only A, [$\Pr(A_i)$].

Then the probability [$\Pr(A_i|B)$] is given by the expression:

$$\Pr\left(A_i|B\right) = \frac{\Pr\left(B|A_i\right)\Pr\left(A_i\right)}{\Pr\left(B\right)} = \frac{\Pr\left(\mathrm{B}|\mathrm{A}_\mathrm{i}\right)\Pr\left(A_i\right)}{\sum_{\mathrm{i}=1}^{\mathrm{n}}\Pr\left(A_i\right)\Pr\left(\mathrm{B}|\mathrm{A}_\mathrm{i}\right)} \qquad \forall\ i = 1,2,\ldots,n$$

Figure 3. Influence diagram for maternal morbidity - Initial State

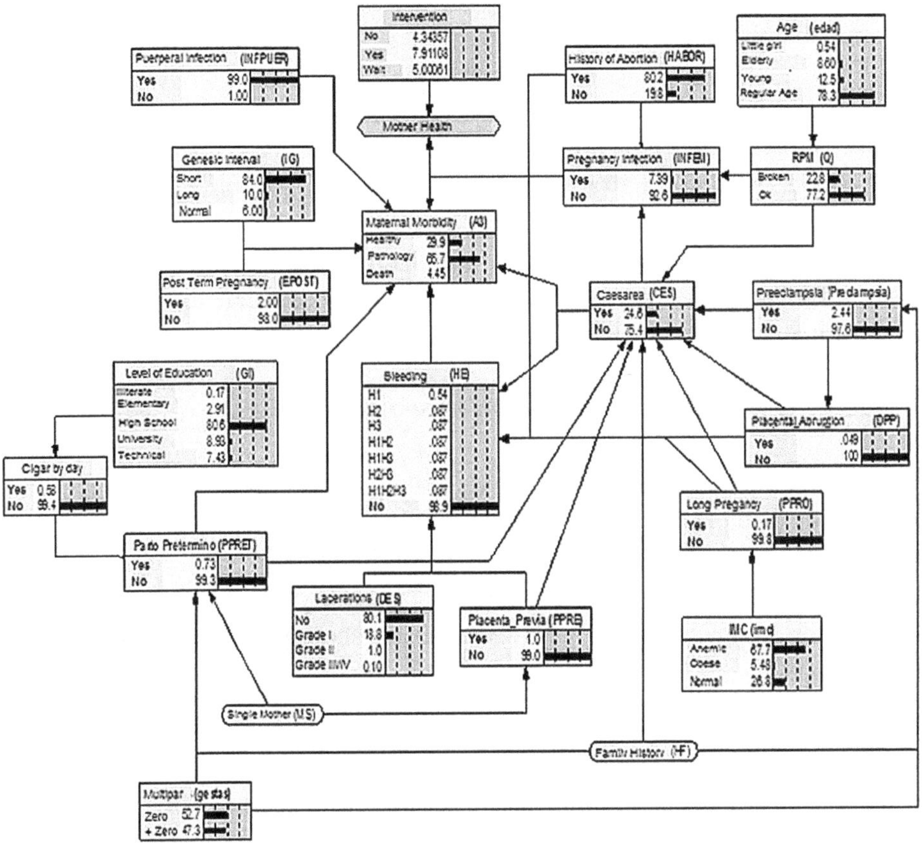

Where:

[Pr(A_i)]: These are the prior probabilities (Indicate a previous probability A)
[Pr($B|A_i$)]: The probability of B conditional on the assumption that there was (Indicate conditional probability B)
[Pr($A_i|B$)]: These are the posterior probabilities (Indicate a post probability).

The present project includes an algorithm coded in C# language (Norsys Software Corp, 2014; Sharp & Jagger, 2002) to find the a priori and a posteriori probabilities of each node. The "pseudocode" of the algorithm is executed in eight steps as follow:

1. The historical data are entered in each node.
2. All combinations of variables are established from all historical data.
3. The execution of all combination of variables.

4. All combinations established in the historical data are counted.
5. Each value of the count is divided by the total sum of the counts, obtaining the conditional probability.
6. The a priori probability is determined, that is the first probability prior to the experiment being conducted.
7. The a-posteriori probability is calculated after the experiment; this explains the relationship of the variables in context of cause and effect.

This probability is inserted into the simulator Netica (Norsys Software Corp, 2014) to find strong correlation between variables. The simulator is also used to select variables and create diagnosis scenarios.

Phase 6: Diagnosis of Maternal Morbidity

In this phase the model diagram is used for the prediction of maternal morbidity based on the medical data of the patient.

Figure 4 shows the diagnosis of maternal morbidity based on the probability of occurrence. In this scenario there is a 95.2% probability that the mother leaves the hospital with complications because she has had a short genesic interval and a post term pregnancy.

Figure 4. Example of a maternal morbidity diagnosis using probability

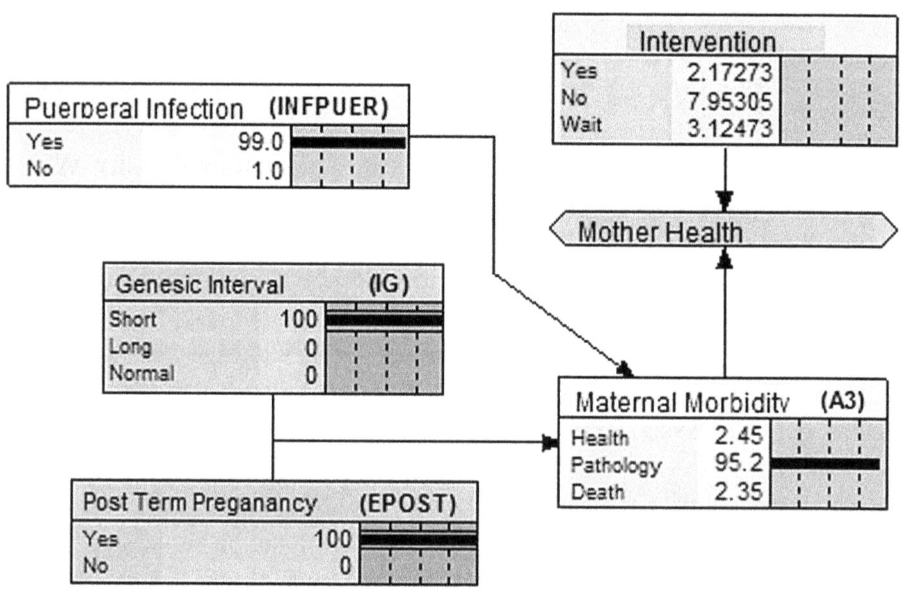

Examples of Diagnosis Scenarios Derived from the Predictive Model

In order to validate the model, it was necessary to organize different meetings with physicians specialized in the healthcare of pregnant women. In the first meetings they validated the variables of the cause-effect model, supporting the influence diagram. It was observed in many cases that the hypotheses proposed by the experts, based on their experience, were not supported; however, after the processing of the data it was observed that many of the hypotheses proposed by the physicians were supported, a confirmation of the validity of the proposed influence diagram model.

Usually physicians organize medical boards in order to analyze complex cases and discuss possible solutions based on their experience. Here, by using the influence diagram model and referring to the knowledge database composed of the medical records of thousands of pregnant women, participating physicians were able to create complex scenarios to derive the probability of success. Ten examples of such diagnosis scenarios are presented next.

Diagnosis Scenario 1: Caesarean Birth and Maternal Morbidity

Scenario 1 investigates the relationships between caesarean birth and maternal morbidity. The results are presented in Figure 5 which analyzed caesarean birth as a risk factor:

A) If caesarean section is not performed, then there is a 29.9% probability of healthy mother, a probability of 65.7% that the mother will have complications, and a 4.45% probability that the mother will die during childbirth or after.

B) However, if the mother decides to give birth by caesarean, then the probability of having complications is 92.8% and the probability of dying is 3.61%.

Figure 5. Caesarean birth and maternal morbidity

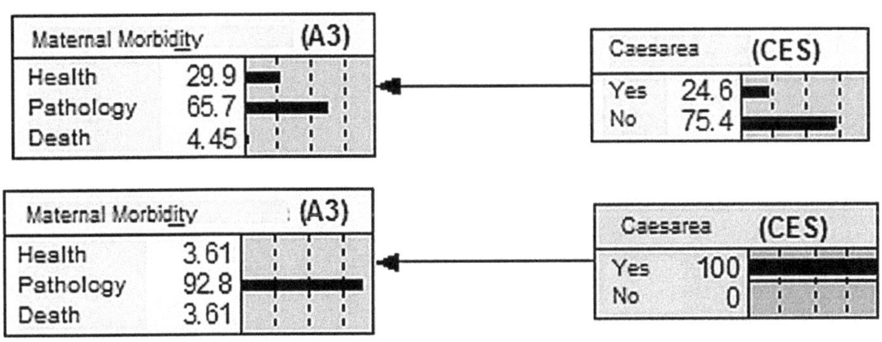

Diagnosis Scenario 2: Maternal Morbidity and Two Risk Factors

Scenario 2 investigates the relationship between the genesic interval and maternal morbidity. Figure 6 shows that if the genesic interval is short, the probability of the mother having complications is 65.7%, the risk of dying is 4.45, and the probability that she leaves the delivery without any complication is 29.9%. It follows that the genesic interval can be a protective factor and if it is short it becomes a risk factor. It is also noted that 98% of mothers give birth within the normal period and only 2% have a post-term pregnancy.

Diagnosis Scenario 3: Maternal Morbidity Based on Genesic Interval

Scenario 3 investigates the relationship between the genesic interval and maternal morbidity. Figure 7 show that if a mother has a long genesic interval, then the probability of being healthy at childbirth or after is 70.2%.

Diagnosis Scenario 4: Maternal Morbidity Based on Genesic Interval and Post-Term Pregnancy

Scenario 4 investigates the relationships between the genesic interval and post-term pregnancy with respect to maternal morbidity. Figure 8 shows that the maternal morbidity risk increases significantly when genesic interval is short and the mother has a post-term pregnancy. If the mother has a short genesic interval and childbirth does not occur at the time expected, the probability of complications is 95.2% and the probability of death is 2.35%

Figure 6. Influence Diagram regarding maternal morbidity with two risk factors

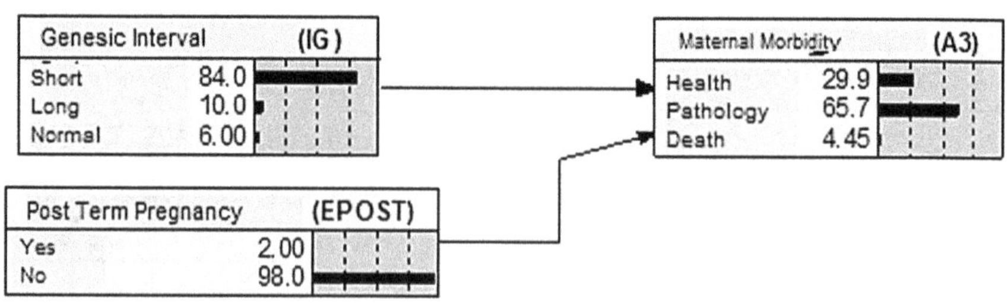

Figure 7. Inference-based maternal morbidity and genesic interval.

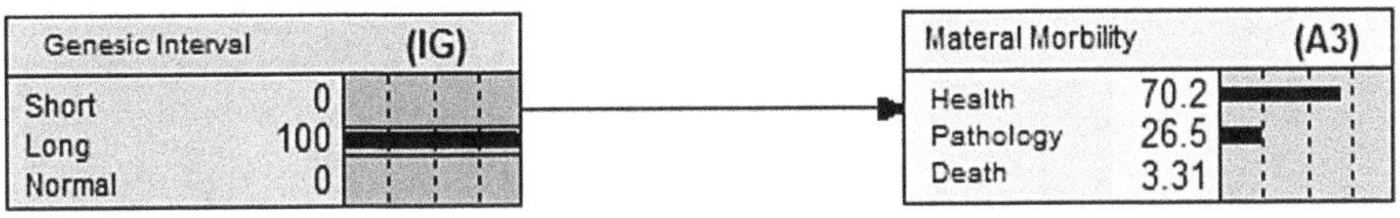

Genesic Interval
(IG)
Short 0
Long 100
Normal 0
Materal Morbility
(A3)
Health 70.2
Pathology 26.5
Death 3.31

Figure 8. Maternal morbidity based on genesic interval and post term pregnancy

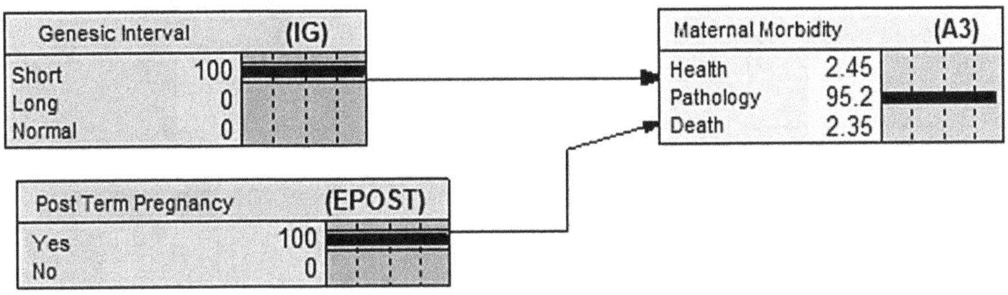

Diagnosis Scenario 5: Maternal Morbidity and Bleeding (1)

Scenario 5 investigates the relationship between bleeding and maternal morbidity. Figure 9 shows that if the mother has no bleeding, the probability of death is 4.45%; in contrast, if the mother is bleeding the probability of death is 26.4%. Therefore, bleeding is a high risk factor in maternal death.

Diagnosis Scenario 6: Maternal Morbidity Risk Factor for Bleeding (2)

Scenario 6 investigates the relationship between bleeding and maternal morbidity. Figure 10 shows that lacerations and placenta previa are risk factors for maternal morbidity. If the mother has grade III or IV lacerations and has placenta previa, the probability of death in childbirth or after is 26.8%. However, if there is no laceration or placenta previa, the probability of death is only of 4.45%, which corresponds to a normal risk.

Diagnosis Scenario 7: Maternal Morbidity and Seven Risk Factors in the Initial State.

Scenario 7 investigates a combination of seven risk factors in the initial state. Figure 11 shows the case when the pregnant woman has complications and physicians have direct intervention. In this scenario, the health status is 7.91 on a scale of 10 (7.91/10); in contrast, if there is no physician intervention, the health status is reduced to 4.34.

Figure 9. Maternal morbidity and bleeding (1)

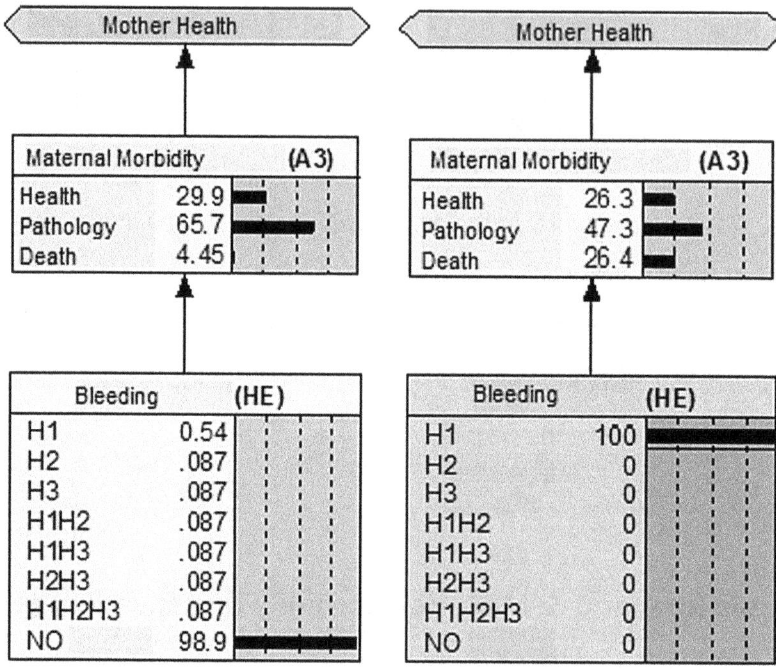

Figure 10. Maternal morbidity and bleeding (2)

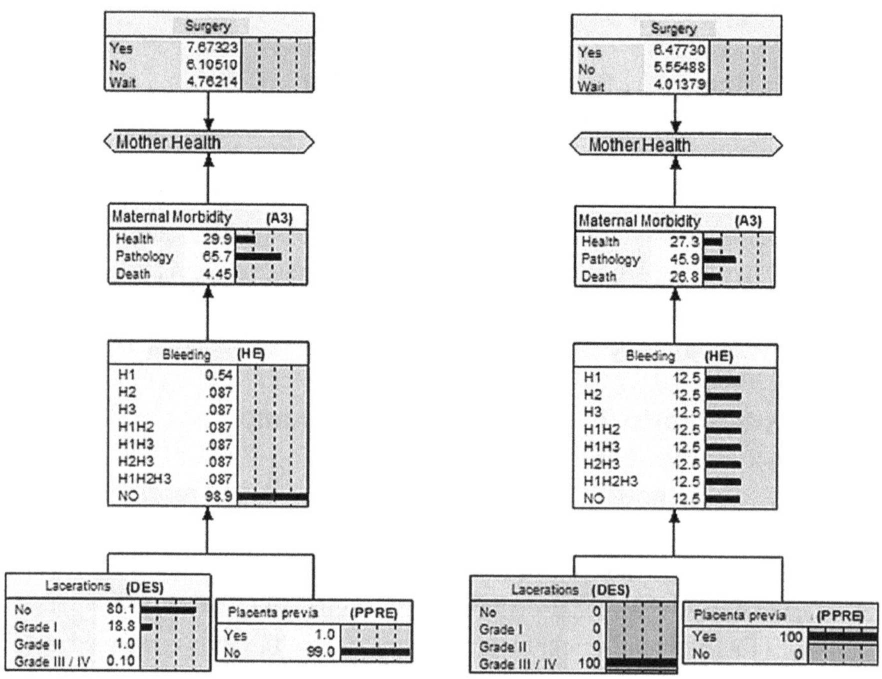

Figure 11. Maternal morbidity and seven risk factors in the initial state

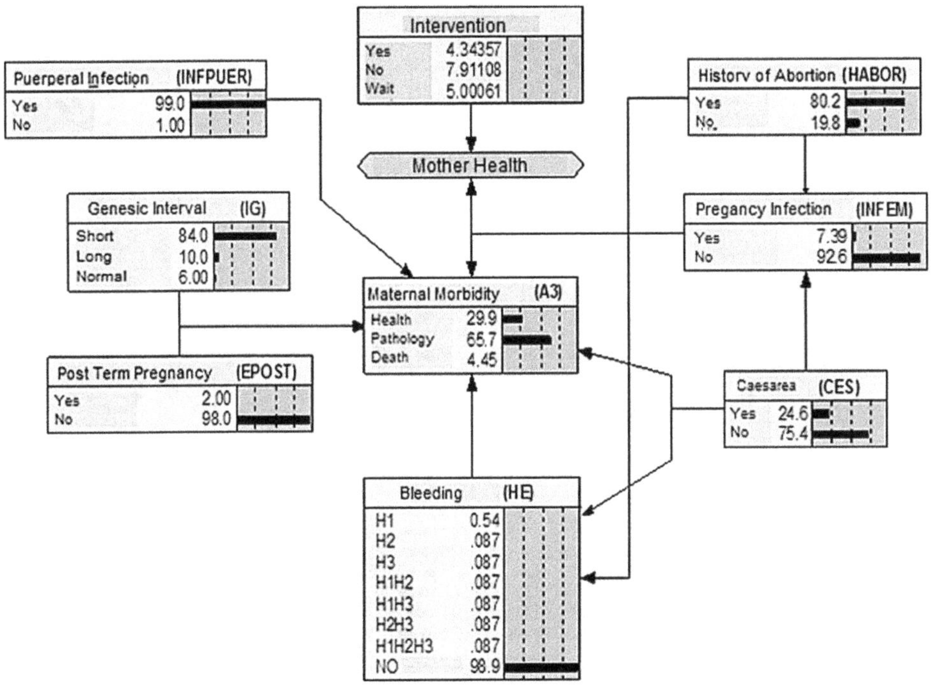

Diagnosis Scenario 8: Maternal Morbidity with Risk Factors of Death

Scenario 8 investigates the death risk factor and maternal morbidity. Figure 12 shows that if the mother suffers lacerations grade III or IV and has a prolonged labor, the probability of death is 27.2%; furthermore if there is no physician intervention, the health deteriorates to 3.98 in a scale of 10.

Diagnosis Scenario 9: Maternal Morbidity with Pathological Risk Factors

Scenario 9 investigates the relationship between pathological risk factors and maternal morbidity. Figure 13 shows that if the pregnant women has a short genesic interval and gives birth after the normal period (post-term pregnancy) the probability of having complications is 95.2%; if the physician does not intervene, the patient's health deteriorates to 2.17 on a scale of 10 (which it may represent coma).

Figure 12. Maternal morbidity with risk factors of death

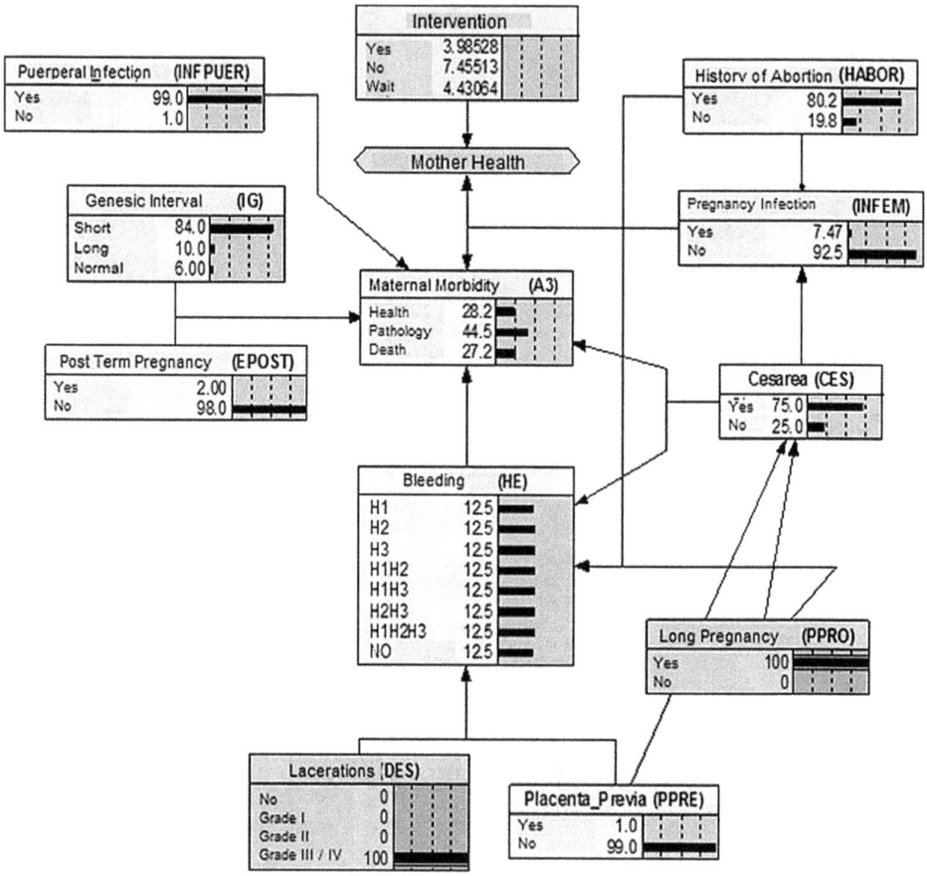

Diagnosis Scenario 10: Maternal Morbidity with Pathologic Risks and Death

Scenario 10 investigates the relationships between pathologic risks and death and maternal morbidity. Figure 14 shows that if the mother has the following conditions:

- Short genesic Interval: Short
- Grade III and IV lacerations
- Placenta Previa

Then the probability of death is 26.3%; however if an intervention is performed, health will be recovered to a level 7.47 on a scale of 10.

Figure 13. Maternal morbidity with pathological risk factors

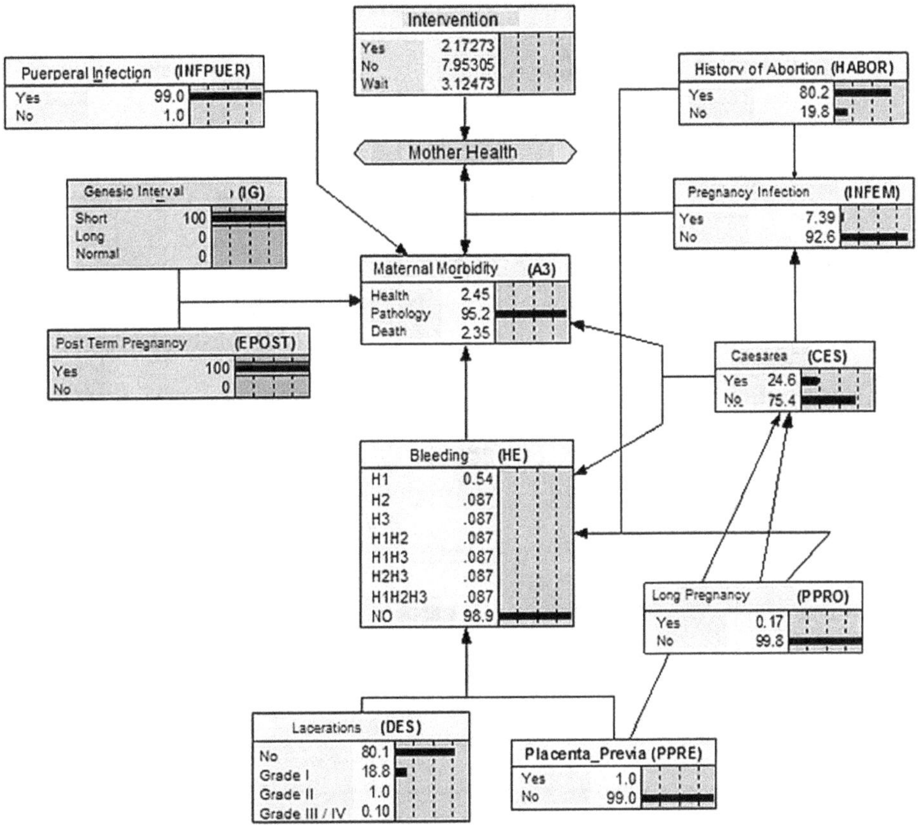

CONCLUSION

The purpose of this research was to build a model based on Influence Diagrams and Bayesian Networks to facilitate physicians' decisions in complex scenarios where maternal morbidity is a high risk.

This chapter has presented the design and implementation of a predictive model of maternal morbidity. The model is based on the application of Influence Diagrams and Bayesian Networks. Influence Diagrams and Bayesian Networks provide a particular advantage in healthcare since they integrate qualitative and quantitative perspectives into single model, in other words, the opinion of physicians regarding particular cases and data recorded in medical records. The model allows the creation of diagnosis scenarios based on a knowledge repository of more than 10 years of medical records at a maternity hospital in Peru.

Figure 14. Maternal morbidity with pathologic risks and death

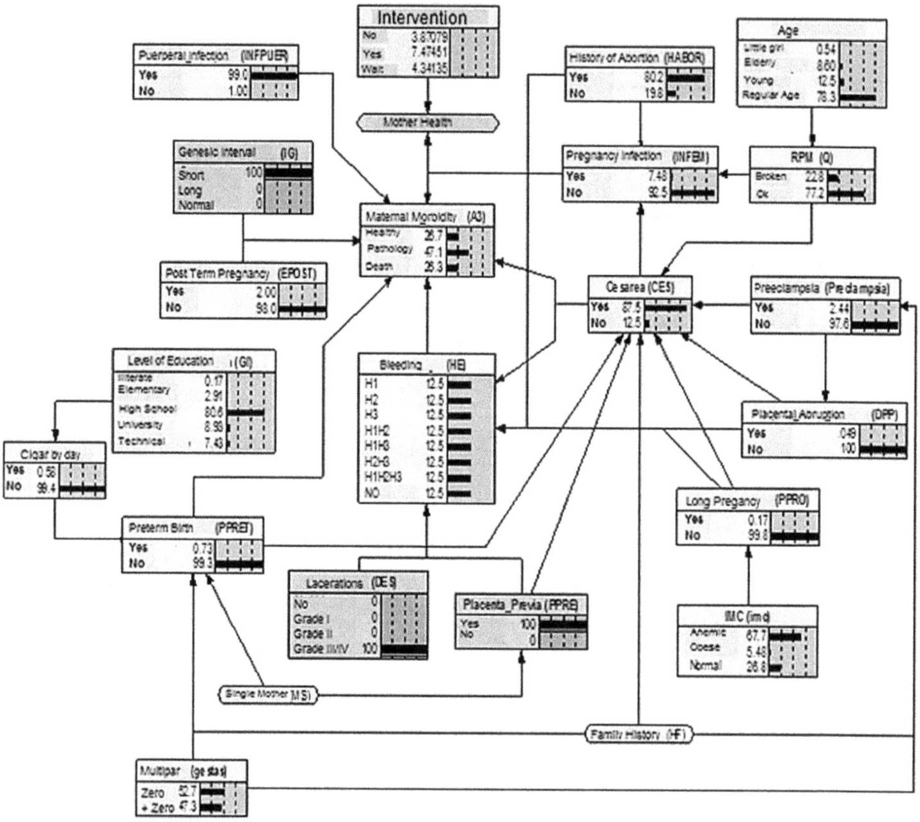

The model enables the physicians to leverage the medical knowledge embedded in cases registered in medical records by analyzing them, creating diagnosis scenarios and facilitating decisions in complex situations. To design and build the model, a population of about 65,000 medical records of pregnant patients collected between 2000 and 2010 was used as the reference knowledge database.

This chapter has presented examples of 10 diagnosis scenarios developed using this predictive model and the knowledge repository available for research purposes. In summary, based on the findings presented in the previous sections, the genesic interval and post-term pregnancy are important risk factors for complications in pregnant women. For example, if the mother has a long birth interval and gives birth within a normal period, then the probability that the mother remains healthy, without any complications after delivery, increases from 29.9% to 71.6%.

Lacerations, placenta previa, prolonged labor and caesarian are risk factors for death. If a mother has one of these complications, the probability of dying in childbirth or after, increases from 4.45% to 29.8%, which is a very high risk.

Furthermore, if a mother has Grade III or IV lacerations and prolonged labor, the probability of death is 27.2%. In such cases physicians must decide on the appropriate intervention. If they decide to intervene, the mother's health status increases to 7.455 on a scale of 10. If the surgery is delayed, the mother's health decreases to 41.43/10, and surgery cannot be done the mother's health status decreases to 3.98/10.

Currently the use of the predictive analytic model is being evaluated at the hospital with the physicians and researchers, while being used concurrently as a learning platform for physician residents (students) in the hospital.

This development and use of such models could be extended to other health specialties where complex risk scenarios and decisions are a challenge. Furthermore, it could be used as a reference for the development and support of public health policies.

REFERENCES

Almond, R. G., Mislevy, R. J., Steinberg, L. S., Yan, D., & Williamson, D. M. (2015). *The Future of Bayesian Networks in Educational Assessment. In Bayesian Networks in Educational Assessment* (pp. 583–599). Springer. doi:10.1007/978-1-4939-2125-6_16

Bain, T. (2003). SQL server 2000 stored procedures handbook. Birmingham, UK: Wrox Press. doi:10.1007/978-1-4302-1125-9

Bulegon, H., Bortoleto, S., & Roman, A. C. (2009). *Developing an Implementation through a Modeling of the Database for Cardiovascular Monitoring*. doi:10.1109/isda.2009.129

Cross, S., Bell, J., & Graham, W. J. (2010). What you count is what you target: The implications of maternal death classification for tracking progress towards reducing maternal mortality in developing countries. *Bulletin of the World Health Organization*, *88*(2), 147–153. doi:10.2471/BLT.09.063537 PMID:20428372

Denison, F., Norwood, P., Bhattacharya, S., Duffy, A., Mahmood, T., Morris, C., ... Scotland, G. (2015). Association Between Maternal Body Mass Index During Pregnancy, Short-term Morbidity, and Increased Health Service Costs: A Population-based Study. *Obstetric Anesthesia Digest*, *35*(1), 18–19. doi:10.1097/01.aoa.0000460386.14360.48

Fernanez, J., Martínez-Selles, M., & Arredondeo, M. T. (2004). *Bayesian Networks and Influence Diagrams as Valid Decision Support Tools in Systolic Heart Failure Management*. Paper presented at the Computers in Cardiology.

Flores, C., & Barros, P., & S, C. (2013). *Leveraging the Learning Process in Health through Clinical Cases Simulator*. Paper presented at the Serious Games and Applications for Health (SeGAH), Vilamoura 10.1109/SeGAH.2013.6665303

In the Belly of the Medical Machine. (2007). *Publishers Weekly*, *254*(7), 72–72.

Kayaalp, M. (2012). *Intensive Care Unit (ICU) Outcome Predictions using Physiologic Trends in the First Two Days. Computing in Cardiology*. CinC.

Mazur, D. J. (2015). Social Pressure on Patient Decision Making through Shifting Mental Models: Presenting Evidence to Patients. *Sociology Mind*, *5*(02), 100–104. doi:10.4236m.2015.52010

Mironov, B. N. (2001). Response to Steven L. Hoch's" BN Mironov and His' Demographic Processes and Problems'. *Slavic Review*, *60*(3), 591–599. doi:10.2307/2696821

Norsys Software Corp. (2014). *Netica Software*. Retrieved from https://norsys.com/netica.html

OMS, UNICEF, UNFPA, & Banco Mundial. (2005). *Mortalidad materna en 2005: estimaciones elaboradas por la OMS, el UNICEF, el UNFPA y el Banco Mundial*. Author.

OMS. (2014). Mortalidad materna. *Salud de la madre, el recién nacido, del niño y del adolescente*. Retrieved from http://www.unfpa.org.mx/ssr_mortalidad_materna.php

Rocha Filho, E. A., Costa, M. L., Cecatti, J. G., Parpinelli, M. A., Haddad, S. M., Pacagnella, R. C., ... Souza, J. P. (2015). Severe maternal morbidity and near miss due to postpartum hemorrhage in a national multicenter surveillance study. *International Journal of Gynaecology and Obstetrics: the Official Organ of the International Federation of Gynaecology and Obstetrics*, *128*(2), 131–136. doi:10.1016/j.ijgo.2014.08.023 PMID:25468058

Say,, L., & Pattinson,, R. C., & Am, G. (2004). WHO Systematic review of maternal morbidity and mortality: the prevalence of severe acute maternal morbidity (near miss). *Reproductive Health* 2004, *1*(4).

Sharp, J., & Jagger, J. (2002). *Microsoft Visual C#. Net step by step*. Redmond, WA: Microsoft Press.

Smith, J. Q. (2011). Bayesian decision analysis: Principles and practice. *Choice: Current Reviews for Academic Libraries*, *48*(11), 2138–2138.

ADDITIONAL READING

Assarag, B., Dujardin, B., Delamou, A., Meski, F.-Z., & De Brouwere, V. (2015). Determinants of maternal near-miss in morocco: Too late, too far, too sloppy? *PLoS ONE*, *10*(1), e0116675. doi:10.1371/journal.pone.0116675 PMID:25612095

Bergh, A.-M., Allanson, E., & Pattinson, R. C. (2015). What is needed for taking emergency obstetric and neonatal programmes to scale? *Best Practice & Research. Clinical Obstetrics & Gynaecology*. doi:10.1016/j.bpobgyn.2015.03.015 PMID:25921973

Bingham, D., & Ruhl, C. (2015). Planning and Evaluating Evidence-Based Perinatal Nurse Staffing. *Journal of Obstetric, Gynecologic, and Neonatal Nursing*, *44*(2), 290–308. doi:10.1111/1552-6909.12544 PMID:25651865

Chaillet, N., Dubé, E., Dugas, M., Audibert, F., Tourigny, C., Fraser, W. D., & Dumont, A. (2006). Evidence-based strategies for implementing guidelines in obstetrics: A systematic review. *Obstetrics and Gynecology*, *108*(5), 1234–1245. doi:10.1097/01.AOG.0000236434.74160.8b PMID:17077251

Declercq, E. (2015). Childbirth in Brazil: Challenging an Interventionist Paradigm. *Birth*, *42*(1), 1-4. 18-19.

Fenwick, J., Toohill, J., Creedy, D., Smith, J., & Gamble, J. (2015). Sources, responses and moderators of childbirth fear in Australian women: A qualitative investigation. *Midwifery*, *31*(1), 239–246. doi:10.1016/j.midw.2014.09.003 PMID:25440298

Ferguson, T. W., Tangri, N., Rigatto, C., & Komenda, P. (2015). Cost-effective treatment modalities for reducing morbidity associated with chronic kidney disease. *Expert review of Pharmacoeconomics & Outcomes Research, 15*(2), 243-252.

Flaherman, V. J., Schaefer, E. W., Kuzniewicz, M. W., Li, S. X., Walsh, E. M., & Paul, I. M. (2015). Early weight loss nomograms for exclusively breastfed newborns. *Pediatrics*, *135*(1), e16–e23. doi:10.1542/peds.2014-1532 PMID:25554815

Glavind, J., & Uldbjerg, N. (2015). Elective cesarean delivery at 38 and 39 weeks: Neonatal and maternal risks. *Current Opinion in Obstetrics & Gynecology*, *27*(2), 121–127. doi:10.1097/GCO.0000000000000158 PMID:25689238

Lundgren, I., Smith, V., Nilsson, C., Vehvilainen-Julkunen, K., Nicoletti, J., Devane, D., ... Begley, C. (2015). Clinician-centred interventions to increase vaginal birth after caesarean section (VBAC): A systematic review. *BMC Pregnancy and Childbirth*, *15*(1), 16. doi:10.118612884-015-0441-3 PMID:25652550

Mallaiah, S., Barclay, P., Harrod, I., Chevannes, C., & Bhalla, A. (2015). Introduction of an algorithm for ROTEM-guided fibrinogen concentrate administration in major obstetric haemorrhage. *Anaesthesia*, *70*(2), 166–175. doi:10.1111/anae.12859 PMID:25289791

Mazur, D. J. (2015). Social Pressure on Patient Decision Making through Shifting Mental Models: Presenting Evidence to Patients. *Sociology Mind*, *5*(02), 100–104. doi:10.4236m.2015.52010

Metz, T. D., Allshouse, A. A., Faucett, A. M., & Grobman, W. A. (2015). Validation of a Vaginal Birth After Cesarean Delivery Prediction Model in Women With Two Prior Cesarean Deliveries. *Obstetrics and Gynecology*, *125*(4), 948–952. doi:10.1097/AOG.0000000000000744 PMID:25751218

Minutolo, A., Esposito, M., & De Pietro, G. (2015). Design and validation of a light-weight reasoning system to support remote health monitoring applications. *Engineering Applications of Artificial Intelligence*, *41*, 232–248.

Mironov, B. N. (2001). Response to Steven L. Hoch's" BN Mironov and His' Demographic Processes and Problems'. *Slavic Review*, *60*(3), 591–599. doi:10.2307/2696821

Nair, M., Kurinczuk, J., Brocklehurst, P., Sellers, S., Lewis, G., & Knight, M. (2015). Factors associated with maternal death from direct pregnancy complications: a UK national case–control study. *BJOG: An International Journal of Obstetrics & Gynaecology*.

Patterson, J., Roberts, C., Isbister, J., Irving, D., Nicholl, M., Morris, J., & Ford, J. (2015). What factors contribute to hospital variation in obstetric transfusion rates? *Vox Sanguinis*, *108*(1), 37–45. doi:10.1111/vox.12186 PMID:25092527

Ragupathy, K. (2015). Commentary: Intra-partum foetal surveillance in high-risk pregnancies. *Archives of Gynecology and Obstetrics*, *291*(1), 9–10. doi:10.100700404-014-3430-2 PMID:25155820

Rocha Filho, E. A., Costa, M. L., Cecatti, J. G., Parpinelli, M. A., Haddad, S. M., Pacagnella, R., & Souza, J. P. (2015). Severe maternal morbidity and near miss due to postpartum hemorrhage in a national multicenter surveillance study. *International Journal of Gynaecology and Obstetrics: the Official Organ of the International Federation of Gynaecology and Obstetrics, 128*(2), 131–136. doi:10.1016/j.ijgo.2014.08.023 PMID:25468058

Semenic, S., Edwards, N., Premji, S., Olson, J., Williams, B., & Montgomery, P. (2015). Decision- making and evidence use during the process of prenatal record review in Canada: A multiphase qualitative study. *BMC Pregnancy and Childbirth, 15*(1), 78. doi:10.118612884-015-0503-6 PMID:25881034

Shapiro-Mendoza, C. K., Tomashek, K. M., Kotelchuck, M., Barfield, W., Nannini, A., Weiss, J., & Declercq, E. (2008). Effect of late-preterm birth and maternal medical conditions on newborn morbidity risk. *Pediatrics, 121*(2), e223–e232. doi:10.1542/peds.2006-3629 PMID:18245397

Thomas, J., Paranjothy, S., & James, D. (2004). National cross sectional survey to determine whether the decision to delivery interval is critical in emergency caesarean section. *bmj, 328*(7441), 665.

von Dadelszen, P., Payne, B., Li, J., Ansermino, J. M., Pipkin, F. B., Côté, A.-M., ... Joseph, K. (2011). Prediction of adverse maternal outcomes in pre-eclampsia: Development and validation of the fullPIERS model. *Lancet, 377*(9761), 219–227. doi:10.1016/S0140-6736(10)61351-7 PMID:21185591

KEY TERMS AND DEFINITIONS

Baysean Theorem: *CRISP-DM methodology*

Influence Diagram: Represents a cause-effect map that allows selection and extraction of data from medical records.

Genesic Interval: It is specified period that the mother rests between two pregnancies.

Preterm Birth: Refers to the childbirth that occurs after 20 weeks and before 37 weeks.

Puerperal Infections: Is also known as postpartum infection. It is referred to bacterial infection of the female reproductive tract following childbirth or miscarriage.

This research was previously published in Improving Health Management through Clinical Decision Support Systems edited by Jane D. Moon and Mary P. Galea; pages 108-126, copyright year 2016 by Medical Information Science Reference (an imprint of IGI Global).

Chapter 10
Scaling the Maternal and Newborn Survival Initiative (MANSI):
Rural India

Deepa Fernandes Prabhu
Massachusetts Institute of Technology, USA

Richard C. Larson
Massachusetts Institute of Technology, USA

ABSTRACT

The infant mortality rate (IMR) and maternal mortality ratio (MMR) are unacceptably high in many parts of rural India. This article focuses on a system analysis approach to the best practices for scaling and replicating of maternal and newborn survival initiative (MANSI), a field-tested pilot program for addressing high IMRs and MMRs. A system dynamics model of the village birthing system is used to understand the resources needed for the viability of scaling or replication, is constructed and incorporated in the analysis. The MANSI program is a public and private partnership between a few key players. Implemented in the Seraikela area of India's Jharkhand state, the program has achieved a 32.7% reduction in neonatal mortality, a 26.5% reduction in IMR, and a 50% increase in hospital births, which tend to have better health outcomes for women and newborns. The authors conclude with a discussion of the prospects for and difficulties of replicating MANSI in other resource-constrained areas, not only in India but in other developing countries as well.

DOI: 10.4018/978-1-7998-2351-3.ch010

INTRODUCTION

IMR (measured per 1000 live births) and MMR (the ratio of the number of maternal deaths during a given time period per 100,000 live births during the same time-period) are widely considered as key indicators of health services, nutrition, poverty and education levels in a country or region. India, despite being one of the fastest growing economies, still lags behind the global IMR and MMR levels. The World Economic Forum ranks India, as among the lowest in gender equality in health and survival in 2014, 141 in a list of 142 countries, only above Armenia ("Global Gender Gap Report 2014," n.d.). India accounts for the largest number of maternal deaths in the world, an estimated 70,000 deaths of new mothers in each year. Of these, almost half are caused by hemorrhage or excessive bleeding (30%) and sepsis or infection (16%), which can be reduced through effective obstetric primary care facilities ("Mother and child," n.d.). Despite the Janani Suraksha Yojna (JSY) program, a scheme started by the Indian government to boost institutional deliveries, just 47% of the deliveries are in hospitals or other healthcare facilities. More than half still take place at home, of which only about 5% are assisted by skilled health personnel. Impediments to health care are directly attributable to the low status of women in society. There is inadequate female knowledge or autonomy to maintain good health and reproductive control. Marriage of young girls and nonuse of contraception further cause gender-specific health vulnerabilities like maternal morbidity and mortality. India has a low life expectancy (68 years in India vs. 78 years in the US), high maternal mortality ratios (~174 per 100,000 in India vs. ~28 per 100,000 in the US) and high infant mortality rates (36 per 1,000 in India vs. 6 per 1,000 in the US) in 2015 (World Health Organization, 2015). In the Seraikela area of Jharkhand, India (see Figure 1), most babies are born in the family's cattle shed. An elder typically cuts the infant's umbilical cord with a sickle that has not been sterilized. The new mother receives no food for three to five days after delivery (three days for a baby boy, five for a girl). The newborn is bathed but not swaddled. He or she is fed honey or goat's milk but not breast milk for the first few days. Initiation of breastfeeding is delayed after birth because of the belief that a mother's milk is "not ready" until two to three days postpartum (Bandyopadhyay, 2009).

These practices show that maternal and infant healthcare in rural parts of India comes after food, livestock's well-being, and religious practices in terms of priority. Few people in such places are aware of the importance of antenatal as well as postnatal care. When it comes to antenatal care, awareness centers on following traditional or superstitious ways. For example, pregnant women are not allowed to eat eggs or take supplements because people fear that such new practices could cause a miscarriage or lead to a birth weight too high for safe delivery. While such worries are understandable, these and other practices ultimately endanger the mother's and baby's health, by making both vulnerable to anemia, sepsis, and pneumonia.

Figure 1. The Seraikela area

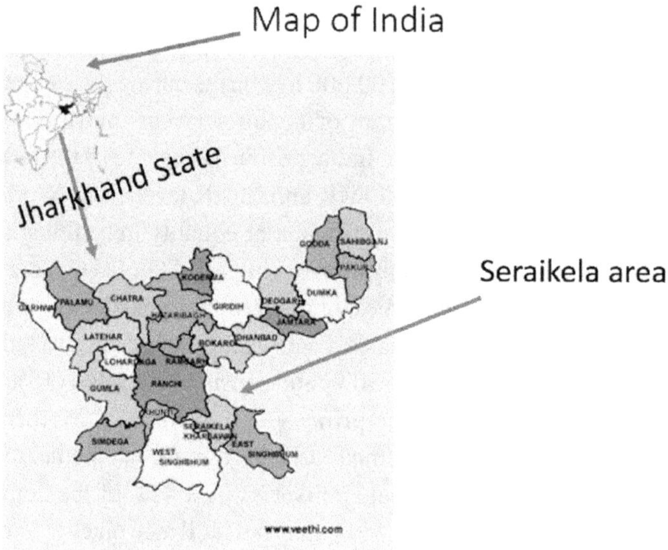

For a maternal and child health program to be effective, it must lower the IMR and MMR. Understanding local cultural practices and beliefs can help program teams design programs that have a better chance of achieving those objectives. A systems analysis of the MANSI system to evaluate best practices of lowering IMR and MMR can be invaluable in scaling or replicating this program in areas where IMR and MMR are very high.

Many Maternal and Child Health (MCH) programs aimed at improving IMR and MMR have been implemented globally. The Literature review section of this paper discusses the MCH programs published in recent years to compare and contrast them and to understand their successes and shortcomings. MANSI as a system segment analyzes the MANSI program in detail from a public health and a systems perspective to understand how all the different parts in the system architecture, design and management functioned together. The system dynamics piece discusses the long-term sustainability, scalability and replicability of the program including a system dynamics model for demonstrating the resources needed for viability. The conclusions section summarizes the findings and makes systems and policy recommendations for scaling or replicating this particular highly successful pilot MCH program.

LITERATURE REVIEW

The World Health Organization's Millennium Development Goals (MDG), defined in 2000 and 2015, include reducing child mortality (goal 4) and improving maternal health (goal 5). (Visit http://www.who.int/topics/millennium_development_goals/en/ to learn more about the goals.) The goals specifically targeted reducing IMRs by 66% and improving MMRs by 75% from 1990 to 2015. With these aims in mind, the WHO published home-based mortality-prevention strategies in 2012. Such strategies included visits from skilled health workers who could promote exclusive breastfeeding (infants receive breast milk only), strategies for keeping infants warm, and hygienic umbilical cord and skin care. These same workers could also identify signs of health problems and infants at risk of death and could encourage families to have infants vaccinated against diseases such as tuberculosis, polio, hepatitis A and B, diphtheria, tetanus, pertussis, infections caused by bacteria, measles, mumps, rubella, pneumonia, severe diarrhea, typhoid, and chickenpox as early as possible.

The WHO's plan called for MDG goals to be attained by 2015 and motivated the launch of many maternal and child health programs around the world.

GLOBAL EFFORTS TO REDUCE IMR AND MMR

As much as 75% of infant deaths occur in the first week of life, caused by low birth weight, infections, asphyxia, and birth trauma. The incidence of such deaths is higher in countries where people have little or no access to health care. Skilled health workers providing effective care at birth and during the first week of life can prevent up to two-thirds of these deaths. As Figure 2 shows, the IMR in most countries and regions has decreased over the last 25 years. However, in 2015, the rate in South East Asia, including India, was 34 per 1,000 live births—significantly higher than the rate of 12.5 in the Americas and 9.8 in Europe.

Maternal deaths are those that occur during pregnancy, as a woman is giving birth, or in the week after a woman has delivered a child. The risk of such deaths increases in places where people have little or no access to routine and emergency care. Immediate causes include hemorrhage, pre-eclampsia, infection, obstructed labor, and delay in seeking or obtaining care and reaching a health-care facility (World Health Organization, 2013). MMRs have also been decreasing around the world, dropping from more than 450 in 1990 to around 200 in 2015. As much as 99% of maternal deaths take place in developing countries, reflecting inequities in income and access to health services between these nations and developed countries.

Figure 2. IMR trends (Global Health Observatory, n.d.)

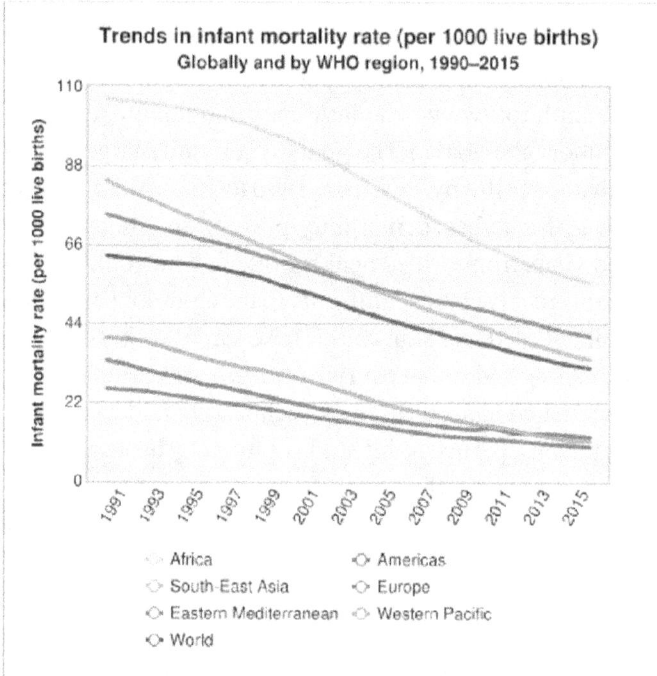

Below, we review outcomes of and lessons learned from maternal and child health programs implemented in sub-Saharan Africa, Pakistan, Nepal, and Vietnam. While sub-Saharan Africa and Pakistan did not achieve MDGs 4 and 5, Nepal and Vietnam were able to meet their targets.

- **Sub-Saharan Africa:** Countries in this region have persistently high IMRs and MMRs owing to a range of biological and social determinants, such as the HIV/AIDS epidemic and civil war (Sartorius, Sartorius, Chirwa, & Fonn, 2011). However, one maternal and child health program executed in the upper-east region of Ghana has been relatively successful in terms of reducing childhood mortality by half in only three years through community-based care. Community engagement was identified as the single most important factor in the program team's ability to scale up the program from the initial three villages to the entire upper east region of Ghana (Awoonor-Williams et al., 2013).
- **Pakistan:** The government of Pakistan launched a maternal, newborn, and child health program in 2005 featuring a new cadre of health workers called community midwives. Officials knew that such community participation would

be necessary for empowering local residents to achieve sustainable quality of healthcare service and to control healthcare costs. But such participation proved limited, owing to lack of adequate governance, and the program is not performing as well as the government hoped. Additional obstacles include insufficient integration between the program and government health facilities, unclear roles of the community-based workers, and political interference from district officials (WHO EMRO 2014).

- **Nepal:** Programs in Nepal launched by government and non-government organizations (NGOs) have focused on addressing declines in fertility, societal changes such as women giving birth to fewer children than in previous years, and the need to enhance both supply of and demand for maternal care. Such programs have reduced the IMR and MMR in that country, putting Nepal on track to meeting WHO goals (Tran, 2013). Indeed, Nepal met these goals by the end of 2015.
- **Vietnam:** Like Nepal, Vietnam was also progressing toward attainment of its MDG 4 and 5 targets in 2013, and met the goals during 2015. It made strides by setting up a special fund in 2003 to give impoverished citizens greater access to healthcare and by implementing more than 50 interventions aimed at improving patient outcomes (Axelson, Gerdtham, Ekman, Hoa, & Alfvén, 2012).

UNDERSTANDING INDIA'S MATERNAL AND CHILD HEALTH CHALLENGES

India's overall IMR in 2015 was 36 (World Bank Data, 2015)—more than double that of Europe or the Americas. The country's MMR was 174 (per 100,000 live births) in 2015, down from 560 in 1990. The number in the United States that year was 14; in Europe, 8. Reasons for the improvement in India's MMR may include improved access to and quality of emergency obstetric care.

One maternal and child health study in India found that regions with lower household incomes and female literacy rates were also likely to see lower infant and child survival rates, regardless of the state where a region is located (Singh, Pathak, Chauhan, & Pan, 2011). Rural communities face particularly daunting challenges. India's 2015 IMR was 18 points higher in the nation's rural areas than its urban centers. Back in 2004, it was 24 points higher.

To improve this and other health indicators in rural India, the Government had formed the National Rural Health Mission (NRHM) in 2005. That same year, the NRHM introduced accredited social health activist (ASHA) workers to enhance use of healthcare services in villages. Each volunteer ASHA is trained in maternal and child health management for 1,000 rural citizens. But despite the training that ASHAs receive, they still lack some important knowledge regarding child health and morbidity (Shrivastava & Shrivastava, 2012). A study found that many ASHAs are not literate. Moreover, nearly 46% of them have less than a secondary-school education level, even though the NRHM requires ASHAs to have achieved at least an eighth-grade level. Supervision of and support for ASHAs have also proved inadequate, resulting in low coverage of health services for mothers, newborns, and children, especially for complicated cases (Modi et al., 2015).

The NRHM also incorporated a home-based neonatal care program, pioneered by SEARCH, into ASHA training in 2007. During that same year, the NRHM launched the Village Health and Nutrition Day program as well. The program provided health and nutrition services and counselling to the community on a pre-designated day, time, and place every month, delivering healthcare services in villages in many states of India.

But efforts in India to improve material and child care had even earlier origins. For instance, in 1960, the Government launched an auxiliary nurse midwife program, which focuses on providing pre- and antenatal checkups and family planning services as well as prescribing supplements for pregnant woman and immunizations for babies. And in 1975, it appointed Anganwadi ("courtyard shelter") workers to be responsible for providing child nutrition, development, and health education for pregnant women in rural areas, with the aim of combating child hunger and malnutrition (Fotso, Higgins-Steele, & Mohanty, 2015).

Despite such efforts, health-care awareness and practice remain meager across India's rural regions (Saxena, Kumar, Kumari, Nath, & Pal, 2015). India's most recent Annual Health Survey, conducted during 2010-2011, still shows higher IMRs and MMRs for the nation's rural areas over its urban centers.

NGOs such as CARE, the United States Agency for International Development (USAID), and The Bill and Melinda Gates Foundation (BMGF) have been running maternal and child health programs in India, suggesting the possibility of future improvement. For instance, CARE partners with local governmental and non-governmental organizations comprising individuals who understand specific locations' cultural, political, and social contexts. The aim is to promote newborn healthcare, including encouraging immunization and reducing malnutrition; to prevent infant and maternal deaths; and to protect those affected by or susceptible to HIV/AIDS and tuberculosis. In 2014, USAID concluded its five-year Maternal and Child Health Integrated Program, which was instrumental in the establishment of five national nodal centers of excellence for nursing and midwifery education across the country.

The BMGF funds maternal and child health programs exclusively in the Indian states of Bihar and Uttar Pradesh. In these initiatives, front-line workers in the state collaborate to meet team-based objectives such as making sure that at least 70% of deliveries included appropriate umbilical cord care (Rotz et al., 2014). The Manthan project, funded by the BMGF, supplied ASHAs with mSakhi, a mobile-phone-based multimedia job aid, to help them update their skills and overcome operational challenges such as lack of access to healthcare information as they carry out their work (Pradesh, Asha, Project, & Play, 2013).

Such programs have greatly reduced IMRs and MMRs in many areas within India. However, much more improvement is needed, on criteria such as health awareness and demand, education, and health-worker training. In both rural and urban India, implementation of the following strategies could help drive these improvements:

- Community-based programs
- Public recognition of successes
- More accessible, sustainable, and low-cost healthcare solutions
- Involvement of local men in maternal and child health programs
- Monitoring of female child sex ratio, to check the alarming decline; the number of girls born per 1,000 boys dropped from 945 in 1991 to 927 in 2001 to 914 in 2011, the year of the last census
- Inclusion of remote and marginalized individuals as beneficiaries in maternal and child health programs
- Solutions aimed at factors affecting MMR; namely, malaria, HIV/AIDS, tuberculosis, and hemorrhage
- Incorporation of mobile technology in programs to improve service utilization

Most important, program leaders must find a way to replicate successful programs in other parts of India and the world afflicted with high IMRs and MMRs, while also tailoring these efforts to each community's unique cultural context. With this imperative in mind, we turn now to a closer examination of the MANSI program.

Methods

We drew on both empirical and theoretical methods for the research presented in this paper. Interviews, observations, and statistics formed the basis of the empirical methods. The first author made two trips to rural India (in 2014 and 2015) to interview MANSI stakeholders and medical officers at primary healthcare centers. The 22 interviews of stakeholders in the MANSI organization and 13 interviews with doctors at the centers illuminated the unique characteristics of and challenges facing the Seraikela area in Jharkhand state. The theoretical methods we used consist of network diagrams and system dynamics (AT, 2012) modeling derived from tools that the first author learned in classes taken at MIT. Together, the field observations and modeling methods enabled us to analyze the MANSI program as a system and consider ways in which the program might be improved and replicated in other needy communities.

Toward these ends, we took the following steps:

1. Gathered information and reviewed scientific knowledge on the problem of high IMRs and MMRs in rural parts of India (Hordijk, 2014).
2. Determined the goals of MANSI stakeholders, including people throughout MANSI's chain of command, community health workers, and doctors at the primary healthcare centers.
3. Identified alternative ways of achieving those goals.
4. Reconsidered the problem in light of the knowledge accumulated.
5. Estimated the impacts of the various courses of action and actions needed to implement them.
6. Assessed possible impacts and consequences of different courses of action.
7. Presented study results in a framework intended to help stakeholders make informed choices about next steps in scaling MANSI.

MANSI AS A SYSTEM

One of India's poorer states, Jharkhand is the only state that saw a decline in institutional births between the last two rounds of the District Level Household Survey (DLHS-2 in 2002 and DHLS-3 in 2007). Jharkhand also has some of the country's highest MMRs (219 per 100,000 live births, versus India's 178), along with large tribal populations afflicted by undernutrition and chronic poverty.

The MANSI program was launched in late 2008 to improve maternal and child health in Jharkhand's Seraikela area. The program trains, empowers, supports, and monitors community health workers called Sahiyas (similar to ASHAs) to perform maternal and child health duties. For instance, MANSI advocates for Sahiyas among community members and healthcare workers, so that people become more willing to follow Sahiyas' guidance. The ultimate goal is to improve IMRs and MMRs.

Figure 3 shows MANSI's organizational structure. Seraikela was divided into four zones, and each zone was assigned a coordinator to manage maternal and neonatal health mobilizers there. A field coordinator managed the Seraikela field office as well as served as a liaison between the zone coordinators and the Tata Steel Rural Development Society (TSRDS) and American Indian Foundation (AIF) program managers. Health mobilizers are local residents familiar with Seraikela's language and customs and appointed to train, support, and monitor Sahiyas across villages in the area.

Figure 3. MANSI organizational structure (Initiative & Lives, n.d.)

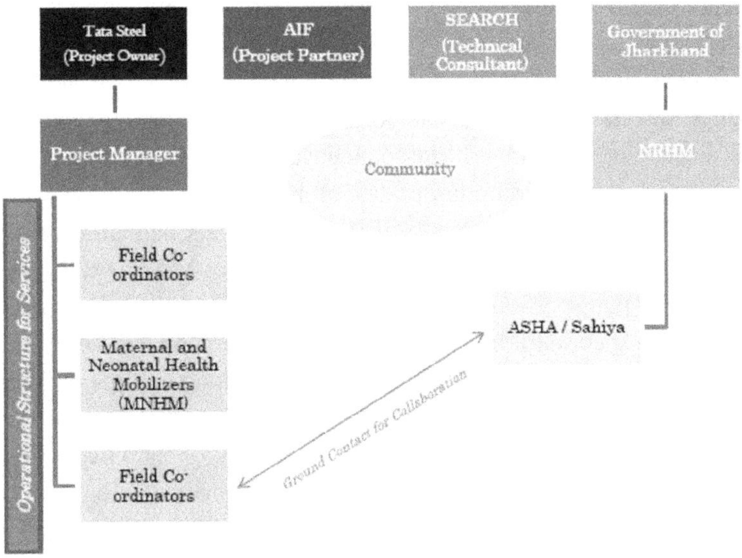

The MANSI pilot program served a population totaling 83,000 across 167 villages and involved 196 Sahiyas. It had 24 people (19 maternal and neonatal health mobilizers, 4 zone coordinators, and 1 field coordinator) on board to manage the area. The MANSI staff interacted with state government health authorities at different levels, to inform them about the program's goals or to get approval to provide services in specific villages, depending on the activities planned. Because the MANSI program was a pilot, TSRDS and AIF closely monitored its execution and invested heavily in building relationships and trust between the MANSI organization and program stakeholders, including SEARCH and community and state government agencies.

The MANSI organization completed a knowledge and skill assessment for Seraikela and each Sahiya before the program started. Assessment results helped MANSI staff design training, build infrastructure capacity, and generate demand for maternal and child healthcare services in the villages. The results also led to ideas for fostering behavior changes such as use of prenatal vitamins, management of supplies such as Sahiya kits, and advocacy of the MANSI program's offerings. The assessment also helped the organization understand major challenges confronting Seraikela; namely, cultural stigmas against feeding a new mother during the first few days after birth, barriers to adoption of new medicines and Sahiya services, discrimination against women, lack of access to healthcare, and community members' lack of trust in government services.

MANSI leaders and Sahiyas regularly met with community members to advocate for acceptance of and requests for Sahiya services by the community. These meetings increased villagers' awareness of the MANSI program, intensified demand for better health services in the area, and fostered dissemination of information about how to access Sahiya services throughout the community. Such meetings, which are still being held, are attended by village heads, panchayat members, and members of village health sanitation and nutrition committees, along with auxiliary nurse midwives, Anganwadi workers, Sahiyas, members of self-help groups, and village residents. At the meetings, Sahiyas discuss what they have learned at MANSI training sessions and explain when people should seek their support. The MANSI representatives highlight Sahiyas' successful interventions to boost demand for their services.

Sahiyas carry a kit, as shown in Figure 4, containing supplies for monitoring, diagnosing, and treating infants in ways that follow home-based newborn care (HBNC) methods. Given the inconsistent quality and reliability of the government supply chain, MANSI decided to supply and manage kit inventories in the pilot program.

At the outset of the MANSI program, staff advocated for improving healthcare access, awareness, and services, starting with making requests to incorporate the more rigorous SEARCH-based form of HBNC. During implementation of the program, the MANSI team needed to persuade local health clinicians to accept use of Sahiyas' services. Staff also advocated for pregnant women and children who needed timely and appropriate services at the local healthcare facility. And if the healthcare representatives demanded bribes to provide services to pregnant women and small children, the staff relayed the issue to higher officials to stop the practice.

Figure 4. Sahiya and kit

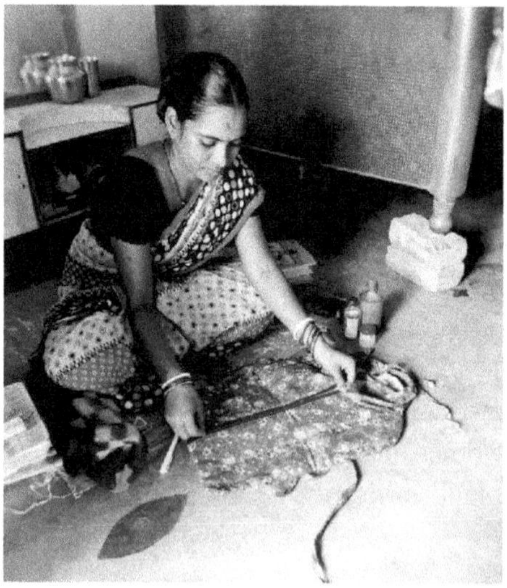

If a pregnant woman's family did not support her following the nutrition and check-up schedule arranged by the Sahiya, then the Sahiya and the maternal and neonatal health mobilizer counseled the woman and her family to support the prenatal plan. If counseling did not change things, then the Sahiya approached a village elder or an auxiliary nurse midwife and asked her to counsel the family on the importance of following the schedule.

MANSI aimed to provide quality in its training, operations, supplies, and support. Toward that end, SEARCH made random visits to villages throughout implementation of the program and assessed delivery of MANSI services. This process played a key role in ensuring the program's effectiveness.

As the Sahiyas' effectiveness, experience, and confidence have increased, so have their status in the eyes of villagers and of local doctors. Indeed, many villagers have begun calling Sahiyas "Doctor Didi" ("Doctor older sister"). Sahiyas are especially proud to show off their rating registers, where people have written appreciative comments. One Sahiya interviewed for this paper, Babita Mahato, stated, "The parents tell me that because I was there the baby survived." Sahiyas receive monetary rewards for bringing pregnant women to the hospital for pre-natal checkups and delivery. The money comes only from the Mukhya Mantri Janani Sishu Suraksha Abhiyan/Janani Suraksha Yojna (MMJSSA/JSY) program, not from the MANSI organization. In lieu of giving cash rewards, MANSI holds an annual meeting to publically recognize and reward Sahiyas' positive contributions to the community. At the meeting, Sahiyas receive non-monetary gifts such as clothing and kitchen items.

SYSTEM ANALYSIS

MANSI's intent was to sustainably improve IMRs and MMRs in Seraikela villages. The intent would be achieved through implementation of rigorous HBNC based on community engagement (Sahiyas using kits) through the existing health system.

Analysis of the MANSI pilot program design shows that it meets the intent, follows rigorous HBNC protocols from SEARCH, and uses the form and tools of the existing health system (Sahiyas and kits). Community engagement in the program was critical to ensure its success in improving IMRs and MMRs. MANSI is also sustainable in financial terms, as it does not give cash incentives to Sahiyas. However, since MANSI supplies the Sahiya kits, and since maternal and neonatal health mobilizers must support and monitor Sahiyas, the system is not sustainable without MANSI's presence. This suggests that replicating and scaling MANSI in other locations will prove difficult unless MANSI can establish an equally strong presence in those other locations.

Figure 5. Information, finance, and supply flows

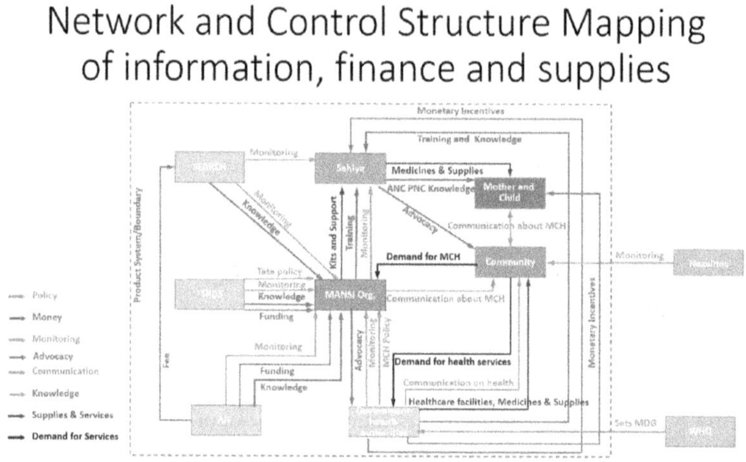

The flow of information, finance, and supplies among the MANSI program's stakeholders is complex, as Figure 5 shows. Sahiyas receive training, goods (such as medicines and kit supplies), services (including advocacy and support), and money, and are monitored closely by other stakeholders such as SEARCH. Members of the community generate demand for quality maternal and child health services and medicines at state government healthcare facilities.

SYSTEM DYNAMICS

Community meetings, Sahiya training sessions, successful advocacy, and empowerment of villagers to seek new pre- and post-natal amenities generated demand for healthcare services in Seraikela. Together, these forces helped elevate Sahiyas' status as well as that of the pregnant women in these villages. This is an example of emergence, a phenomenon that occurs when a system's elements interact in ways that create value greater than the sum of those elements.

Indeed, we usually cannot understand a system's behavior merely by understanding its elements (Meadows, 2008), because those elements interact in complex, dynamic ways. System dynamics modeling can shed light on how a system's elements are changing and interacting, and how such dynamics are affecting the quality of the system's output. Such modeling can therefore help system designers identify ways to make the system as effective as possible.

Figure 6. System dynamics model of Sahiya interactions

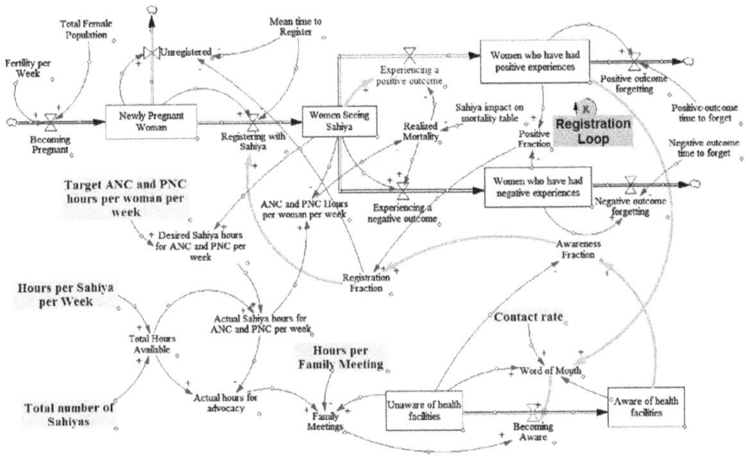

With these benefits in mind, we developed a simplified system dynamics model of MANSI that emphasized Sahiyas' impact on the program's effectiveness. In particular, the model tested the impact of one variable critical to scaling and replicating the program in other locations: total number of Sahiyas. This variable affects Sahiyas' interactions with members of the local communities where they provide services. By understanding the optimum number of Sahiyas for MANSI to achieve its intent, program leaders can make informed choices about key elements of the system, such as training, support, and logistics. Figure 6 shows the modeling of Sahiya interactions in the MANSI system.

Because Sahiyas' interactions with members of the community directly affect mortality of women and children, this model focuses on the relationship between the number of Sahiyas and IMR and MMR. The system's exogenous variables include the following:

- **Total number of Sahiyas:** This variable was set at 100, 150, 196, and 250 during runs of the simulation.
- **Hours per Sahiya per week:** This variable denotes the number of hours that a Sahiya devotes to her work per week, set at 20 for the simulation.
- **Contact rate:** This is the number of times a week that a woman or family who has had a positive experience with a Sahiya is likely to meet other members of the community who are unaware of the health facilities and Sahiya services in the area and to positively influence their perception of these resources. For the simulation, the rate was set at 3 people per week per woman or family.

- **Target antenatal care (ANC) and postnatal care (PNC) hours per woman per week:** This variable denotes the number of hours that a Sahiya interacts with each pregnant woman for ANC and PNC per week. The variable directly influences Seraikela's IMRs and MMRs. A normal pregnancy lasts about 36 weeks, and PNC is usually provided for 6 weeks after that. Over the 42 weeks covered by ANC and PNC, the Sahiya meets the pregnant woman 1 time per month for ANC and then 7 times during the 6 weeks of PNC. We thus calculate this variable as 9 (ANC) + 7 (PNC) / 42 (weeks) = 0.38 hours/woman/week.
- **Hours per family meeting:** This variable, set at 0.25 for the simulation, denotes the number of hours per week per family that a Sahiya needs to advocate ANC and PNC methods.

Closed-loop models comprise two basic types of loops: reinforcing and balancing. Reinforcing loops produce growth or decay, as they compound change in one direction with even more change. Balancing loops (also called goal-seeking processes) try to bring specific aspects of a system to a desired state. In the Sahiya-interactions system, the Registration loop, shown in greater detail in Figure 7, is an example of a reinforcing loop.

As the value of each variable in this loop increases, the next variable increases as well, creating the reinforcing dynamic. Figure 8 depicts how changing number of Sahiyas affects two other variables: number of families who are aware of health facilities, and registration fraction (number of pregnant women who register with the Sahiya and avail themselves of her healthcare services).

Figure 7. Registration as a reinforcing loop

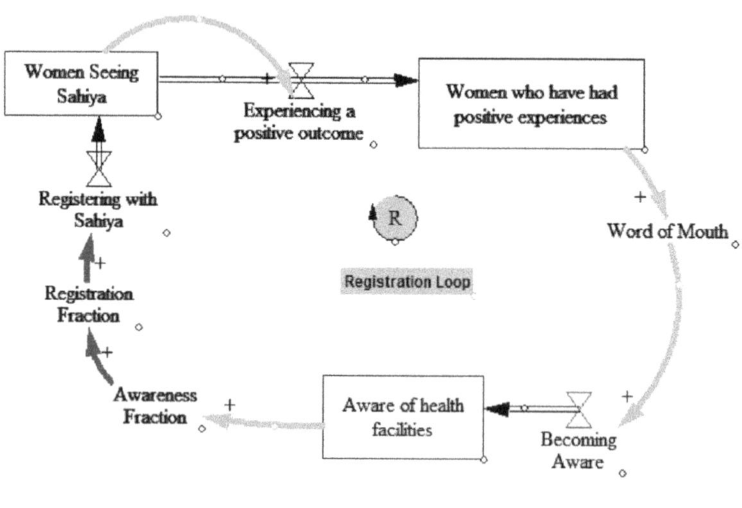

Figure 8. Variables in the Registration reinforcing loop

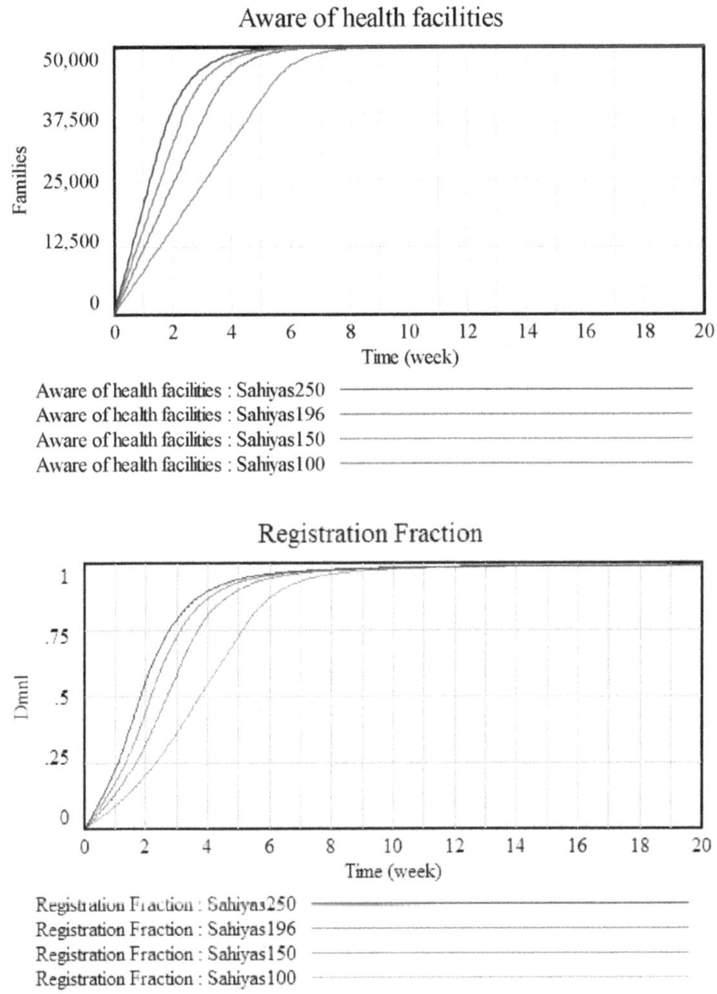

The simulation's results suggest that 150 Sahiyas is the optimum number for maximizing both awareness of health facilities and registration fraction.

All system dynamic models rest on assumptions that the model designers make, drawing on their knowledge of the defining characteristics of the system in question. In the MANSI system, such characteristics include how human beings interact in rural communities. The assumptions underlying the Sahiya-interaction model could be refined through additional research and a sensitivity analysis. We could also make the model more realistic and thus gain additional insights from it by expanding the system's boundaries to include the public-private partnership elements as well as availability of supplies and training.

IMPLEMENTING MANSI IN INDIA

India is home to a largely patriarchal society with significant inequities along dimensions of gender, caste, literacy, religion, and locality ("Social determinants of health in India: progress and inequities across stat...: BartonPlus," n.d.). Such inequities powerfully affect who has access to good healthcare. The MANSI program works well in Seraikela because it makes basic healthcare available to rural women regardless of their caste and religion. Moreover, caste and gender discrimination are not as strong in Seraikela as it is in other parts of India. In places where women have low status and where caste matters much more, any community-based program would have to be backed by strong advocacy in order to succeed.

In India, access to healthcare is also constrained by corruption in the public sector, which creates an environment characterized by lack of trust between healthcare service providers and patients (Berger, 2014). Moreover, in many parts of India, the public and private sectors are not inclined to work together because of bureaucracy and politics. But the PPP model works well for the MANSI program in Seraikela. There, Tata Steel has earned local citizens' trust and has forged good relationships with local government authorities to overcome corruption in healthcare delivery and to ensure accountability of healthcare providers for quality of services, facilities, and medicines. A social audit of potential new locations for a MANSI-type program could help uncover issues of low accountability, lack of trust, and corruption, setting the stage for designing an effective program.

RECOMMENDATIONS FOR SUCCESS

Consistent availability of training, supplies, monitoring, and a focus on the community's welfare appear crucial to the MANSI program's success. Program teams seeking to launch similar efforts in other areas could learn much from this insight, and possibly avoid failures experienced by maternal and child health programs implemented in Pakistan.

With these points in mind, Table 1 lists policy recommendations for each program stakeholder during each phase of a similarly intended program, along with a rough indication of cost.

To improve the MANSI program in areas with different cultural, political, and infrastructure characteristics from Seraikela's, we offer the following system design and management recommendations:

Table 1. Recommendations for stakeholders, per phase

Stakeholders/ Timeline	Planning	Implementation : Phase 1 (first 6 months)	Implementation : Phase 2 (6 months to 3 years)	Implementation :Phase 3 (3 years and beyond)
Women and children	Assess needs and traditional practices $	Register, educate, set up ANC and PNC, advocate, empower $$$	Register, educate, set up ANC and PNC, advocate, empower $$	Register, educate, set up ANC and PNC, advocate, empower $$
Sahiyas	Assess training needs $	Train on rigorous HBNC methods, empower $$	Provide refresher training, support, supplies; reward and monitor $$	Provide refresher training, support, supplies; reward and monitor $$
Community	Assess needs and traditional practices $	Generate demand, advocate, train, build trust and accountability $$	Advocate, train, empower, build trust and accountability $$	Advocate, empower, build trust and accountability $
Government	Assess needs, infrastructur e, and policies $	Set up and implement policy, training, infrastructure, and supplies; build trust and accountability $$$	Manage infrastructure, supplies, program; generate demand; build trust and accountability $$	Manage infrastructure, technology, supplies, analytics, education; generate demand; build trust and accountability $$
Non-	Assess needs	Set up and	Monitor	Hand governance over to local

Build Community

- Include public sector and village health authorities in Sahiya training.
- Integrate fathers and mothers-in-law in new-mother education.
- Support better education and livelihoods for poor and rural families.
- Reinforce child health practices through regular community meetings.

Boost Empowerment

- Encourage women, families, and community members to speak up for their newborns and to challenge assumptions that infant deaths are inevitable.

Ensure Continuity of Healthcare

- Monitor children from birth to 5 years of age.
- Regulate, qualify, and integrate non-degree allopathic practitioners (NDAPs) as part of the existing public health care system in India (May, Roth, & Panda, 2014).
- Increase the number of health workers with skills required for delivering high-quality care for newborns as well as mothers and children (Mason et al., 2014).

Leverage Technology

- Use electronic medical records in partnership with primary healthcare clinics to collect and use healthcare data to improve patient outcomes.
- Use audio visual aids to educate women and families on needed behavioral changes.

Provide Ongoing Sahiya Training

- In Sahiya training sessions, emphasize high-risk cases requiring prompt referral (Shrivastava & Shrivastava, 2012).

Generate Demand for Program Services

- Use songs to teach families about healthcare methods.
- Involve revered film stars and cricketers in advocating for better health outcomes for women and children.
- Create comics and stories relaying the importance of improving health outcomes.

Step Up Political Involvement

- Focus political leaders' attention on the importance of addressing high mortality rates among pregnant women and infants.
- Include governance at the panchayat level, the most local level of governance in India.

Improve Financing

- Focus on investing in better mortality outcomes and harmonized funding (Akseer et al., 2015) between public and private partners, so funds reach the right programs, in the right areas, and programs meet state and local goals.
- Franchise the existing MANSI model to other government or nonprofit groups to facilitate scaling.

CONCLUSION

In 2015, every day, as many as 16,000 children in Southern and Central Asia and in sub-Saharan Africa and Oceania died, most of them from preventable causes (UNICEF 2015). The global MMR decreased 45% during 1990-2013, but it needs to drop another 50% to meet MDG 5 targets. In 2013, an estimated 289,000 women died (roughly 800 each day), primarily in Southern Asia and sub-Saharan Africa.

These numbers are unacceptable. A repeatable, scalable, low-cost program similar to MANSI could reduce neonatal mortality by nearly 33% and lead to a 50% increase in hospital births, further improving newborns' chances of survival.

MANSI saves lives at a cost of just $25 per mother and child. The program works by giving Sahiyas the training, support, and supplies needed for them to ensure that women and their children get appropriate antenatal, childbirth, and postnatal care. During 2013-2015, the program saved an estimated 1,800 newborns' lives. Sahiyas always encourage women to give birth at a healthcare facility whenever possible. But if that is not possible, they make sure that new mothers deliver in a clean room. They cut the infant's umbilical cord with a new, sterile single-edge blade to avoid infection. And they help the mother to start breastfeeding her baby as soon as possible. If this program can be scaled and replicated in other parts of India and around the world, untold thousands of additional lives could be saved.

Future research directions will include systems analyses of scaled or replicated MANSI systems in India and other countries to add to the collective wisdom of best practices in reducing IMR and MMR. A similar analysis approach on other successful programs for reducing IMR and MMR needs to be conducted as well.

REFERENCES

Akseer, N., Lawn, J. E., Keenan, W., Konstantopoulos, A., Cooper, P., Ismail, Z., ... Bhutta, Z. A. (2015). Ending preventable newborn deaths in a generation. *International Journal of Gynaecology and Obstetrics, 131*, S43–S48. doi:10.1016/j.ijgo.2015.03.017 PMID:26433505

Awoonor-Williams, J. K., Sory, E. K., Nyonator, F. K., Phillips, J. F., Wang, C., & Schmitt, M. L. (2013). Lessons learned from scaling up a community-based health program in the Upper East Region of northern Ghana. *Global Health, Science and Practice, 1*(1), 117–133. doi:10.9745/GHSP-D-12-00012 PMID:25276522

Axelson, H., Gerdtham, U.-G., Ekman, B., Hoa, D. T., & Alfvén, T. (2012). Inequalities in reproductive, maternal, newborn and child health in Vietnam: A retrospective study of survey data for 1997–2006. *BMC Health Services Research, 12*(1), 456. doi:10.1186/1472-6963-12-456 PMID:23237475

Bandyopadhyay, M. (2009). Impact of ritual pollution on lactation and breastfeeding practices in rural West Bengal, India. *International Breastfeeding Journal, 4*(1), 2. doi:10.1186/1746-4358-4-2 PMID:19323839

Berger, D. (2014). Corruption ruins the doctor-patient relationship in India. *BMJ (Clinical Research Ed.), 348*, g3169.

Cowling, K., Dandona, R., & Dandona, L. (2014). Social determinants of health in India: Progress and inequities across states. *International Journal for Equity in Health, 13*(1), 88.

Fotso, J. C., Higgins-Steele, A., & Mohanty, S. (2015). Male engagement as a strategy to improve utilization and community-based delivery of maternal, newborn and child health services: Evidence from an intervention in Odisha, India. *BMC Health Services Research, 15*(Suppl. 1), S5. doi:10.1186/1472-6963-15-S1-S5 PMID:26062910

Hordijk, L. (2014). What is Systems Analysis. Retrieved October 20, 2015, from http://www.iiasa.ac.at/web/home/about/whatisiiasa/whatissystemsanalysis/what_is_systems_analysis.html

Intrahealth International. (2013, September). mSakhi: An interactive mobile phone-based job aid for accredited social health activists (ASHAs).

Mason, E., McDougall, L., Lawn, J. E., Gupta, A., Claeson, M., Pillay, Y. ..., & Chopra, M. (2014). From evidence to action to deliver a healthy start for the next generation. *Lancet, 384*(9941), 455–467. doi:10.1016/S0140-6736(14)60750-9 PMID:24853599

May, C., Roth, K., & Panda, P. (2014). Non-degree allopathic practitioners as first contact points for acute illness episodes: Insights from a qualitative study in rural northern India. *BMC Health Services Research, 14*(1), 182. doi:10.1186/1472-6963-14-182 PMID:24755399

Meadows, D. H. (2008). *Thinking in systems: A primer*. Chelsea Green Publishing.

Modi, D., Gopalan, R., Shah, S., Venkatraman, S., Desai, G., Desai, S., & Shah, P. (2015). Development and formative evaluation of an innovative mHealth intervention for improving coverage of community-based maternal, newborn and child health services in rural areas of India. *Global Health Action, 8*(1), 26769. doi:10.3402/gha.v8.26769 PMID:25697233

Nagarajan, R. (2011). Mother and child: Survival not guaranteed. *The Times of India*. Retrieved November 25, 2015, from http://timesofindia.indiatimes.com/india/Mother-and-child-Survival-not-guaranteed-/articleshow/8796351.cms?referral=PM

Rotz, D., Rangarajan, A., Borkum, E., Sridharan, S., Sethi, S., & Manoranjini, M. (2014). *Promising findings from the frontline health worker team-based goals and incentives intervention in Bihar*. Mathematica Policy Research.

Sartorius, B. K., Sartorius, K., Chirwa, T. F., & Fonn, S. (2011). Infant mortality in South Africa - distribution, associations and policy implications, 2007: An ecological spatial analysis. *International Journal of Health Geographics, 10*(1), 61. doi:10.1186/1476-072X-10-61 PMID:22093084

Saxena, V., Kumar, P., Kumari, R., Nath, B., & Pal, R. (2015). Availability of Village Health and Nutrition Day services in Uttarakhand, India. *Journal of Family Medicine and Primary Care, 4*(2), 251–256. doi:10.4103/2249-4863.154667 PMID:25949976

Shrivastava, S. R., & Shrivastava, P. S. (2012). Evaluation of trained Accredited Social Health Activist (ASHA) workers regarding their knowledge, attitude and practices about child health. [pii]. *Rural and Remote Health, 12*(4), 2099. PMID:23198703

Shrivastava, S. R., & Shrivastava, P. S. (2012). Evaluation of trained Accredited Social Health Activist (ASHA) workers regarding their knowledge, attitude and practices about child health. *Rural and Remote Health, 12*(4), 2099. PMID:23198703

Singh, A., Pathak, P. K., Chauhan, R. K., & Pan, W. (2011). Infant and child mortality in India in the last two decades: A geospatial analysis. *PLoS One*, *6*(11), e26856. doi:10.1371/journal.pone.0026856 PMID:22073208

Tran, P. (2013). Analysis: Nepal's maternal mortality decline paradox. *IRIN Asia*. Retrieved September 22, 2015, from http://www.irinnews.org/report/97667/analysis-nepal-s-maternal-mortality-decline-paradox

WHO EMRO. (2014). Community participation eludes Pakistan's maternal, newborn and child health programme. *EMHJ*, *20*(1). Retrieved September 20, 2015, from http://www.emro.who.int/emhj-vol-20-2014/volume-20-issue-1/community-participation-eludes-pakistans-maternal-newborn-and-child-health-programme.html

World Economic Forum. (n.d.). Global Gender Gap Report 2014. Retrieved November 25, 2015, from http://reports.weforum.org/global-gender-gap-report-2014/part-1/the-global-gender-gap-index-results-in-2014/country-results/

World Health Organisation. (2013). Maternal mortality. Retrieved from http://www.who.int/gho/maternal_health/mortality/maternal_mortality_text/en/

This research was previously published in the International Journal of System Dynamics Applications (IJSDA), 8(1); edited by Ahmad Taher Azar; pages 94-111, copyright year 2019 by IGI Publishing (an imprint of IGI Global).

Chapter 11
Sustainable Development Goal 3 and Maternal Health in Nigeria:
Any Hope of Meeting the Target by 2030?

Idongesit Eshiet
University of Lagos, Nigeria

ABSTRACT

This chapter addresses the feasibility of Nigeria achieving Target 3.1 of Sustainable Development Goal 3, which aims at reducing maternal deaths to less than 70 per 100,000 live births by 2030. Maternal deaths occur due to lack of access to maternal healthcare, which encompasses the healthcare dimensions of family planning, preconception, prenatal, and postnatal care for women. Nigeria is presently the second largest contributor to maternal deaths globally, having a maternal mortality ratio of 814 per 100,000 live births. Will Nigeria achieve this goal by 2030? This chapter assesses the maternal health landscape of Nigeria and the measures taken by the government to address maternal health from the perspective of the feasibility of achieving SDG 3, Target 3.1 by 2030.

DOI: 10.4018/978-1-7998-2351-3.ch011

INTRODUCTION

Maternal morbidity and mortality have remained an endemic health issue for women through the ages. However, to stem the tide of maternal mortality, the United Nations had as its fifth Millennium Development Goal - a commitment to improve maternal health. The goal targeted a reduction in maternal mortality ratio by three-quarters between 1990 and 2015, as well as the achievement of universal access to reproductive health by the same year (United Nations (UN), 2005). Subsequently, the goal spurred up commitments by various national governments to maternal healthcare. This led to a reduction in maternal deaths. Thus, maternal mortality ratio declined globally by about 44 per cent - from 385 deaths to 216 deaths per 100,000 live births. Similarly, the approximate global lifetime risk of maternal death fell considerably from 1 in 73 in 1990 to 1 in 180 in 2015 (WHO, 2015). Statistically, this meant a 2.3 per cent annual rate reduction - a remarkable progress, but it unfortunately failed to meet the estimated 5.5 per cent annual rate reduction that was needed to achieve the targeted three-quarters reduction in 2015 (WHO, 2015).

This progress in stemming maternal deaths is however, unevenly distributed among the different regions of the world. While the developed world has been freed from the shackles of maternal deaths, the developing world is still grappling with the challenge. A majority of the deaths still occurs in the developing world. For example, the developing world accounted for approximately 99% (302,000) of the deaths in 2015, and had a maternal mortality ratio of 239. This was 20 times higher than the 12 deaths per 100,000 live births that occurred in the developed world. Similarly, the estimated lifetime risk of maternal death in the developing world stands at 1 in 3,300, as compared with 1 in 41in the developing world (WHO, 2015).

Regionally, sub-Saharan Africa has the highest maternal mortality ratio. It accounted for about 66% (201,000) of the deaths in 2015 with a maternal mortality ratio of 546. Equally, a woman's life time risk of dying during or following a pregnancy in sub-Saharan Africa, is estimated at 1 in 36 as compared to 1 in 4,900 for the developed world (WHO, 2015). At the country level, Nigeria and India are estimated to account for over one third of all maternal deaths globally. Nigeria accounted for 19% (58,000) with a maternal mortality ratio of 814 in 2015, while India accounted for 15% (45,000) of the deaths (WHO, 2015).

The Millennium Development Goal 5 has been rested, as the target year (2015) for its achievement had come and gone. Although, its targets of reducing maternal mortality ratio by three-quarters and the achievement of a universal access to reproductive health were not achieved, nevertheless, the progress made as a result of the goal is quite remarkable. Field findings reveal that all regions of the world that implemented the Millennium Development Goals have experienced considerable reductions in maternal mortality rate (UN, 2015). In view of this, the Sustainable

Development Goals (SDGs) (which replaced the Millennium Development Goals), have established a transformative new agenda for maternal health, towards ending preventable maternal mortality. Thus, Target 3.1 of SDG 3 (Ensure Healthy Lives and Promote well-being for all at all Ages), aims at reducing the global Maternal Mortality Ratio (MMR) to less than 70 per 100,000 live births by 2030 (UN, 2016).

Will Nigeria achieve this target with a current maternal mortality ratio of 814 deaths per 100,000 live births? What policies and actions has the Nigerian state taken to address the problem of high maternal mortality ratio, in line with the World Health Organization's advice to countries to identify and address the barriers that limit access to quality maternal healthcare? These are some of the contending issues that this chapter interrogates.

BACKGROUND

Maternal health refers to the health of women during pregnancy, childbirth and the postpartum period. It encompasses the health care dimensions of family planning, preconception, prenatal and postnatal care, which aims at reducing maternal morbidity and mortality (World Health Organization (WHO), 2012[a]).

- **Family Planning:** Refers to a conscious effort by a couple to limit their family size or space their children through the use of contraceptives. According to the World Health Organization (WHO), a vital issue in tackling maternal morbidity and mortality is the prevention of unwanted and too-early pregnancies. Thus, the Organization observes that satisfying the unmet need for family planning of women alone could reduce the number of maternal deaths by almost a third (WHO, 2012[b]). The Organization therefore, advocates that all women including adolescents should be given access to family planning (WHO, 2012[a]).
- **Antenatal Care (ANC):** Refers to the medical care of a woman during pregnancy. The major objective of antenatal care is to ensure optimal health outcomes for the mother and child. Antenatal care from a trained healthcare provider helps to monitor the pregnancy and reduce morbidity risks for mother and child during pregnancy and delivery. It has been observed that ANC provides the following benefits for mother and child:

(a) it enables early detection of complications and prompt treatment (for example, detection and treatment of sexually transmitted infections, malaria, high blood pressure, etc.) (b) it enables the prevention of diseases through immunization and micronutrient supplementation (c) it enables birth preparedness and complication

readiness and (d) it enables health promotion and disease prevention through health messages and counselling. (National Population Commission & ICF International, 2014, p. 128)

The World Health Organization recommends a minimum of four ANC visits for every pregnant woman who has no complications. The first visit should occur by the end of 16 weeks of pregnancy, the second visit should be between 24 and 28 weeks of pregnancy, while the third visit should be by 32 weeks and the fourth visit by 36 weeks. However, women with complications, special needs or conditions beyond the scope of basic care may require additional visits (National Population Commission & ICF International, 2014). Nigeria's ANC policy aligns with that of the WHO.

- **Delivery Care:** Entails delivery in a health facility and by a skilled attendant – skilled attendance at delivery encompasses the presence of health professionals such as doctors, midwives, and nurses as well as an enabling environment, where the equipment, drugs and other resources required for effective and efficient management of complications are available. Evidence from the developed world shows that delivery in health facility and by a skilled attendant are the factors that have aided the drastic reduction in maternal deaths (Adamu, 2011; Kruk, Galea, Prescott, & Freedman, 2007).
- **Postnatal Care (PNC):** The postnatal period is the time from immediately after birth up to 40 days. The postpartum period is particularly important for women, because during this period, they may develop serious life-threatening complications, especially in the interval immediately after delivery. Evidence shows that a large proportion of maternal and neonatal deaths occur during the first 48 hours after delivery (National Population Commission & ICF International, 2014; Adamu, 2011). Thus, receiving postnatal care is critical in making a difference between life and death for mother and child (WHO, 2012[a]). Postnatal care visits also provide opportunity to learn and acquire information on issues such as family planning, maternal and child nutrition, immunization, hygiene and sanitation, etc. (USAID, 2009). WHO recommends that all women receive a health check within three days of giving birth.

Factors Influencing Uptake of Maternal Healthcare

Healthcare solutions to prevent or manage maternal health issues are well known, according to the World Health Organization (WHO, 2012[a]). Thus, all that a woman needs is to have access to antenatal care in pregnancy, skilled care during childbirth, and care and support in the weeks after childbirth, in order to escape an unnecessary death (WHO, 2012[a]). However, there are certain factors that may impede access to maternal healthcare. These factors include socio-economic, demographic, cultural and geographical factors.

Studies reveal mother's age at child birth as influencing utilization of maternal healthcare, although there are contradictory findings with regard to the direction of the effect of mother's age and utilization of maternal healthcare services. While some studies show a lack of association between mother's age and utilization of maternal healthcare services (Magadi et al., 2007; Celik & Hotchkiss, 2000), some others show higher utilization for younger women than older women (Abou-Zahr & Wardlaw, 2001), yet some others show a higher utilization for older women than younger women (Tsawe, Moto, Netshivhera, Ralesego, Nyathi, & Susuman, 2015; Reynolds, Wong, & Tucker, 2006).

Similarly, birth order is shown as a predictor of maternal healthcare services utilization. Evidence shows that women who have more than three living children are more confident about their ability to handle their maternal health issues and so do utilize maternal health services less frequently than those who have had less than three children (Tsawe, Moto, Netshivhera, Ralesego, Nyathi, & Susuman, 2015; Raj Baral, Lyons, Skinner, & van Teijlingen, 2012; Simkhada, Teijlingen, Porter, & Simkhada, 2008). Maternal education is also shown as a factor influencing the utilization of maternal healthcare services. Studies reveal that the higher a woman's level of education, the more likely she is to access and use maternal healthcare services (Tsawe, Moto, Netshivhera, Ralesego, Nyathi, & Susuman, 2015; Ononokpono & Odimegwu, 2014: Ayele, Belayihun, Teji, & Ayana, 2014). However, some other studies do question the independent effect of education on maternal health utilization, arguing that some other factors such as husband's educational level, socio-economic environment do mediate on the association between education and utilization of maternal healthcare services (Gage & Calixte, 2006; Raghupathy, 1996).

Studies similarly show a relationship between women's employment status and access to and utilization of maternal healthcare services. While it could be assumed that working women who earn income would have more autonomy and the financial wherewithal to seek maternal healthcare services, in reality this is not always so, as the context in which women are employed does impact on their access to maternal healthcare services. Thus, the contextual differences in women's employment have given rise to different findings on the association between employment and access to and utilization of maternal health services. Studies reveal a positive relationship between a woman's formal employment and utilization of maternal healthcare services as such healthcare provisioning are part of the official employment benefits (Ononokpono & Odimegwu, 2014; Dalal, Shabnam, Andrews-Chavez, Mårtensson & Timpka, 2012). However, in context where women have no control over their earnings and where women do not earn money for the work they do or where employment is poverty-induced, employment is found not to be associated with maternal healthcare services utilization (Lowe, Chen, & Huang, 2016; Furuta & Salway, 2006; Addai, 2000; Nwakoby 1994).

The place of residence similarly plays a significant role in access to and utilization of maternal healthcare services. Studies show that women who reside in urban areas are more likely to have access to and utilize maternal healthcare services than those who reside in the rural areas (Muchabaiwa, Mazambani, Chigusiwa, Bindu, & Mudavanhu, 2012; Dagne, 2010; Babalola & Fatusi, 2009). This may be attributed to the lopsided healthcare provisioning in developing countries in which sophisticated health facilities are often situated in the urban areas (Peltzer, Skinner, Mfecane, Shisana, Nqeketo, & Mosala, 2005). Thus, issues of accessibility and affordability have been critical factors in determining maternal healthcare utilization as rural women often have to travel long distances before accessing the nearest heath facility (Tsawe & Susuman, 2014; Silal, Penn-Kekana, Harris, Birch, & McIntyre, 2012; Ensor & Cooper, 2004).

Household wealth quintile is also associated with the use of maternal healthcare services. This is however, not surprising, as the use of maternal healthcare services entails some monetary costs such as cost of transportation, medication, user fees, etc. Thus, women from rich families are more likely to utilize maternal healthcare services than women from poor families (Gabrysh & Campbell, 2009). Likewise, the use of maternal healthcare also increases with the wealth quintile of women themselves, thus women from the rich quintile use maternal healthcare services more than those from the poor quintile (Fotso, Ezeh, Madise, Ziraba & Ogollah, 2009).

Religion also mediates access to and utilization of maternal healthcare services. For example, studies reveal a higher use of maternal healthcare services by non-Muslim women, and a lower rate of use by Muslim women (Babalola & Fatusi, 2009; Ethiopian Society of Population Studies, 2008; Addai, 2000). Similarly, cultural factors such as the traditional gender division of labour, patriarchy, which denies women autonomy in decision making, etc. are associated with non-utilization of maternal healthcare services (Lowe, Chen, & Huang, 2016; Ayele, Belayihun, Teji, & Ayana, 2014).

The World Health Organization however, advises countries to identify and address these barriers that limit access to quality maternal healthcare, in order to improve maternal health of their women (WHO, 2012a).

THEORECTICAL FRAMEWORK

The chapter situates its analysis within the functionalist perspective in Sociology. The functionalist perspective derives its analysis from the works of Sociologists such as Herbert Spencer, Emile Durkheim, Talcott Parsons and Robert Merton (Haralambos & Holborn, 2013). Functionalists argue that the society could be viewed as a unified system that is made up of differentiated but interrelated parts that work together for the effective functioning of the whole. These parts are the social institutions such as the family, government, economy, education, health, religion, media, etc., which provide different functions to the society. Since the parts work together for the effective functioning of the whole society, a dysfunction in any of these parts, affects the effective functioning of the whole society.

From this vein, the family institution is one of the component parts of the society that ensures societal continuity by reproducing its members, while the health institution ensures system maintenance by taking care of the sick and health needs of societal members. The family adequately reproduces her members through a functional healthcare system. Therefore, a dysfunctional health institution affects the family's reproductive role and this in turn disrupts the societal functioning.

Maternal death therefore, goes beyond being an individual problem to a societal problem. High maternal deaths such as that, which occur in Nigeria, impede human and societal development. And these deaths cannot be curbed unless the health system and the other institutions of the society are functioning effectively. Empirical evidence shows an association between the level of a country's development and maternal mortality rate (World Economic Forum, 2017a). Thus, in a context of poverty, patriarchy, poor healthcare delivery, poor education, ineffective transportation system and a general atmosphere of underdevelopment, maternal deaths will be high. This explains the difference between the developed and developing world where maternal mortality ratio is 12 and 239 per 100,000 live births respectively and the estimated lifetime risk of maternal death is 1 in 3,300 and 1 in 41for the developed and developing world respectively (UN, 2015). Therefore, from the functionalist perspective, achieving Sustainable Development Goal 3, Target 3.1, in Nigeria requires having a viable healthcare system, as well as a general development of the society that is the effective functioning of all the other social institutions.

METHODOLOGY

The study utilises secondary sources for its analysis. Extant literature in textbooks, journals, government's reports and records as it pertains to the research topic serve as the source materials for the chapter.

MAIN FOCUS OF THE CHAPTER

Maternal Health Landscape in Nigeria

The indicators measuring the different components of maternal health in Nigeria reveal a rather gloomy picture. Findings of the National Demographic and Health Survey (NDHS) 2013 reveal that contraceptive prevalence among Nigerian women stands at 16%, while only 15% of married women use a contraceptive and 16% has an unmet need for family planning. This poor access to family planning has resulted in a high fertility rate, which stands at 5.6 children per woman. With regards to antenatal visits, the survey reveals that only 51% of pregnant women have four antenatal visits while 34% have no antennal care. In terms of delivery care, only 38% of births are delivered by a skilled health provider (midwife, doctor or nurse) and only 36% of them are delivered in a health facility while 63% are delivered at home. For postnatal care, about 58% of women do not have postnatal check-up. Similarly, there is a high prevalence (23%) of teenage (15-19 years) pregnancy, which is a major health concern due to its association with higher morbidity and mortality for both mother and child (National Population Commission & ICF International, 2014).

These statistics reveal a poor maternal health landscape in Nigeria, hence Nigeria's present status as the second largest contributor to maternal deaths globally, accounting for 19 per cent (58,000) of the overall deaths with a Maternal Mortality Ratio (MMR) of 814 (WHO, 2015).

In view of this high maternal mortality rate, what steps has Nigeria taken (as a signatory to the Millennium Development Goals and now Sustainable Development Goals) to stem the tide of maternal deaths?

Measures Taken to Address Maternal, Newborn and Child Health Since the Adoption of Millennium Development Goals 4 and 5 by the Nigerian Government

Nigeria was one of the signatories to the Millennium Development Goals (MDGs) in 2000. Thus, it adopted the Goals as a strategy for achieving sustainable human development by the target year 2015. In view of this, Goals 4 and 5 were adopted to address Maternal, Newborn and Child Health (MNCH). Goal 4 aimed at reducing under-five mortality to 71 per 1,000 live births while Goal 5 aimed at reducing maternal mortality ratio by three-quarters between 1990 and 2015. Nigeria's efforts yielded a positive result as there was a consistent decrease in child and maternal mortality ratio from 1990 to 2015.

A key strategy adopted by the federal government towards the implementation of MDGs 4 and 5 was the Integrated Management of Newborn, Infant, and Childhood Health (IMNCH) strategy - an all-encompassing evidence-based approach, which incorporates all aspects of maternal and child healthcare system, including material and human resources, health governance, health information, strengthening of clinical services and community engagement (Findley, Uwemedimo, Doctor, Green, Adamu, & Afenyadu, 2013). The strategy was adopted under the auspices of the Federal Ministry of Health in 2007 (Federal Ministry of Health, 2007).

The implementation of the IMNCH strategy led to the following actions by the federal government:

- **Institutionalization of a Bi-Annual Maternal, Newborn and Child Health Week (MNCHW):** This is a week celebrated twice yearly in all states of the federation. MNCHW was introduced in 2010 as a strategic action to accelerate the reduction of child mortality and improve maternal health through improved access to maternal and child healthcare services. During the week, integrated high-impact and no-cost package of protective and preventive services are rendered to the whole family by taking services to the communities (UNICEF, 2016). The Week's interventions complement routine health services by ensuring that basic maternal and child healthcare reaches all mothers and children.
- **Strengthening Institutional Capacity and Infrastructure:** This led to the building of more Primary Health Centers (PHCs). In fact, PHCs are located in every local government in order to enable an extended coverage of maternal and child healthcare interventions (UNICEF, 2013). Equally, tertiary health facilities were refurbished and provided with equipment for emergency obstetric and newborn care, while supplies of Reproductive, Maternal, Newborn and Child Health (RMNCH) commodities such as midwifery kits, magnesium sulphate, treated mosquito nets, contraceptives, anti-retroviral (ARV) drugs, etc. was strengthened (and this is continuous and on-going) (Onyebuchi Chukwu, 2015).
- **Midwives Service Scheme (MSS):** Similarly, to improve and increase the number of personnel at the PHCs, the Midwives Service Scheme (MSS) was introduced in 2009. The MSS focuses on ensuring the availability of skilled attendance at birth in order to reduce maternal, infant and child mortality through increased recruitment and training (National Primary Healthcare Development Agency, 2010). Equally, capacity building of the existing health workers was carried out (this is continuous and on-going).

Thus, midwives and nurses were trained in Life Saving Skills (LSS) and in Integrated Management of Child Illness (IMCI) strategy. This was done in order to equip them with the requisite skills needed to save lives (National Primary Healthcare Development Agency (NPHDA), 2010).

- **Improved Health Financing:** This has been done through various measures such as the MDGs (now SDGs) conditional grant scheme, which is a scheme in which States and Local Governments are availed the opportunity to access funds annually from the Federal Government through counterpart contribution for the execution of projects, in line with the objectives of MDGs (SDGs) (Federal Republic of Nigeria, 2012). Also, health financing is made available through the Community Based Social Health Insurance Programme (CBSHIP), which is a programme under the auspices of the National Health Insurance Scheme (NHIS). The CBSHIP is targeted at the informal sector groups, which comprise a substantial proportion of the Nigerian population. The aim of CBSHIP is to address the critical problem of financial and geographical access to healthcare services by the informal groups. The CBSHIP has been implemented in some selected states. Similarly, to increase health financing, the budgetary allocation to the health sector was increased. For example, from 5% in 2006 to 7% in 2011 (Onyebuchi Chukwu, 2015). However, in recent times, the budgetary allocation has been decreasing, from 5.78% in 2015 to 4.23% in 2016 and further down to 4.17% in 2017 (Ifijeh, 2017).
- **Development and Review of Reproductive, Maternal, Newborn and Child Health (RMNCH) Policy Guidelines:** The various policies regulating RMNCH in Nigeria were reviewed. In 2010, the *National Reproductive Health (RH) Policy,* which was formulated in 2001 was reviewed in line with the objectives of the IMNCH strategy. The Reproductive Health Policy is a comprehensive framework, designed to address the reproductive health needs of Nigerians by designing and implementing appropriate programmes that would result in a well-functioning healthcare delivery system that guarantees access to affordable good quality care at all levels (Federal Ministry of Health, 2001).

Similarly, in 2010, *Training Manuals (Trainer and Trainee's versions) on the Use of Magnesium Sulphate in the Management of Severe Pre-Eclampsia and Eclampsia* was developed for the training of health workers. The manuals provide hands-on, detailed, descriptive and practical instructions and tips necessary to respond to obstetric emergencies (pre-eclampsia and eclampsia), the avoidable cause of maternal and child deaths (Federal Ministry of Health, 2010a; 2010b).

Also, the *National Family Planning/Reproductive Health Service Protocols* formulated in 2004 was reviewed in 2010. The National Family Planning/Reproductive Health Service Protocols is a framework for facilitating the provision of reproductive health services and quality care at service delivery points (Federal Ministry. of Health, 2010c). The review was done in response to new global trends in family planning and reproductive health practices.

Equally, the World Health Organization's Integrated Management of Childhood Illness (IMCI) strategy was adopted and this led to the development of the *Integrated Management of Childhood Illness Health Facility and Community Guidelines and Protocols* in 2011. The IMCI strategy is designed to reduce child mortality and morbidity in developing countries. The approach focuses on the major causes of death in children through improving case management skills of health workers, strengthening the health system and addressing family and community practices (Ketsela, Habimana, Martines, Mbewe, Williams, & Sabiiti, 2012).

- **Tapping into the Support of Multi and Bilateral Agencies, Non-Governmental Organizations (NGOs) and the Private Sector:** Through partnerships with multi and bilateral agencies as well as with NGOs and the private sector, a lot of interventions were carried out (this is continuous and on-going) in the health sector (Onyebuchi Chukwu, 2015). Such partners include UNICEF, DFID, Pathfinder, etc.
- **Enactment of the National Health Act (2014):** Which is a comprehensive framework for the development and management of a national health system in Nigeria. The Act provides free basic healthcare services for children under-age five, and pregnant women. This would grant more pregnant women access to maternal healthcare services, especially delivery services. However, regrettably, three years down the line, the Act is yet to be translated from law into reality. The Act is yet to be implemented.
- **Actions by State Governments:** Taking a cue from the steps taken by the Federal Government to address MCNH, some State Governments (Lagos, Akwa Ibom, etc.) became more sensitive to maternal and child health issues. This resulted in increased budgetary allocations to the health sector, as well as the abolition of user fees for rendering of basic health services to mother and child.

These steps culminated in a downward trend in MMR from 1350 per 100,000 live births in 1990 to 814 per 100,000 live births in 2015, as depicted in Table 1.

Table 1. Trend of maternal deaths in Nigeria (1990 to 2015)

Year	Maternal Mortality Ratio (MMR) per 100, 000 live births	Number of Deaths
1990	1350	57,000
1995	1250	59,000
2000	1170	62,000
2005	946	56,000
2010	867	57,000
2015	814	58,000

Source: World Health Organization, 2015

In terms of the annual rate of reduction, statistics in Table 2 reveal that there was a 2% reduction between 1990 – 2015. Similarly, there was a 1.4% reduction between 1990 – 2000 while there was 1.5% reduction between 2000 – 2015. These statistics reveal that the progress has not only been slow but retrogressing in recent times.

The progress made by Nigeria in reducing maternal deaths, as depicted in Tables 1 and 2 was not significant to meet the target of MDG 5. Thus, MDG 5 was a missed goal for Nigeria, just as it was globally. Till date, a lot of women still die during pregnancy or due to complications associated with child birth. Hence, Nigeria still remains the second largest contributor to maternal death globally. So is Nigeria poised to achieve SDG 3 Target 3.1 by 2030?

BARRIERS TO ACHIEVING SDG 3 IN NIGERIA AND SOLUTIONS

Although the achievement of MDG 5 was a missed goal for Nigeria, the most worrisome part is that Nigeria still remains the second and third largest contributor to maternal and child deaths respectively globally. This raises some salient questions – 'why is Nigeria still the second and third largest contributor to maternal and child deaths respectively, despite the implementation of an Integrated Management of

Table 2. Annual rate of reduction of maternal deaths in Nigeria

Years	%
1990 – 2015	2
1990 – 2000	1.4
2000 – 2015	1.5

Source: World Health Organization, 2015

Newborn, Infant, and Childhood Health (IMNCH) strategy?' 'Will Nigeria achieve Sustainable Development Goal 3, Target 3.1, by the year 2030?' This section of the chapter attempts to answer these questions by identifying the barriers to achieving SDG 3, Target 3.1 and proffering solutions.

A critical factor influencing maternal health is the level of a country's development. Evidence shows an association between the level of a country's development and maternal mortality rate (World Economic Forum, 2017a). For example, the global reduction in maternal deaths by about 44 per cent (from 385 deaths in 1990 to 216 deaths in 2015 per 100,000 live births) as a result of commitments by national governments to achieving MDG 5, was not evenly distributed between the developed and developing countries. While maternal deaths have reduced significantly in the developed world, a high number of maternal deaths still occur in the developing countries. In 2015, an approximately 99% (302,000) of the global maternal deaths took place in developing countries. Similarly, the maternal mortality ratio of 239 per 100,000 live births for the developing world is 20 times higher than the 12 deaths per 100,000 live births for the developed world. Equally, the estimated lifetime risk of maternal death in the developing world is 1 in 3,300, as compared to1 in 41in the developing world (WHO, 2015). These statistics clearly show that there is a relationship between the level of a country's development and maternal mortality rate. A core reason accountable for this differential in maternal mortality rate is the disparity in the healthcare systems of both climes. While the developed world has a viable healthcare and referral system in which pregnant women can receive emergency obstetric care when needed, this is absent in most of the developing world.

It must however, be noted that the burden of maternal deaths is also not evenly borne by developing countries. Evidence shows that among the developing countries, progress in stemming maternal and infant deaths in response to the then MDGs 4 and 5 did vary widely. Thus, some Low and Middle Income Countries (LMICs) did make significant progress more than others (World Health Organization & United Nations Children's Fund, 2014). Some had fast-track progress, while others had slow progress. Thus, to ascertain the causes of this differential in progress, a consortium of development agencies (World Health Organization, World Bank, Partnership for Maternal, Newborn and Child Health and Alliance for Health Policy and Systems) undertook some studies in 144 Low and Middle Income Countries. The objective was to ascertain the success factors responsible for the fast-track progress of some LMICs (Kuruvilla, Schweitzer, Bishai, Chowdhury, Caramani, & Frost, 2014). Findings reveal that the key to progress is the improvement across a range of health determinants, both within and beyond the health sector. Thus, apart from reforms within the health sector, factors such as good governance, improved levels of education, women's political and socio-economic participation, environmental management (access to clean water, sanitation, etc.), reduced levels of fertility and poverty among others, were some of the identified success factors. In essence, countries that made fast-track progress were those who addressed a range of factors within and beyond the health sector.

Good governance, especially the control of corruption (as measured by the World Bank's World Governance Indicators (World Bank, 2017) and women's political and socio-economic empowerment were found to be key critical success factors. Thus, ensuring value for money in project interventions (a key indicator of good governance) was a key success factor. Therefore, countries with fast-track progress have improved health outcomes, despite having relatively low levels of investment and an environment of political and economic challenges. This finding confirmed the finding of an earlier study, which reveals that health can be achieved with relatively low resources, if the resources are used efficiently and strategically (Balabanova, Mills, Conteh, Akkazieva, Banteyerga, & Dash, 2013).

In terms of women's political and socio-economic empowerment, findings of the studies also affirmed findings of earlier studies (World Economic Forum, 2017[b]; Bishai, Cohen, Alfonso, Adam, Kuruvilla, & Schweitzer, 2014; Caramani & Eugster, 2014; PMNCH WHO, World Bank, & AHPSR, 2014; Options Consultancy Services/ Evidence for Adam & Franz-Vasdeki, 2012). The studies unravel the relationships between education, protection of women's rights, women's political empowerment, women's participation in socio-economic activities and improved maternal and child health. Countries with fast-track progress were those who recognized and addressed these factors. Such countries have a significant number of women in their parliaments and labour force (WHO, 2014; World Bank, 2017; Asian Development Bank and World Bank, 2012).

Nigeria's readiness to meet SDG 3 Target 3.1 is assessed in this chapter in the light of these success factors. Nigeria is categorized among the Low Human Development Countries (LHDC) with a Human Development Index (HDI) of 0.527, ranking 152 out of the 188 countries in the Index (UNDP, 2016). Nigeria has 50.9% of her population being multi-dimensionally poor, while 18.4% live near multi-dimensional poverty. (Multidimensional poverty refers to multiple overlapping deprivations suffered by individuals in three dimensions of - education, health and living standards) (UNDP, 2016). Nigeria does not have a viable healthcare system. The ratio of doctors per 10,000 population is 4.0, while that of nurses and midwives is 16.1. Similarly, the number of hospital beds per 10,000 population is 5. These are far below the World Health Organization's standards, which prescribes for example, one doctor to 600 patients (WHO, 2016).

In terms of literacy, Nigeria has a literacy rate of 59.6%. Gender disparity of literacy level reveals that 69.2% males are literate as compared to 49.7% females (Central Intelligence Agency, 2017). The unemployment rate in Nigeria is high. The National Bureau of Statistics reports that 18.8% of Nigerians are unemployed, while 40.0% are both unemployed and underemployed. Among the unemployed, females constitute 21.2%, while males constitute 16.5%. Similarly, 24.2% of females are underemployed while 17.9% of males are similarly underemployed. In terms of rural/urban dichotomy, 16.4% of rural dwellers are unemployed while 23.4% of urban dwellers are similarly unemployed (National Bureau of Statistics, 2017). The NBS also reports that Nigeria has a poverty rate of 60.9% with 61.8% of urban dwellers being poor, while 73.2% of rural dwellers are similarly poor (NBS, 2012). According to UNICEF (2017) about 70 million Nigerians lack access to safe drinking water, and over 110 million lacked access to improved sanitation in 2013. Similarly, open defecation rate at 28.5%, poses grave public health risks. UNICEF estimates the economic impact of poor sanitation and hygiene, as costing the Nigerian economy about 1.3 per cent of her Gross Domestic Product (GDP).

Nigeria is plagued with bad governance. Corruption is at its peak. Transparency International Corruption Perceptions Index (2016) ranks Nigeria 136 out of 176 countries with a score of 28%. Nigeria has been ranked in this position consecutively for the past four years. In terms of political participation, women have a marginal representation of 5.6% in parliament as compared to 94.4% for men. Similarly, only 12.0% women are in ministerial positions as compared to 28.9% for men. In terms of out of school children, Nigeria has 10.5 million out-of-school children with 40.0% being females, while 28.9% are males. On the overall, Nigeria ranks 122 out of 144 countries in the Global Gender Gap Index (World Economic Forum, 2017[b]).

These indicators show that Nigeria has not done much to address maternal health determinants both in the health sector and beyond the health sector. As the evidence of the success factors has shown, tackling maternal health challenges involves much more than addressing issues within the health sector. It entails a commitment to address a range of factors both within and beyond the health sector.

SOLUTIONS AND RECCOMMENDATIONS

To achieve SDG 3, Target 3.1 by 2030, there is a need for a total overhauling of the Nigerian State. However, this cannot be done with the present crop of political leadership, but with a new set of visionary and purpose driven leadership who are committed to using the common wealth of Nigeria to improve the well-being of all Nigerians. Such leaders should be elected through free and fair elections. This also calls for an overhauling of the electoral process, to allow for free and fair elections devoid of violence and rigging, which currently characterise the Nigerian electoral landscape. Such visionary leaders when instituted to power should carry out reforms that address the following issues both within and beyond the health sector.

Beyond the Health Sector

- Practice good governance. This should be done based on the yard sticks of good governance as measured by the World Bank (2017).
- Control of corruption. This leadership should control corruption by a demonstration of the political will to legislate, prosecute and punish offenders to serve as a deterrent to others.
- Gender parity in political and socio-economic participation. They should take deliberate steps to increase the enrolment of women in education, especially higher education. Also, the political space and labour force should be opened to more women to be involved in decision-making. A start up point can be through deliberate policies in line with the thirty-five percent prescription of the Beijing Platform of Action (1995).
- Intensive environmental management through the provision of access to clean water, sanitation, adequate housing, etc.
- Reduction of the level of poverty through provision of direct employment and employment opportunities such as trainings, micro credit, business tools, etc.
- Provision of critical infrastructures such as electricity, security, transportation, etc.

Within the Health Sector

- Immediate implementation of the National Health Act (2014), which is yet to be implemented since its promulgation in 2014.
- Ensuring value for money in project interventions. This should be done through laid down procedures that enable transparency and accountability in projects' execution.
- Reduction in fertility rate through targeted campaigns, using diverse means (drama, songs, jingles, bill boards, fliers, door to door, etc.) to create awareness on the dangers of high fertility.
- Provision of free contraceptives and family planning to poor women and adolescents who are actively engaged in sex.

FUTURE RESEARCH DIRECTION

The diverse factors associated with the achievement of quality maternal and infant health as unravelled by this study calls for the conduct of more studies, especially empirical studies that will address a range of factors within and beyond the health sector that impact on maternal health in Nigeria. Such studies should focus on issues such as poverty, women socio-economic and political empowerment, governance, corruption, cultural practices, environmental management, health expenditure, etc.

CONCLUSION

In response to the then MDG 4 and 5, the Nigerian government took deliberate steps to stem maternal and infant mortality. The Integrated Maternal, Newborn and Child Heath (IMNCH) strategy was adopted as a radical measure to curb the very high rate of maternal and infant mortality. This led to a revitalization of the then weak and moribund primary healthcare system characterized by - insufficient health centres, insufficient, unskilled and poorly motivated staff, none or outdated equipment, lack of drugs, etc. The introduction of the strategy led to the building of more primary health centres, improved supply management, enhanced capacity of health personnel and support of high impact intervention packages by development partners. These actions led to a consistent reduction in maternal deaths from 1350 per 100,000 live births in 1990 to 814 per 100,000 live births in 2015. However, the progress made was painfully slow. The rate of reduction was a far cry from the stipulated 5.5% reduction target for MDG 5 by 2015.

Evidence shows that the failure of Nigeria to make fast-track progress was due to her failure to address other health determinants beyond the health sector. Health sector reforms were not accompanied by reforms or fundamental changes in other sectors, such as governance, education, women's political and socio-economic empowerment, environmental management, poverty alleviation, etc.

Millennium Development Goal 5 was rested in 2015 (its target year). However, the goal has been replaced by another transformative agenda for maternal health - Sustainable Development Goal 3 (Target 3.1). Nigeria has also adopted this goal, but an observation of the health and related landscape shows that Nigeria has done nothing radically different with a view to meet the target of this goal by 2030. Health financing is still very low and in fact depreciating over the years. For example, budgetary allocation to the health sector has been decreasing from 5.8% in 2015 to 4.2% in 2016 and further down to 4.1% in 2017. These figures are far below the 13% allocation recommended by the World Health Organization or the 15% recommended by the Abuja Declaration of the African Union. Furthermore, in a socio-political context characterized by bad governance and high level of corruption, the situation is even worse, as the money may not be spent for value in project interventions but may end up in the private pockets of government officials, leaving the health sector worst for it.

Similarly, poverty, a key determinant of health including maternal health is on the increase. The unemployment rate is rising on a daily basis. Many are losing their jobs, while only few new jobs are created. At the same time, those in employment go without salaries for months. In the midst of high rate of poverty, people will hold unto traditional values such as depriving the girl child of education and giving her out in an early marriage. Women will prefer to patronize the nearby community traditional birth attendant rather than expend scarce resource to travel to a primary health centre located far from the community. Also, pregnant women will have no access to the required nutrition due to lack of income, etc. In sum, the current development indicators of Nigeria, as highlighted in this study, tell it all. Therefore, if Nigeria does not take radical steps to address a range of health determinants, both within and beyond the health sector as recommended by this study, SDG 3 Target 3.1 will remain a missed goal by 2030 just like MDG 5.

REFERENCES

AbouZahr, C., & Wardlaw, T. (2001). Maternal Mortality at the End of the Decade: What Signs of Progress? *Bulletin of the World Health Organization*, *79*(6), 561–573. PMID:11436479

Adam, T., & Franz-Vasdeki, J. (2012). *Success Factors for Women's and Children's Health*. Background Paper. A Quantitative Mapping of Trends in Reductions of Maternal and Child Mortality in the High Mortality-Burden countdown to 2015 Countries. Alliance for Health Policy and Systems Research and the Partnership for Maternal, Newborn & Child Health. Retrieved on July 8, 2017 from http://www.who.int/pmnch/knowledge/publications/adam.pdf

Adamu, H. A. (2011). *Utilization of Maternal Health Care Services in Nigeria: An Analysis of Regional differences in the Patterns and Determinants of Maternal Health Care Use* (Master of Public Health Dissertation). University of Liverpool.

Addai, I. (2000). Determinants of Use of Maternal-Child Health Services in Rural Ghana. *Journal of Biosocial Science*, *32*(1), 1–15. PMID:10676056

Asian Development Bank and World Bank. (2012). *Country Gender Assessment for Lao People's Democratic Republic: Reducing Vulnerability and Increasing Opportunity*. Asian Development Bank and World Bank.

Ayele, D. Z., Belayihun, B., Teji, K., & Ayana, D. A. (2014). Factors Affecting Utilization of Maternal Health Care Services in Kombolcha District, Eastern Harare Zone, Oromia Regional State, Eastern Ethiopia. *International Scholarly Research Notices*. Retrieved from https://www.hindawi.com/journals/isrn/2014/917058/

Babalola, S., & Fatusi, A. (2009). Determinants of Use of Maternal Health Services in Nigeria - Looking Beyond Individual and Household Factors. *BMC Pregnancy and Childbirth*, *9*(43), 1–13. PMID:19754941

Balabanova, D., Mills, A., Conteh, L., Akkazieva, B., Banteyerga, H., Dash, U., ... McKee, M. (2013). Good Health at Low Cost 25 years on: Lessons for the Future of Health Systems Strengthening. *Lancet*, *381*(9883), 2118–2133. doi:10.1016/S0140-6736(12)62000-5 PMID:23574803

Bishai, D. M., Cohen, R., Alfonso, Y. N., Adam, T., Kuruvilla, S., & Schweitzer, J. (2016). Factors Contributing to Maternal and Child Mortality Reductions in 146 Low- and Middle-Income Countries between 1990 and 2010. *PLoS One*, *11*(1), e0144908. doi:10.1371/journal.pone.0144908 PMID:26783759

Caramani, D., & Eugster, B. (2014). *Which Factors are necessary and/or Sufficient for Accelerated Reduction of Maternal and Child Mortality in Low and Middle Income Countries? Results from a Boolean, Qualitative Comparative Analysis (QCA)*. Partnership for Maternal, Newborn & Child Health and Partners Technical Paper. Geneva: World Health Organization. Retrieved on October 3, 2017 from http://www.who.int/pmnch/knowledge/publications/success_factors.pdf

Celik, Y., & Hotchkiss, D. R. (2000). The Socio-Economic Determinants of Maternal Healthcare Utilization in Turkey. *Social Science & Medicine*, *50*(12), 1797–1806. doi:10.1016/S0277-9536(99)00418-9 PMID:10798333

Central Intelligence Agency. (2017). *World Fact Book*. Retrieved on November, 2017 from https://www.cia.gov/library/publications/the-world-factbook/geos/ni.html

Dagne, E. (2010). *Role of Socio-Demographic Factors on Utilization of Maternal Healthcare Services in Ethiopia*. UMEA University Dissertation.

Dalal, K., Shabnam, J., Andrews-Chavez, J., Mårtensson, L. B., & Timpka, T. (2012). Economic Empowerment of Women and Utilization of Maternal Delivery Care in Bangladesh. *International Journal of Preventive Medicine*, *3*(9), 628–636. PMID:23024852

Ensor, T., & Cooper, S. (2004). Overcoming Barriers to Health Service Access: Influencing the Demand Side. *Health Policy and Planning*, *19*(2), 69–79. doi:10.1093/heapol/czh009 PMID:14982885

Ethiopian Society of Population Studies. (2008). *Maternal Healthcare seeking Behavior in Ethiopia: Findings from EDHS 2005.* Retrieved from http://ethopia.unfpa.org/drive/Maternal Health.pdf

Federal Government of Nigeria (2012). *MDGs Conditional Grants Scheme: Implementation Manual (Revised).* Abuja, Nigeria: Office of the Senior Special Assistant to the President on MDGs.

Federal Ministry of Health. (2001). *National Reproductive Health Policy and Strategy to Achieve Quality Reproductive and Sexual Health for all Nigerians.* Abuja, Nigeria: Federal Government of Nigeria.

Federal Ministry of Health. (2007). *Integrated Maternal, Newborn and Child Health Strategy Nigeria.* Abuja, Nigeria: Federal Ministry of Health.

Federal Ministry of Health. (2010a). Training Manuals (Trainee's Version) on the use of Magnesium Sulphate in the Management of severe Pre-Eclampsia and Eclampsia. Abuja, Nigeria: Federal Government of Nigeria, Population Council & MacAurthur Foundation.

Federal Ministry of Health. (2010b). Training Manuals (Trainer's Version) on the use of Magnesium Sulphate in the Management of severe Pre-Eclampsia and Eclampsia. Abuja, Nigeria: Federal Government of Nigeria, Population Council & MacAurthur Foundation.

Federal Ministry of Health. (2010c). National Family Planning/Reproductive Health Service Protocols. Abuja, Nigeria: Federal Government of Nigeria.

Federal Ministry of Health. (2014). *National Health Act.* Abuja, Nigeria: Federal Government of Nigeria.

Findley, S. E., Uwemedimo, O. T., Doctor, H. V., Green, C., Adamu, F., & Afenyadu, G. (2013). Early Results of an Integrated Maternal, Newborn and Child Health Program, Northern Nigeria, 2009 to 2011. *BMC Public Health, 13*(1), 1034. doi:10.1186/1471-2458-13-1034 PMID:24175944

Fotso, J. C., Ezeh, A., Madise, N., Ziraba, A., & Ogollah, R. (2009). What does Access to Maternal Care Mean among the Urban Poor? Factors Associated with Use of Appropriate Maternal Health Services in the Slum Settlements of Nairobi, Kenya. *Maternal and Child Health Journal, 13*(1), 130–137. doi:10.100710995-008-0326-4 PMID:18297380

Furuta, M., & Salway, S. (2006). Women's Position within the Household as a Determinant of Maternal Health Care Use in Nepal. *International Family Planning Perspectives*, *32*(1), 17–27. doi:10.1363/3201706 PMID:16723298

Gabrysch, S., & Campbell, O. M. (2009). Still too Far to Walk: Literature Review of the Determinants of Delivery Service Use. *BMC Pregnancy and Childbirth*, *9*(1), 34. doi:10.1186/1471-2393-9-34 PMID:19671156

Gage, A. J., & Calixte, M. G. (2006). Effects of Physical Accessibility of Maternal Health Services on their Use in Rural Haiti. *Population Studies*, *60*(3), 271–288. doi:10.1080/00324720600895934 PMID:17060054

Haralambos & Holborn. (2013). Sociology Themes and Perspectives (8th ed.). London: Harper Collins Publishers limited.

Ifijeh, M. (2017, February 9). Nigeria's Grossly Inadequate 2017 Health Budget. *This Day Newspaper*. Retrieved on November 12, 2017 from https://www.thisdaylive.com/index.php/2017/02/09/nigerias-grossly-inadequate-2017-health-budget/

Ketsela, T., Habimana, P., Martines, J., Mbewe, A., Williams, A., & Sabiiti, J. N. (2012). *Integrated Management of Childhood Illness (IMCI)*. Retrieved on August 3, 2017 from http://www.who.int/pmnch/media/publications/aonsectionIII_5.pdf

Kruk, M. E., Galea, S., Prescott, M. R., & Freedman, L. P. (2007). Healthcare Financing and Utilization of Maternal Health Services in Developing Countries. *Health Policy and Planning*, *22*(5), 303–310. doi:10.1093/heapol/czm027 PMID:17681975

Kuruvilla, S., Schweitzer, J., Bishai, D., Chowdhury, S., Caramani, D., … Frost, L. (2014). Success factors for reducing maternal and child mortality. *Bulletin of the World Health Organization*, *92*, 533-544. Retrieved on November 29, 2017 from http://www.who.int/bulletin/volumes/92/7/14-138131/en/

Lowe, M., Chen, D. R., & Huang, S. L. (2016). Social and Cultural Factors Affecting Maternal Health in Rural Gambia: An Exploratory Qualitative Study. *PLoS One*, *11*(9), e0163653. doi:10.1371/journal.pone.0163653 PMID:27661617

Magadi, M. A., Agwanda, A. O., & Obare, F. O. (2007). A Comparative Analysis of the Use of Maternal Health Services between Teenagers and Older Mothers in sub-Saharan Africa: Evidence from Demographic Health Surveys. *Social Science & Medicine*, *64*(6), 1311–1325. doi:10.1016/j.socscimed.2006.11.004 PMID:17174017

Muchabaiwa, L., Mazambani, D., Chigusiwa, L., Bindu, S., & Mudavanhu, V. (2012). Determinants of Maternal Healthcare Utilization in Zimbabwe. *International Journal of Economic Science Application Res.*, *5*(2), 145–162.

National Bureau of Statistics (NBS). (2012). *Nigeria Poverty Profile 2010*. Abuja, Nigeria: Federal Government of Nigeria.

National Bureau of Statistics (NBS). (2017). *Unemployment/Underemployment Report. Q4 2016*. Abuja, Nigeria: Federal Government of Nigeria.

National Population Commission & ICF International. (2014). *Nigeria Demographic and Health Survey 2013*. Abuja, Nigeria: NPC & ICF International.

National Primary Healthcare Development Agency (NPHCDA). (2010). *Midwives Service Scheme*. Retrieved on August 10, 2017 from https://www.nphcda.org/programmes/midwives-service-scheme/

Nwakoby, B. N. (1994). Use of Obsteric Services in Rural Nigeria. *Journal of the Royal Society of Health, 114*(3), 132–136. doi:10.1177/146642409411400304 PMID:7932482

Ononokpono, D. N., & Odimegwu, C. O. (2014). Determinants of Maternal Health Care Utilization in Nigeria: A Multilevel Approach. *The Pan African Medical Journal, 17*(1), 2. Retrieved from http://www.panafrican-med-journal.com/content/series/17/1/2/full on 6/7/2017 PMID:24643545

Onyebuchi Chukwu, C. O. (2015). *Maternal, Newborn and child Health in Nigeria: Where are we now?* Presentation by the Honorable Minister of Health, Nigeria. Retrieved on October 26, 2017 from http://www.who.int/pmnch/about/steering_committee/B11_11_02_nigeriapresentation.pdf

Options Consultancy Services/Evidence for Action, Cambridge Economic Policy Associates, & the Partnership for Maternal, Newborn and Child Health. (2013). *Success Factors for Women's and Children's Health: Country Specific Review of Data and Literature on 10 Fast-Track Countries' Progress Towards MDGs 4 and 5*. Retrieved on July 10, 2017 from http://www.who.int/pmnch/knowledge/publications/country_data_review.pdf

Peltzer, K., Skinner, D., Mfecane, S., Shisana, O., Nqeketo, A., & Mosala, T. (2005). Factors Influencing the Utilization of Prevention of Mother-to-Child-Transmission Services by Pregnant Women in the Eastern Cape, South Africa. *Health SA Gesondheid, 10*(1), 26–40. doi:10.4102/hsag.v10i1.186

PMNCH, WHO, World Bank, & AHPSR. (2014). Success Factors for Women's and Children's Health: Policy and Programme Highlights from 10 Fast-Track Countries. Geneva: Authors.

Raghupathy, S. (1996). Education and the Use of Maternal Health Care in Thailand. *Social Science & Medicine*, *43*(4), 459–471. doi:10.1016/0277-9536(95)00411-4 PMID:8844947

Raj Baral, Lyons, & Skinner, & van Teijlingen. (2012). Maternal Health Services Utilization in Nepal: Progress in the New Millennium? *Health Science Journal*, *6*(4), 618–633.

Reynolds, H. W., Wong, E. L., & Tucker, H. (2006). Adolescents Use of Maternal and Child Health Services in Developing Countries. *International Family Planning Perspectives*, *32*(1), 6–16. doi:10.1363/3200606 PMID:16723297

Silal, S., Penn-Kekana, L., Harris, B., Birch, S., & McIntyre, D. (2012). Exploring Inequalities in Access to and Use of Maternal Health Services in South Africa. *BMC Health Services Research*, *12*(1), 120. doi:10.1186/1472-6963-12-120 PMID:22613037

Simkhada, B., Teijlingen, E. R., Porter, M., & Simkhada, P. (2008). Factors Affecting the Utilization of Antenatal Care in Developing Countries: Systematic Review of the Literature. *Journal of Advanced Nursing*, *61*(3), 244–260. doi:10.1111/j.1365-2648.2007.04532.x PMID:18197860

Tsawe, M., Moto, A., Netshivhera, T., Ralesego, L., Nyathi, C., & Susuman, A. S. (2015). Factors Influencing the Use of Maternal Healthcare Services and Childhood Immunization in Swaziland. *International Journal For Equity in Health*. Retrieved from https://www.ncbi.nlm.nih.gov/pmc/articles/PMC4391603/

Tsawe, M., & Susuman, A. S. (2014). Determinants of Access to and Use of Maternal Health Care Services in the Eastern Cape, South Africa: A Quantitative and Qualitative Investigation. *BioMed Central Research Notes, 7*, 723. Retrieved from https://www.ncbi.nlm.nih.gov/pmc/articles/PMC4203863/

United Nations. (2005). *The Millennium Development Goals Report 2005*. New York: United Nations.

United Nations. (2016). *Transforming Our World: The 2030 Agenda for Sustainable Development. ARES/70/1*. Retrieved on August 2, 2017 from sustainabledevelopment.org

United Nations Children's Fund (UNICEF). (2013). *Maternal and Child Mortality*. Retrieved on May 1, 2013 from http://www.unicef.org/nigeria/children_1926.html

United Nations Children's Fund (UNICEF). (2016). *Evaluation of the Maternal, Newborn and Child Health Week in Nigeria*. Abuja, Nigeria: UNICEF Nigeria Country Office.

United Nations Children's Fund (UNICEF). (2017). *Water Sanitation and Hygiene*. Retrieved on November 29, 2017 from https://www.unicef.org/nigeria/wes.html

United Nations Development Programme. (2016). *Human Development Report*. Washington, DC: United Nations Development Programme.

USAID. (2009). *Maternal and Child Health*. Retrieved on August,2, 2017 from http://www.usaid.gov/our_work/global_health/mch/mh/techareas/post.html

World Bank. (2014). *The Worldwide Governance Indicators (WGI) project*. Washington, DC: World Bank. Retrieved on October 4, 2017 from http://info.worldbank.org/governance/wgi/index.aspx

World Bank. (2017). *World Governance Indicators*. Retrieved on November 29, 2017 from https://data.worldbank.org/data-catalog/worldwide-governance-indicators

World Economic Forum. (2017a). *The Global Competitiveness Report*. Geneva, Switzerland: World Economic Forum.

World Economic Forum. (2017b). *The Global Gender Gap Report*. Geneva, Switzerland: World Economic Forum.

World Health Organization. (2012a). Trends in Maternal Mortality: 1990-2010. WHO, UNICEF, UNFPA, World Bank Estimates. Geneva: World Health Organization.

World Health Organization. (2012b). *MDG 5: Improve Maternal Health*. Retrieved on May 31, 2013 from http://www.who.int/topics/maternal_health/en/

World Health Organization. (2014). *Success Factors for Women's and Children's Health: Country Multistakeholder Policy Reviews*. Geneva: World Health Organization. Retrieved on September18, 2017 from http://www.who.int/pmnch/knowledge/publications/successfactors/en/index2.html

World Health Organization. (2014). *Success Factors for Women's and Children's Health: Multisector Pathways to Progress*. Geneva: World Health Organization.

World Health Organization. (2015). *Trends in Maternal Mortality: 1990-2015. WHO, UNICEF, UNFPA, World Bank Estimates*. Geneva, Switzerland: World Health Organization.

World Health Organization. (2016). *Global Health Workforce Statistics*. Retrieved on November 29, 2017 from http://www.who.int/hrh/statistics/hwfstats/

World Health Organization & United Nations Children's Fund. (2014). *Countdown to 2015 and beyond: Fulfilling the Health Agenda for Women and Children*. Geneva: World Health Organization & United Nations Children's Fund.

KEY TERMS AND DEFINITIONS

Antenatal: Healthcare given to a pregnant woman before childbirth.

Child: A person who is under five years.

Childbirth: The act of bringing to the world a new life (person).

Death: The end of the existence of an individual in the world.

Family Planning: The act of preventing unwanted pregnancies.

Federal Ministry of Health, Nigeria: The institutional framework that regulates healthcare in Nigeria.

Mortality: The ratio of deaths per certain number of population.

Pregnancy: The act of conception of a new life in the womb by a woman.

Postnatal: Healthcare given to a woman immediately after childbirth and within 40 days of delivery.

Postpartum: The period immediately after childbirth and health issues that occur during this period.

World Health Organization: The international body that provides regulatory guide for healthcare practices globally.

This research was previously published in Human Rights, Public Values, and Leadership in Healthcare Policy edited by Augustine Nduka Eneanya; pages 247-271, copyright year 2019 by Medical Information Science Reference (an imprint of IGI Global).

Chapter 12
Health Effects of Pesticides on Pregnant Women and Children

Mudasir Youssouf
Central University of Punjab, India

Arun Kalia
Central University of Punjab, India

Zahid Nabi
Central University of Jammu, India

Zubair A. Malik
Government HSS, India

ABSTRACT

Pesticides, along with hybrid seeds and fertilizers, are an integral part of the green revolution and are used to control and eradicate disease vectors for the improvement of agricultural production. Pesticides is an umbrella term for insecticides, nematocides, fungicides, herbicides, fumigants, repellents, and attractants. Pesticides are used against unwanted plants and animals to control diseases and losses. Efforts at different levels may help to reduce the impact of pesticides on newborn babies and on pregnant women. Different efforts can be considered at clinical, educational, and policymaking institutes. Use of risk assessment tools, encouragement of organic diets, educating parents working in agricultural fields from hazards of pesticides particularly in pregnancy and breast feeding, implementation of integrated pest management (IPM) programs, and encouraging policies supporting IPM can help in tackling the menace of pesticide hazards.

DOI: 10.4018/978-1-7998-2351-3.ch012

INTRODUCTION

Drinking water is classified among the most precious resources of the earth, however by anthropogenic activities both the quality and quantity of available water is continuously deteriorating (Benner *et al.*, 2013). A large part of world's population is forced to use contaminated drinking water (WHO, 2010). Millions of deaths mostly in developing countries could be prevented if people adhere to reliable safe drinking water sources. Around 2.4 million deaths occur annually, mostly in developing countries by living in unhygienic conditions and having no access to potable water (Pruss-Ustun *et al.*, 2008). Among the two basic drinking water sources, surface water receives high extent of pollutants as compared to groundwater which is less exposed though groundwater can act as pollution source for decades due to higher residence times of pesticides and lower microbial activity as compared to surface water (Rodrigo *et al.*, 2014). With the varying pollutants and contaminants, the traditional water testing and monitoring processes and techniques (for microbial contamination) have also shifted to include the health risks of chemical contaminants, mostly when associated with chronic exposures (Fawell & Nieuwenhuijsen, 2003; Thompson *et al.*, 2007).

Due to widespread distribution, toxicity and persistence, pesticides are now the important class of water pollutants, even at very low concentrations pesticides can be hazardous to aquatic life because of bioconcentration process. Out of 22 identified POPs, 15 of them are pesticides mainly aldrin, dieldrin, endrin, chlordane, DDT, hexachlorobenzene, mirex, heptachlor, toxaphene, etc. Considering the severity of POPs a separate international environmental treaty (Stockholm conference) was signed in 2001 to eliminate or restrict the production and use of POPs (Xu *et al.*, 2013; Ali *et al.*, 2014). Properties like persistence in degradation process, ability to travel long distances, bioaccumulation, carcinogenic, hormone disruption and causing immunological and reproductive disorders has increased public concerns towards POPs (Vos *et al.*, 2000; Buccini, 2003; Sanpera *et al.*, 2003). Across the globe, 884 million people (13% of the world's population) depend on unprotected and distant water sources for drinking water collection and 3.6 billion people have well developed piped water system. However, in many low and middle-income countries, piped water system work for few hours and also are not safe, for example in Asian cities, more than one in five water supply schemes fail to meet national water quality standards (Bartram and Cairncross, 2010).

Pesticide contamination of surface water and groundwater can occur from both point sources (spill sites, disposal sites) and non-point sources which are the dominant source of pesticide pollution includes agricultural or urban runoff, infiltration from application sites, etc. (Fig. 1).

Figure 1. Schematic diagram depicting possible routes of pesticides into streams and groundwater
Thodal et al., 2009.

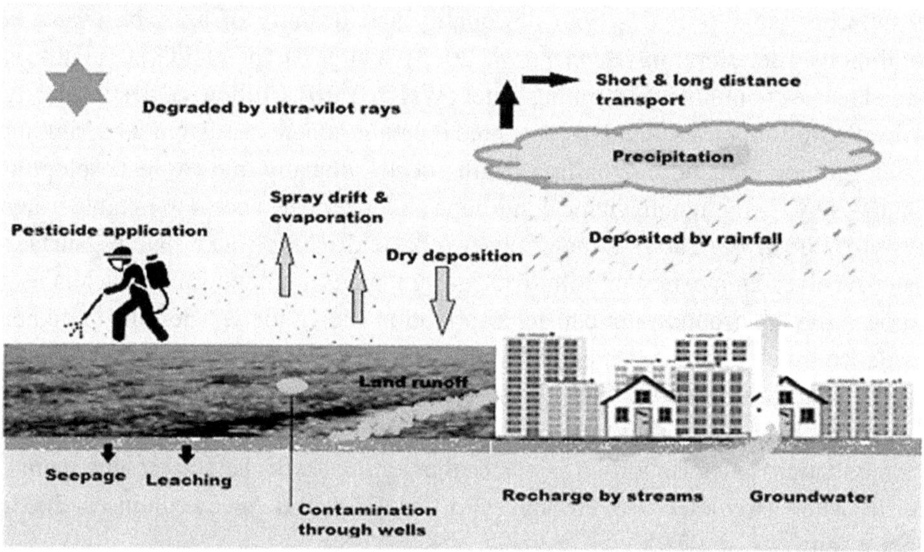

The importance and threat to freshwater ecosystem services were also highlighted in Millennium Ecosystem Assessment (MEA) report which identified heavy metals and pesticides as anthropogenic pollutants of extensive importance (Assessment, 2005).

For proper risk assessment and mitigation, information of the actual concentration of pesticides in the environment is fundamental. The most important matter of concern is the human exposure to pesticides by food and water (De Gerónimo *et al.*, 2014).The occurrence of pesticides in drinking water is related to high treatment costs, different toxicological incidences and hindrance in water usage. To restrict toxicological effects on human population and environmental pollution drinking water regulations are required (Lehmann *et al.*, 2017). There is a variation of regulatory limits for pesticide residues in drinking water from one regulating agency to another and it depends on different parameters like the type of water, type of residue, the analytical method followed and other environmental factors (Hamilton *et al.*, 2003). Each country must establish its own pesticide residue limits according to its actual environmental, economic and technological situation and shouldn't copy standards without considering the conditions under which they have been framed. The standard and guideline values for pesticide residues in drinking water by different agencies is given in Table 1

Table 1. Comparison of standards by different agencies for pesticide residues in drinking water

<table>
<tr><th rowspan="2">Pesticide</th><th rowspan="2">GV*
µg/l
(WHO)</th><th colspan="2">USEPA</th><th rowspan="2">USA Health Advisory, Lifetime
µg/l</th><th rowspan="2">BIS</th></tr>
<tr><th>MCL**
µg/l</th><th>MCLG***
µg/l</th></tr>
<tr><td>Alachlor</td><td>20</td><td>2</td><td>0</td><td>-</td><td rowspan="26">Desirable limit for pesticides is given as “absent” In absence of alternate source the permissible limit is 0.001mg/l (1µg/l</td></tr>
<tr><td>Aldicarb</td><td>10</td><td>7</td><td>7</td><td>7</td></tr>
<tr><td>Aldicarb sulfone</td><td>-</td><td>7</td><td>7</td><td>7</td></tr>
<tr><td>Aldicarb sulfoxide</td><td>-</td><td>7</td><td>7</td><td>7</td></tr>
<tr><td>Aldrin/ Dieldrin</td><td>0.03</td><td>-</td><td>-</td><td>-</td></tr>
<tr><td>Atrazine</td><td>2</td><td>3</td><td>3</td><td>200</td></tr>
<tr><td>Carbofuran</td><td>7</td><td>40</td><td>40</td><td>40</td></tr>
<tr><td>Chlordane</td><td>0.2</td><td>2</td><td>0</td><td>-</td></tr>
<tr><td>2,4-D</td><td>30</td><td>70</td><td>70</td><td>70</td></tr>
<tr><td>DDT</td><td>2</td><td>-</td><td>-</td><td>-</td></tr>
<tr><td>1,2-Dibromo-3-chloropane</td><td>1</td><td>0.2</td><td>0</td><td>-</td></tr>
<tr><td>Diquat</td><td>10</td><td>20</td><td>20</td><td>-</td></tr>
<tr><td>EDB</td><td>0.4-15</td><td>0.05</td><td>0</td><td>-</td></tr>
<tr><td>Fenoprop (2,4,5-TP)</td><td>9</td><td>50</td><td>50</td><td>50</td></tr>
<tr><td>Glyphosate</td><td>unnec</td><td>700</td><td>700</td><td>700</td></tr>
<tr><td>Hexachlorobenzene</td><td>1</td><td>1</td><td>0</td><td>-</td></tr>
<tr><td>Lindane</td><td>2</td><td>0.2</td><td>0.2</td><td>0.2</td></tr>
<tr><td>Methoxychlor</td><td>20</td><td>40</td><td>40</td><td>40</td></tr>
<tr><td>Molinate</td><td>6</td><td>-</td><td>-</td><td>-</td></tr>
<tr><td>Pentachlorophenol</td><td>9</td><td>1</td><td>0</td><td>-</td></tr>
<tr><td>Permethrin</td><td>20</td><td>-</td><td>-</td><td>-</td></tr>
<tr><td>Picloram</td><td>-</td><td>500</td><td>500</td><td>500</td></tr>
<tr><td>Propanil</td><td>20</td><td>-</td><td>-</td><td>-</td></tr>
<tr><td>Simazine</td><td>2</td><td>4</td><td>4</td><td>4</td></tr>
<tr><td>2,4,5-T</td><td>9</td><td>-</td><td>-</td><td>70</td></tr>
<tr><td>Trifluralin</td><td>20</td><td>-</td><td>-</td><td>5</td></tr>
</table>

Hamilton et al., 2003; BIS, 2012.

***GV:** Guideline Value, the concentration of a contaminant which doesn’t show any significant risk to health over lifetime consumption.

****MCL:** Maximum Contaminant Level, allowed is drinking water and are enforceable standards set as closely possible to MCLGs taking technology and cost into consideration.

*****MCLG:** Maximum Contaminant Level Goal, level of the contaminant in drinking water below which there is no known or expected risk to health and are non-enforceable standards.

Also, there is an increasing need for the implementation of a scientifically efficient pesticide registration programme that filters out banned and damage causing pesticides (Teklu *et al.*, 2015). Sharing of information, cooperation and coordination between pesticide importing and exporting countries can help in accomplishing a single regional or international framework and compilation of a regional database (Islam *et al.*, 2017). Different countries have different regulations for pesticide consumption, for example, in India The Insecticide Act 1968 and Rules 1971 was enacted to regulate pesticide usage in the country and Central Insecticides Boards and registration Committee (CIB & RC), is responsible for granting or refusing registration to pesticides, also it gives detailed account of banned pesticides in the country, as is given in Table 2 (CIBRC, 2015).

In this chapter, we emphasized the possible routes of pesticide entry into drinking water and also discussed the effects of pesticide exposure to pregnant women and children. A very few studies has been carried out which discusses effects of pesticides on pregnant women and newborn children. Fetuses and children are the weakest age group to pesticide exposure and better understanding pesticide pollution and its control can help to lower health hazard incidences.

ENVIRONMENTAL FATE AND INPUT PATHWAYS OF PESTICIDES INTO DRINKING WATER

Once pesticides are accidentally or deliberately released into the environment, they either find their way directly into aquatic ecosystems or indirectly by atmospheric deposition during spray drift or by volatilization after their application (Schafer *et al.*, 2011). There are two sources by which pesticides enter water bodies which include diffused or by point sources. Leaching through the upper soil and vadose zone (unsaturated zone), and infiltration through river banks and beds are some of the examples of pesticide diffuse pathways into groundwater. Point source includes pesticide contamination from agricultural runoff, accidental spills, leaking or faulty equipment, storage canisters etc. (Reichenberger *et al.*, 2007).

The basic aim of drinking water schemes should be public health protection and can be delivered by constructing a regulatory framework encompassing health-based targets, proper and adequate treatment for every type of contaminant species and performing extensive monitoring (WHO, 2010). Once pesticides come in contact with the environment they are prone to degradation by biotic and abiotic sources. Pesticide degradation may start right from their application to their absorption/sink sites, however, degradation process may be slow due to the persistence of pesticides and variety of new compounds are formed as transformation products or degradates (Parsons *et al.*, 2008). The transformation products may be less or more toxic and

Table 2. List of pesticides which are banned and restricted in use in India: (As on 20th October 2015)

S. No.	Pesticides Banned for Manufacture, Import and Use	Pesticides Restricted for Use in the Country	Pesticides Refused Registration
1	Aldicarb	Aluminium Phosphide	2,4, 5-Trichloro phenoxy acetic acid
2	Aldrin	Captafol	Ammonium Sulphamate
3	Benzene Hexachloride	Cypermethrin	Azinphos Ethyl
4	Calcium Cyanide	Dazomet	Azinphos Methyl
5	Chlorbenzilate	Diazinon	Binapacryl
6	Chlordane	Dichloro Diphenyl Trichloroethane (DDT)	Calcium Arsenate
7	Chlorofenvinphos	Fenitrothion	Carbophenothion
8	Copper Acetoarsenite	Fenthion	Chinomethionate (Morestan)
9	Dibromochloropropane	Methoxy Ethyl Mercuric Chloride	Dicrotophos
10	Dieldrin		EPN
11	Endrin		Fentin Acetate
12	Ethyl Mercury Chloride		Fentin Hydroxide
13	Ethyl Parathion		Lead Arsenate
14	Ethylene Dibromide (EDB)		Leptophos (Phosvel)
15	Heptachlor		Mephosfolan
16	Lindane (Gamma-HCH)		Mevinphos (Phosdrin)
17	Maleic Hydrazide		Thiodemeton / Disulfoton
18	Menazon		Vamidothion
19	Metoxuron		
20	Nitrofen		
21	Paraquat Dimethyl Sulphate		
22	Pentachloro Nitrobenzene		
23	Pentachlorophenol		
24	Phenyl Mercury Acetate		
25	Sodium Methane Arsonate		
26	Tetradifon		
27	Toxaphene(Camphechlor)		
28	Trichloro acetic acid (TCA)		

stable than its base compound (Andreu and Pico, 2004). Pesticide and its degradation products follow different paths before they reach to major surface or groundwater sources, so there are optimal chances of pesticides contamination in water abstracted for drinking purposes (Damalas and Eleftherohorinos, 2011).

Conventional water treatment facilities (coagulation/flocculation, sedimentation, filtration and disinfection) are not able to remove or reduce pesticide residue concentration, so there should some specific treatment facilities for removal of entire pesticide classes (Rodrigo *et al.*, 2014). Over the past few decades, different water treatment technologies including chemical, physical and biologic processes have been developed for pesticide removal. A brief account of different treatment processes and their limitations used in pesticide removal in drinking water is expressed in Figure 2.

PESTICIDE TOXICITY AND HEALTH PROBLEMS IN PREGNANT WOMEN AND NEWBORN BABIES

Pesticides were considered as a blessing for human life for enhancing agricultural productivity and wiping out infectious diseases but their large-scale use has caused numerous hazards to the ecosystem and human life (Mostafalou and Abdollahi, 2013). The extent or ability of pesticides to cause disease, injury or illness in living organisms is called the pesticide toxicity. The pesticide toxicity is studied by subjecting test animals to different doses of the active ingredient and at the same time each of its formulated products (Asghar *et al.*, 2016). On the basis of severity and time duration of toxicity symptoms two types of toxicity are acute and chronic (Gao and Lu, 2015).

Figure 2. Common practices used for pesticide removal in drinking water

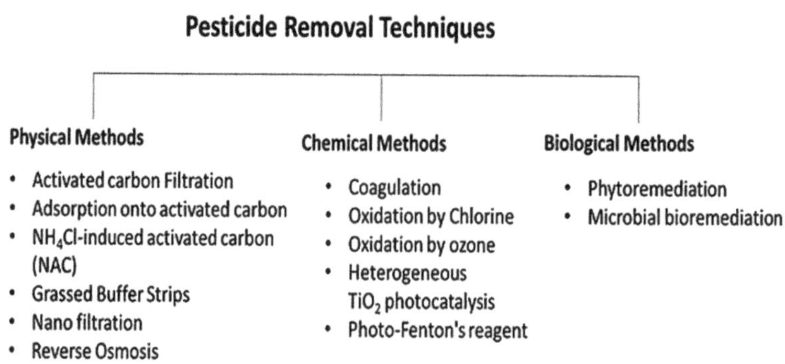

There is no complete date available on toxicity of every pesticide, a brief account of acute oral and dermal toxicity of some pesticides is given in Table 3. However, chronic toxicity can't be identified at the same lethal doses (Criswell *et al.*, 2014).

Acute toxicity of pesticides results from mild to devastating and lethal consequences like a headache, vomiting, abdominal pain, respiratory problems, ulceration in the upper gastrointestinal tract, etc. (Roberts and Karr, 2012). Chronic effects (described by gradual progression and long-term pesticide contact) which are diagnosed in epidemiological studies are worse than acute effects and include adverse neurobehavioral and cognitive problems, cardiovascular diseases, respiratory problems like asthma, pediatric cancer, acute lymphocytic leukemia, preterm birth, low birth weight and hormonal imbalance etc (Souza *et al.* 2011; Mostafalou and Abdollahi 2012; Mostafalou and Abdollahi, 2013).

Table 3. Acute oral and dermal lethal doses of different pesticides for humans

Common Name	Trade Name	Acute Oral LD50 mg/kg	Acute Dermal LD50 mg/kg
aldicarb	Temik	1	20
allethrin	(many)	480	11,200
azadirachtin	Aza-Direct, Ecozin, others	>5,000	>2,000
Carbaryl	Sevin	246-283	4,000
chlorfenapyr	Phantom, Pylon	560	>2,000
chlorpyrifos	Lorsban, Dursban, Durap	96-270	2,000
DDT	–	113	2,510
diazinon	Diazinon, Spectracide	300-400	3,600
dichlorvos	DDVP, Vapona	80	105-107
dictotophos	Bidrin	17-22	224
diquat	Diquat, Reglone	215-235	>400
dienochlor	Pentac	3,160	>3,160
dimethoate	Dimethoate, Cygon	235	400
endosulfan	Thiodan, Phaser	160	359
hydroprene	Gen Trol	>34,000	5,100
lindane	Lindane, others	200	2,000
malathion	Cythion, Malathion	2,800	4,100
methoprene	Altosid, Precor, others	>34,000	>3,000
methoxfendozide	Intrepid	>5,000	>2,000
methyl bromide	(many)	214	–

continues on following page

Table 3. Continued

Common Name	Trade Name	Acute Oral LD50 mg/kg	Acute Dermal LD50 mg/kg
permethrin	Ambush, Astro, others	2,215`	>2,000
phorate	Thimet, GX-118	4	6
phosphoric acid	Foray	1,530	2,740
potassium salts	M-Pede	>5,000	>2,000
propargite	Omite, Comite	4,029	2,940
pyrethrin	(many)	1,500	>1,800
pyriproxyfen	Distance	>5,000	>2,000
rotenone	(many)	350	940
sulfur	Microthiol, Thiodex	>2,000	2,000
sulfotepp	Bladafum	10	65
tebufenozide	Confirm	>5,000	>5,000
tebupirimphos	Aztec	132	>2,000
thiamethoxam	actara, Cruiser, others	>5,000	>2,000
thiodicarb	Larvin	166	>2,000
diuron	Karmex	3,40	2,000
fenac	Fenatrol	1,780	>3,160
glyphosate	Rodeo, Roundup	5,000	>5,000
hexazinone	Velpar	1,690	5,278
methazole	Probe	2,501	>12,500
metolachlor	Dual	2,780	>10,000
paraquat	Grmoxone, Cyclone	150	–
propachlor	Ramrod	500-1,700	–
simazine	Princep	>5,000	>3,100

Criswell et al., 2014.

Although all age groups are vulnerable to pesticide toxicity but considering the stage of developing fetus and the children, they are more sensitive to chemicals as most of the organ systems are in developing stage, for example, their immune system may not be able to safeguard them against disease-causing agents or environmental threats (Weselak *et al.*, 2007). Children's behaviour and inability to understand their physical environment can place them at greater risk of exposure. Also, children for their weight, consume more food, drinks and air, increasing their possible dietary exposure. Therefore special attention should be paid to children's exposure to pesticides from food, water, inhalation, playground, etc. and the fetus can be exposed to pesticides across the placenta, amniotic fluid and ovarian follicular fluid (Colborn, 2006; Gilden *et al.*, 2010). Different studies have proved the vulnerability of fetuses to pesticides as they can pass through the placenta and blood-brain barrier and were also found in amniotic fluid (Bradman *et al.*, 2003). In comparison to pregnant women, children are more susceptible to pesticide poisoning due to their high respiratory and heart rate, higher metabolism, food consumption pattern and hand-to-mouth behaviour (Garry, 2004). Exposure to pesticides during fetal and early child development stages has been correlated with different diseases which will be briefly discussed in this chapter.

Pesticides and Birth Abnormalities

Exposure to toxicants during early stages of fetal development is associated with an increased risk of birth-related defects which are detectable at birth or within few years of childhood. The two common birth related deformities caused by pesticide exposure of fetuses are preterm birth or low birth weight (LBW), children born with these disorders experience higher rates of morbidity through the perinatal period as compared to normal ones (Stillerman *et al.*, 2008; Windham and Fenster, 2008). Household pesticide exposures through different sources on the time of pregnancy have adverse impacts on birth outcomes. Suppression of neurite outgrowth is associated with pesticide exposure as these inhibit acetylcholinesterase, down-regulate muscarinic receptors, inhibit the adenylate cyclase signalling cascade and leads to decrease brain DNA and RNA synthesis (Das and Barone, 1999; Yang *et al.*, 2008). Many studies have claimed a positive association between pesticide exposure with spontaneous abortions or fetal death (Petrelli *et al.*, 2000). Assessment of fetal growth is usually derived by surrogate measures at delivery, including gestation period, fetal size and birth weight. Dichlorodiphenyltrichloroethane (DDT) is an organochlorine pesticide and prototype persistent environmental chemical with endocrine disrupting effects. Longnecker *et al.* (2001) reported that dichlorodiphenyltrichloroethane use increases preterm births, small-for-gestational age which is a major contributor to infant mortality in a sampling subset of more than 44 000 eligible children born between 1959 and 1966 and measured the DDE concentration in their mothers' serum samples. Siddiqui *et al.*, (2003) examined the association between dichlorodiphenyltrichloroethane exposure and intra-uterine growth retardation and found that exposure of pregnant women to organochlorine pesticides elevate the risk of intra-uterine growth retardation, which is one of the factors for increased infant mortality in India. Curtis *et al.*, (1999) studied that application of pesticides was associated with a long time to pregnancy, resulting in a fecundability ratio of 0.46 and low spraying velocity resulted in a fecundability ratio of 0.47. Perera et al. (2005) reported that cord chlorpyrifos, and combined mixtures of cord chlorpyrifos, diazinon and propoxur-metabolite are associated with birth weight and length, indicating that prenatal chlorpyrifos exposures have impaired fetal growth among this minority cohort and that diazinon exposures may have contributed to the effects.

Neurologic and Neurobehavioral Effects

Susceptibility of fetuses and young children to potential neurotoxic effects of pesticides is higher than adults as their brains are developing rapidly (Eskenazi *et al.*, 2007). Different pesticides act as acetylcholinesterase (AChE) inhibitors and during developmental stages, pesticide exposure even at low levels can be detrimental to neurologic functioning (Munoz-Quezada *et al.*, 2013). Pesticides inhibit acetylcholinesterase enzyme (which is already lower during pregnancy) and prevent breakdown of the neurotransmitter acetylcholine, increasing its concentration and time in the neuronal junction. This acetylcholinesterase suppression disturbs synaptogenesis, and axonogenesis, cell replication and differentiation (Dam *et al.*, 2003; Tadeo, 2008). Eskenazi et al. (2007) reported that exposure of organophosphate (OP) pesticides is adversely impacting the mental development and pervasive developmental problems in newborns. Rauh *et al.* (2006) also studied the Prenatal Chlorpyrifos Exposure on Neurodevelopment by relating the maternal blood levels of a diethyl phosphate pesticide during pregnancy and performance on the Bayley Scales of Infant Development. They reported that in initial three years of life with high prenatal chlorpyrifos is directly related to delays in psychomotor and mental development and it also affected the mothers with symptoms of pervasive developmental problems. In another study, Rauh *et al.* (2011) highlighted the widespread use of chlorpyrifos and investigated that prenatal exposure of chlorpyrifos at 7 years of age is associated with deficits in Working Memory Index and Full-Scale IQ. Berkowitz *et al.* (2004) reported the relationship between paraoxonase (PON1) polymorphisms and enzyme activity and its effects on infant growth and neurodevelopment and reported that chlorpyrifos has deleterious effect on fetal neurodevelopment among mothers with low paraoxonase (PON1) activity.

Hormonal Imbalance and Endocrine Disruption Abnormalities

Reports of pesticides acting as endocrine disrupters were reported as early as 1949 when the aerial application of DDT was found as the main cause in low sperm count of men (Singer 1949). Pesticides interfere with the hormonal functioning of females, which lead to negative effects on the reproductive system through disordering the hormonal balance necessary for proper functioning (Bretveld et.

al. 2006). Cell receptors become susceptible to the action of exogenous chemicals due to which imbalance of the endocrine system in female adversely affects the menstrual cycle and fertility (Figure 3) (Nicolopoulou-Stamati and Pitsos, 2001). Pesticides come under the class of endocrine-disrupting contaminants (EDC) that exert hormonal activity and when delivered during a specific period of embryonic development, have the potential to modify the organization of the reproductive, immune and nervous systems permanently (Guillette *et al.*, 1995). EDCs mimic the action of natural hormones by binding to different hormone receptors interfere with the synthesis, transport, metabolism and elimination of hormones. There has been enough research that reported certain pesticides acting as potential EDCs (Table 4). During the periods of gestation and breastfeeding fetuses and babies get larger doses of EDCs due to the mobilization of maternal fat reserves (Balabanic *et al.*, 2011). EDC's having estrogenic properties can also block ovulation in females, by affecting the luteinizing hormone surge, like the contraceptive pills do (Ashby *et al.*, 2002). Different studies have suggested even adverse endocrine-disrupting effects, like cryptorchidism, hypospadias and different birth defects on children and fetuses exposed to pesticides (Carbone *et al.*, 2006). Farr *et al.* (2004) studied the relationship between pesticide exposure and menstrual function and reported that use of carbamate pesticides was linked with an increased chance of long cycles and with a lesser risk of irregular cycles.

Pediatric Cancer

Cancer is considered as the second leading cause for children's death after accidents and among the 12 different types of cancer Leukemia has the highest rate of incidence, whereas childhood brain tumours (CBT) and lymphomas are respectively on second and third most frequent groups (Nasterlack, 2007). Fetuses are more sensitive to harm from environmental toxicants and their prenatal exposures have been associated with adverse health impacts (Selevan, 2000). Various epidemiologic studies conducted all over the globe indicate that current pesticide exposures are

Figure 3. Potential effects of pesticides on female reproduction
Bretveld et al., 2006.

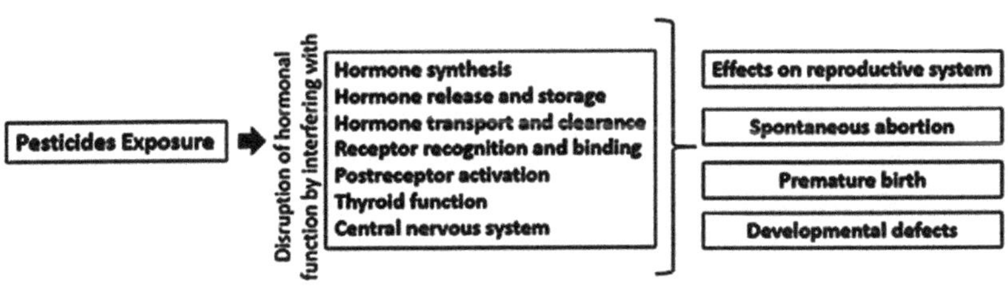

Table 4. Common endocrine-disrupting pesticide groups: their effects and modes of action

Pesticide Group	Hormones Affected	Mechanisms	References
Organochlorines	Oestrogens, androgens, prolactin	Inhibition of androgen receptor, oestrogen-sensitive reporter, binding to androgen receptors, interruption in induction of aromatase	Daxenberger, 2002; Lemaire *et al.*, 2004
Organophosphates	Oestrogens	Onset of oestrogen-related genomic activity	Gwinn *et al.*, 2005
Carbamates	Steroids, androgens, oestrogens	Oestrogen receptor interruption with cellular microtubule formation in oestrogen-sensitive cells	Lu *et al.*, 2006; Goad *et al.*, 2004
Triazines	Androgens	Inhibition of androgen receptors, binding to androgen-binding receptors, induction or inhibition of aromatase	Ishihara *et al.*, 2003
Pyrethrins	Progesterone, oestrogens	Inhibition or potentiation of oestrogen action by interfering progesterone action	Kim *et al.*, 2007

associated with increased risks of childhood leukaemia, brain cancer, neuroblastoma, non-Hodgkin's lymphoma, Wilms' tumour, and Ewing's sarcoma. Pesticides of different groups including organochlorines, organophosphates, carbamates and pyrethroids are classified as possible carcinogens by USEPA and IARC (George and Shukla, 2011). Infante-Rivard and Weichenthal (2007) reported that parental occupational exposure to pesticides during pregnancy contribute to children's cumulative burden. Shim *et al.* (2009) diagnosed brain cancer cases at <10 years of age and reported the associations between parental exposure to pesticides and risk of astrocytoma in offspring from statewide cancer registries of four U.S. Atlantic Coast states. Turner *et al.* (2011) confirmed the positive association between unspecified residential pesticides, insecticides and herbicides exposures during pregnancy with childhood leukaemia in a meta-analysis of previous observational epidemiologic studies. Greenop *et al.* (2013) suggested that pesticide exposure during pregnancy was related to an increase in childhood brain tumours (CBT). Similarly, Chen *et al.* (2015) observed a positive relationship between exposure to pesticides and paediatric cancer and the strongest relation was found between from exposure to indoor pesticides and acute childhood leukaemia.

Many different diseases that are supposed to occur by the pesticide exposure, but lack of consistent evidence and ongoing investigations are major limitations to put those diseases on the list. We will give a brief account some of such astounding diseases. Pesticides as endocrine disrupters are believed to affect the development of the male reproductive system. Several studies revealed male children of women who were exposed to pesticides in early pregnancy showed signs of reduced genital size and change in hormone level (Andersen *et al.*, 2008; Wohlfahrt-Veje *et al.*, 2012a). Other scientists reported early breast development in female offspring of pregnant greenhouse workers who were exposed to non-persistent pesticides. Breast development started 1-1.5 years earlier in daughters of pesticide-exposed pregnant women as compared to daughters of unexposed pregnant women (Wohlfahrt-Veje *et al.*, 2012b). A very few reports showed a positive association of maternal pesticide exposure with Neural tube defects (NTDs), which occur during neurulation when neural tube remains open and is not closed in 21 to 28 days of postconception (Brender *et al.*, 2010; Yang *et al.*, 2014). But in other studies, the association of maternal pesticide exposure with NTDs has not consistently been ascertained (Lacasana *et al.*, 2006; Makelarski *et al.*, 2014). Shelton *et al.* (2012) reviewed that parental exposure to pesticides may or may not influence the trend of increasing Autism, which is composite behaviourally specified condition is usually found in children below the age of 3 years. Asthma, a paediatric widespread respiratory disease has been associated with foetal or early life exposure to pesticides by many researchers. Raanan *et al.* (2015) suggested pesticide exposure in early life stage is associated with different respiratory diseases and Salameh *et al.* (2006) revealed chronic respiratory symptoms and asthma were influenced by pesticide exposure and also found asthma in adult Lebanese caused by pesticide exposure.

CONCLUSION

In this study, we attempted to find the potential health effect of pesticide-contaminated drinking water on pregnant women (fetuses) and children. We tried to explore different routes of pesticide exposure into drinking water and also discussed different diseases caused in most risk-prone age groups. Stringent laws and regulations can help in tackling the pollution of drinking water with pesticides. There should be the monitoring and regulatory authorities to maintain safe and desirable drinking water supply. Also, utilization of biopesticides instead or chemical pesticide formulations and organic farming practices can lower the chemical pesticide load in the environment. Biopesticides are an eco-friendly alternative to synthetic chemical pesticides, which involves a broad array of biologically originated pesticides from microbes, nematodes, secondary metabolites of plants and also involves the exploitation of predatory or parasitic relation of organisms to control the pest population. Biopesticides are easily degradable as compared to conventional pesticides and also less hazardous to ecosystems. There is also a growing stress for the adoption of agricultural practices which depends on the use of biological inputs rather than synthetic chemical fertilizers and pesticides. Organic farming practices can provide better food quality without pesticide and nutrient pollution also the ecological soil quality can be maintained. In conclusion awareness about the pesticide contamination in drinking water and health hazards of these pesticide residues can help in minimizing the deleterious impacts of pesticides.

REFERENCES

Ali, U., Syed, J. H., Malik, R. N., Katsoyiannis, A., Li, J., Zhang, G., & Jones, K. C. (2014). Organochlorine pesticides (OCPs) in South Asian region: A review. *The Science of the Total Environment*, *476*, 705–717. doi:10.1016/j.scitotenv.2013.12.107 PMID:24522007

Andersen, H. R., Schmidt, I. M., Grandjean, P., Jensen, T. K., Budtz-Jørgensen, E., Kjaerstad, M. B., & Main, K. M. (2008). Impaired reproductive development in sons of women occupationally exposed to pesticides during pregnancy. *Environmental Health Perspectives*, *116*(4), 566–572. doi:10.1289/ehp.10790 PMID:18414644

Andreu, V., & Pico, Y. (2004). Determination of pesticides and their degradation products in soil: Critical review and comparison of methods. *Trends in Analytical Chemistry*, *23*(10), 772–789. doi:10.1016/j.trac.2004.07.008

Asghar, U., Malik, M. F., & Javed, A. (2016). Pesticide exposure and human health: A review. *Journal of Ecosystem and Ecography*, 5-12.

Ashby, J., Tinwell, H., Stevens, J., Pastoor, T., & Breckenridge, C. B. (2002). The effects of atrazine on the sexual maturation of female rats. *Regulatory Toxicology and Pharmacology*, *35*(3), 468–473. doi:10.1006/rtph.2002.1571 PMID:12202059

Assessment, M. E. (2005). *Ecosystems and human well-being: wetlands and water*. Washington, DC: World Resources Institute.

Balabanic, D., Rupnik, M., & Klemencic, A. K. (2011). Negative impact of endocrine-disrupting compounds on human reproductive health. *Reproduction, Fertility, and Development*, *23*(3), 403–416. PMID:21426858

Bartram, J., & Cairncross, S. (2010). Hygiene, sanitation, and water: Forgotten foundations of health. *PLoS Medicine*, *7*(11), e1000367. doi:10.1371/journal.pmed.1000367 PMID:21085694

Benner, J., Helbling, D. E., Kohler, H. P. E., Wittebol, J., Kaiser, E., Prasse, C., & Springael, D. (2013). Is biological treatment a viable alternative for micropollutant removal in drinking water treatment processes? *Water Research*, *47*(16), 5955–5976. doi:10.1016/j.watres.2013.07.015 PMID:24053940

Berkowitz, G. S., Wetmur, J. G., Birman-Deych, E., Obel, J., Lapinski, R. H., Godbold, J. H., & Wolff, M. S. (2004). In utero pesticide exposure, maternal paraoxonase activity, and head circumference. *Environmental Health Perspectives*, *112*(3), 388–391. doi:10.1289/ehp.6414 PMID:14998758

BIS IS10500. (2012). *Indian Standard Drinking Water–Specification (Second revision)*. Bureau of Indian Standards (BIS).

Bradman, A., Barr, D. B., Henn, B. G. C., Drumheller, T., Curry, C., & Eskenazi, B. (2003). Measurement of pesticides and other toxicants in amniotic fluid as a potential biomarker of prenatal exposure: A validation study. *Environmental Health Perspectives*, *111*(14), 1779–1782. doi:10.1289/ehp.6259 PMID:14594631

Brender, J. D., Felkner, M., Suarez, L., Canfield, M. A., & Henry, J. P. (2010). Maternal pesticide exposure and neural tube defects in Mexican Americans. *Annals of Epidemiology*, *20*(1), 16–22. doi:10.1016/j.annepidem.2009.09.011 PMID:20006272

Bretveld, R. W., Thomas, C. M., Scheepers, P. T., Zielhuis, G. A., & Roeleveld, N. (2006). Pesticide exposure: The hormonal function of the female reproductive system disrupted? *Reproductive Biology and Endocrinology*, *4*(1), 30. doi:10.1186/1477-7827-4-30 PMID:16737536

Buccini, J. (2003). The Development of a Global Treaty on Persistent Organic Pollutants (POPs). In Persistent Organic Pollutants. The Handbook of Environmental Chemistry (vol. 3, pp. 13-30). Springer.

Carbone, P., Giordano, F., Nori, F., Mantovani, A., Taruscio, D., Lauria, L., & Figa-Talamanca, I. (2006). Cryptorchidism and hypospadias in the Sicilian district of Ragusa and the use of pesticides. *Reproductive Toxicology (Elmsford, N.Y.)*, *22*(1), 8–12. doi:10.1016/j.reprotox.2006.01.006 PMID:16530380

Chen, M., Chang, C. H., Tao, L., & Lu, C. (2015). Residential exposure to pesticide during childhood and childhood cancers: A meta-analysis. *Pediatrics*, *136*(4), 719–729. doi:10.1542/peds.2015-0006 PMID:26371195

CIBRC. (2015). *List of pesticides which are banned, refused registration and restricted in use*. Retrieved March 8, 2018, from http://cibrc.nic.in/ibr2012.doc

Colborn, T. (2006). A case for revisiting the safety of pesticides: A closer look at neurodevelopment. *Environmental Health Perspectives, 114*(1), 10–17. doi:10.1289/ehp.7940 PMID:16393651

Criswell, J. T., Shelton, K., & Luper, C. (2014). *Toxicity of pesticides. Pesticide Applicator Certificate Series.* Oklahoma Cooperative Extension Service EPP-7457-8. Available from: http://www.dasnr22.dasnr.okstate.edu/docushare/dsweb/get/.../EPP-7457web.pdf

Curtis, K. M., Savitz, D. A., Weinberg, C. R., & Arbuckle, T. E. (1999). The effect of pesticide exposure on time to pregnancy. *Epidemiology (Cambridge, Mass.), 10*(2), 112–117. doi:10.1097/00001648-199903000-00005 PMID:10069244

Dam, K., Seidler, F. J., & Slotkin, T. A. (2003). Transcriptional biomarkers distinguish between vulnerable periods for developmental neurotoxicity of chlorpyrifos: Implications for toxicogenomics. *Brain Research Bulletin, 59*(4), 261–265. doi:10.1016/S0361-9230(02)00874-2 PMID:12464398

Damalas, C. A., & Eleftherohorinos, I. G. (2011). Pesticide exposure, safety issues, and risk assessment indicators. *International Journal of Environmental Research and Public Health, 8*(5), 1402–1419. doi:10.3390/ijerph8051402 PMID:21655127

Das, K. P., & Barone, S. Jr. (1999). Neuronal differentiation in PC12 cells is inhibited by chlorpyrifos and its metabolites: Is acetylcholinesterase inhibition the site of action? *Toxicology and Applied Pharmacology, 160*(3), 217–230. doi:10.1006/taap.1999.8767 PMID:10544056

Daxenberger, A. (2002). Pollutants with androgen-disrupting potency. *European Journal of Lipid Science and Technology, 104*(2), 124–130. doi:10.1002/1438-9312(200202)104:2<124::AID-EJLT124>3.0.CO;2-T

De Gerónimo, E., Aparicio, V. C., Bárbaro, S., Portocarrero, R., Jaime, S., & Costa, J. L. (2014). Presence of pesticides in surface water from four sub-basins in Argentina. *Chemosphere, 107*, 423–431. doi:10.1016/j.chemosphere.2014.01.039 PMID:24548646

Eskenazi, B., Marks, A. R., Bradman, A., Harley, K., Barr, D. B., Johnson, C., & Jewell, N. P. (2007). Organophosphate pesticide exposure and neurodevelopment in young Mexican-American children. *Environmental Health Perspectives, 115*(5), 792–798. doi:10.1289/ehp.9828 PMID:17520070

Farr, S. L., Cooper, G. S., Cai, J., Savitz, D. A., & Sandler, D. P. (2004). Pesticide use and menstrual cycle characteristics among premenopausal women in the agricultural health study. *American Journal of Epidemiology*, *160*(12), 1194–1204. doi:10.1093/aje/kwi006 PMID:15583372

Fawell, J., & Nieuwenhuijsen, M. J. (2003). Contaminants in drinking waterEnvironmental pollution and health. *British Medical Bulletin*, *68*(1), 199–208. doi:10.1093/bmb/ldg027 PMID:14757718

Gao, F., & Lu, X. (2015). Detection of pesticides in foods by enzymatic biosensors. In *Improving and Tailoring Enzymes for Food Quality and Functionality*. Cambridge, UK: Woodhead publishing. doi:10.1016/B978-1-78242-285-3.00007-7

Garry, V. F. (2004). Pesticides and children. *Toxicology and Applied Pharmacology*, *198*(2), 152–163. doi:10.1016/j.taap.2003.11.027 PMID:15236951

George, J., & Shukla, Y. (2011). Pesticides and cancer: Insights into toxicoproteomic-based findings. *Journal of Proteomics*, *74*(12), 2713–2722. doi:10.1016/j.jprot.2011.09.024 PMID:21989265

Gilden, R. C., Huffling, K., & Sattler, B. (2010). Pesticides and health risks. *Journal of Obstetric, Gynecologic, and Neonatal Nursing*, *39*(1), 103–110. doi:10.1111/j.1552-6909.2009.01092.x PMID:20409108

Goad, R. T., Goad, J. T., Atieh, B. H., & Gupta, R. C. (2004). Carbofuran-induced endocrine disruption in adult male rats. *Toxicology Mechanisms and Methods*, *14*(4), 233–239. doi:10.1080/15376520490434476 PMID:20021136

Greenop, K. R., Peters, S., Bailey, H. D., Fritschi, L., Attia, J., Scott, R. J., & Milne, E. (2013). Exposure to pesticides and the risk of childhood brain tumors. *Cancer Causes & Control*, *24*(7), 1269–1278. doi:10.100710552-013-0205-1 PMID:23558445

Guillette, L. J. Jr, Crain, D. A., Rooney, A. A., & Pickford, D. B. (1995). Organization versus activation: The role of endocrine-disrupting contaminants (EDCs) during embryonic development in wildlife. *Environmental Health Perspectives*, *103*(Suppl 7), 157–164. doi:10.1289/ehp.95103s7157 PMID:8593864

Gwinn, M. R., Whipkey, D. L., Tennant, L. B., & Weston, A. (2005). Differential gene expression in normal human mammary epithelial cells treated with malathion monitored by DNA microarrays. *Environmental Health Perspectives*, *113*(8), 1046–1051. doi:10.1289/ehp.7311 PMID:16079077

Hamilton, D. J., Ambrus, A., Dieterle, R. M., Felsot, A. S., Harris, C. A., Holland, P. T., & Wong, S. S. (2003). Regulatory limits for pesticide residues in water (IUPAC Technical Report). *Pure and Applied Chemistry*, *75*(8), 1123–1155. doi:10.1351/pac200375081123

Infante-Rivard, C., & Weichenthal, S. (2007). Pesticides and childhood cancer: An update of Zahm and Ward's 1998 review. *Journal of Toxicology and Environmental Health. Part B*, *10*(1-2), 81–99.

Ishihara, A., Sawatsubashi, S., & Yamauchi, K. (2003). Endocrine disrupting chemicals: Interference of thyroid hormone binding to transthyretins and to thyroid hormone receptors. *Molecular and Cellular Endocrinology*, *199*(1), 105–117. doi:10.1016/S0303-7207(02)00302-7 PMID:12581883

Islam, M. N., Bint-E-Naser, S. F., & Khan, M. S. (2017). Pesticide Food Laws and Regulations. In *Pesticide Residue in Foods*. Cham, Switzerland: Springer. doi:10.1007/978-3-319-52683-6_3

Kim, S. D., Cho, J., Kim, I. S., Vanderford, B. J., & Snyder, S. A. (2007). Occurrence and removal of pharmaceuticals and endocrine disruptors in South Korean surface, drinking, and waste waters. *Water Research*, *41*(5), 1013–1021. doi:10.1016/j.watres.2006.06.034 PMID:16934312

Lacasana, M., Vazquez-Grameix, H., Borja-Aburto, V. H., Blanco-Muñoz, J., Romieu, I., Aguilar-Garduño, C., & García, A. M. (2006). Maternal and paternal occupational exposure to agricultural work and the risk of anencephaly. *Occupational and Environmental Medicine*, *63*(10), 649–656. doi:10.1136/oem.2005.023333 PMID:16873458

Lehmann, E., Turrero, N., Kolia, M., Konaté, Y., & De Alencastro, L. F. (2017). Dietary risk assessment of pesticides from vegetables and drinking water in gardening areas in Burkina Faso. *The Science of the Total Environment*, *601*, 1208–1216. doi:10.1016/j.scitotenv.2017.05.285 PMID:28605838

Lemaire, G., Terouanne, B., Mauvais, P., Michel, S., & Rahmani, R. (2004). Effect of organochlorine pesticides on human androgen receptor activation in vitro. *Toxicology and Applied Pharmacology*, *196*(2), 235–246. doi:10.1016/j.taap.2003.12.011 PMID:15081270

Longnecker, M. P., Klebanoff, M. A., Zhou, H., & Brock, J. W. (2001). Association between maternal serum concentration of the DDT metabolite DDE and preterm and small-for-gestational-age babies at birth. *Lancet*, *358*(9276), 110–114. doi:10.1016/S0140-6736(01)05329-6 PMID:11463412

Lu, C., Toepel, K., Irish, R., Fenske, R. A., Barr, D. B., & Bravo, R. (2006). Organic diets significantly lower children's dietary exposure to organophosphorus pesticides. *Environmental Health Perspectives, 114*(2), 260–263. doi:10.1289/ehp.8418 PMID:16451864

Makelarski, J. A., Romitti, P. A., Rocheleau, C. M., Burns, T. L., Stewart, P. A., Waters, M. A., & Olney, R. S. (2014). Maternal periconceptional occupational pesticide exposure and neural tube defects. *Birth Defects Research. Part A, Clinical and Molecular Teratology, 100*(11), 877–886. doi:10.1002/bdra.23293 PMID:25124525

Mostafalou, S., & Abdollahi, M. (2012). Concerns of environmental persistence of pesticides and human chronic diseases. *Journal of Clinical and Experimental Pharmacology, 2*(3), 1–2.

Mostafalou, S., & Abdollahi, M. (2013). Pesticides and human chronic diseases: Evidences, mechanisms, and perspectives. *Toxicology and Applied Pharmacology, 268*(2), 157–177. doi:10.1016/j.taap.2013.01.025 PMID:23402800

Munoz-Quezada, M. T., Lucero, B. A., Barr, D. B., Steenland, K., Levy, K., Ryan, P. B., & Vega, C. (2013). Neurodevelopmental effects in children associated with exposure to organophosphate pesticides: A systematic review. *Neurotoxicology, 39*, 158–168. doi:10.1016/j.neuro.2013.09.003 PMID:24121005

Nasterlack, M. (2007). Pesticides and childhood cancer: An update. *International Journal of Hygiene and Environmental Health, 210*(5), 645–657. doi:10.1016/j.ijheh.2007.03.001 PMID:17434797

Nicolopoulou-Stamati, P., & Pitsos, M. A. (2001). The impact of endocrine disrupters on the female reproductive system. *Human Reproduction Update, 7*(3), 323–330. doi:10.1093/humupd/7.3.323 PMID:11392379

Parsons, S. A., Boxall, A. B. A., Sinclair, C. J., & Ramwell, C. (2008). *Pesticide degradates of concern to the drinking water community*. Denver, CO: AWWA Research Foundation.

Perera, F. P., Rauh, V., Whyatt, R. M., Tang, D., Tsai, W. Y., Bernert, J. T., & Diaz, D. (2005). A summary of recent findings on birth outcomes and developmental effects of prenatal ETS, PAH, and pesticide exposures. *Neurotoxicology, 26*(4), 573–587. doi:10.1016/j.neuro.2004.07.007 PMID:16112323

Petrelli, G., Figa-Talamanca, I., Tropeano, R., Tangucci, M., Cini, C., Aquilani, S., & Meli, P. (2000). Reproductive male-mediated risk: Spontaneous abortion among wives of pesticide applicators. *European Journal of Epidemiology, 16*(4), 391–393. doi:10.1023/A:1007630610911 PMID:10959949

Pruss-Ustun, A., Bos, R., Gore, F., & Bartram, J. (2008). *Safer water, better health: costs, benefits and sustainability of interventions to protect and promote health.* Geneva: World Health Organization.

Raanan, R., Harley, K. G., Balmes, J. R., Bradman, A., Lipsett, M., & Eskenazi, B. (2015). Early-life exposure to organophosphate pesticides and pediatric respiratory symptoms in the Chamacos cohort. *Environmental Health Perspectives, 123*(2), 179. PMID:25369257

Rauh, V., Arunajadai, S., Horton, M., Perera, F., Hoepner, L., Barr, D. B., & Whyatt, R. (2011). Seven-year neurodevelopmental scores and prenatal exposure to chlorpyrifos, a common agricultural pesticide. *Environmental Health Perspectives, 119*(8), 1196–1201. doi:10.1289/ehp.1003160 PMID:21507777

Rauh, V. A., Garfinkel, R., Perera, F. P., Andrews, H. F., Hoepner, L., Barr, D. B., & Whyatt, R. W. (2006). Impact of prenatal chlorpyrifos exposure on neurodevelopment in the first 3 years of life among inner-city children. *Pediatrics, 118*(6), e1845–e1859. doi:10.1542/peds.2006-0338 PMID:17116700

Reichenberger, S., Bach, M., Skitschak, A., & Frede, H. G. (2007). Mitigation strategies to reduce pesticide inputs into ground-and surface water and their effectiveness; a review. *The Science of the Total Environment, 384*(1), 1–35. doi:10.1016/j.scitotenv.2007.04.046 PMID:17588646

Roberts, J. R., & Karr, C. J. (2012). Pesticide exposure in children. *Pediatrics, 130*(6), e1765–e1788. doi:10.1542/peds.2012-2758 PMID:23184105

Rodrigo, M. A., Oturan, N., & Oturan, M. A. (2014). Electrochemically assisted remediation of pesticides in soils and water: A review. *Chemical Reviews, 114*(17), 8720–8745. doi:10.1021/cr500077e PMID:24983494

Salameh, P., Waked, M., Baldi, I., Brochard, P., & Saleh, B. A. (2006). Respiratory diseases and pesticide exposure: A case-control study in Lebanon. *Journal of Epidemiology and Community Health, 60*(3), 256–261. doi:10.1136/jech.2005.039677 PMID:16476757

Sanpera, C., Ruiz, X., Jover, L., Llorente, G., Jabeen, R., Muhammad, A., & Fasola, M. (2003). Persistent organic pollutants in little egret eggs from selected wetlands in Pakistan. *Archives of Environmental Contamination and Toxicology, 44*(3), 360–368. doi:10.100700244-002-2044-z PMID:12712296

Schafer, R. B., Van den Brink, P. J., & Liess, M. (2011). Impacts of pesticides on freshwater ecosystems. *Ecological Impacts of Toxic Chemicals*, 111-137.

Selevan, S. G., Kimmel, C. A., & Mendola, P. (2000). Identifying critical windows of exposure for children's health. *Environmental Health Perspectives*, *108*(Suppl 3), 451–455. doi:10.1289/ehp.00108s3451 PMID:10852844

Shelton, J. F., Hertz-Picciotto, I., & Pessah, I. N. (2012). Tipping the balance of autism risk: Potential mechanisms linking pesticides and autism. *Environmental Health Perspectives*, *120*(7), 944–951. doi:10.1289/ehp.1104553 PMID:22534084

Shim, Y. K., Mlynarek, S. P., & van Wijngaarden, E. (2009). Parental exposure to pesticides and childhood brain cancer: US Atlantic coast childhood brain cancer study. *Environmental Health Perspectives*, *117*(6), 1002–1006. doi:10.1289/ehp.0800209 PMID:19590697

Siddiqui, M., Srivastava, S., Mehrotra, P., Mathur, N., & Tandon, I. (2003). Persistent chlorinated pesticides and intra-uterine foetal growth retardation: A possible association. *International Archives of Occupational and Environmental Health*, *76*(1), 75–80. PMID:12592586

Singer, P. L. (1949). Occupational oligospermia. *Journal of the American Medical Association*, *140*, 1249.

Souza, A. D., Medeiros, A. D. R., Souza, A. C. D., Wink, M., Siqueira, I. R., Ferreira, M. B. C., & Torres, I. L. D. S. (2011). Evaluation of the impact of exposure to pesticides on the health of the rural population: Vale do Taquari, State of Rio Grande do Sul (Brazil). *Ciencia & Saude Coletiva*, *16*(8), 3519–3528. doi:10.1590/S1413-81232011000900020 PMID:21860952

Stillerman, K. P., Mattison, D. R., Giudice, L. C., & Woodruff, T. J. (2008). Environmental exposures and adverse pregnancy outcomes: A review of the science. *Reproductive Sciences (Thousand Oaks, Calif.)*, *15*(7), 631–650. doi:10.1177/1933719108322436 PMID:18836129

Tadeo, J. L. (Ed.). (2008). *Analysis of pesticides in food and environmental samples*. CRC Press. doi:10.1201/9781420007756

Teklu, B. M., Adriaanse, P. I., Ter Horst, M. M., Deneer, J. W., & Van den Brink, P. J. (2015). Surface water risk assessment of pesticides in Ethiopia. *The Science of the Total Environment*, *508*, 566–574. doi:10.1016/j.scitotenv.2014.11.049 PMID:25481716

Thodal, C. E., Carpenter, J., & Moses, C. W. (2009). *Monitoring for Pesticides in Groundwater and Surface Water in Nevada, 2008 (No. 2009-3093)*. US Geological Survey.

Thompson, T., Fawell, J., Kunikane, S., Jackson, D., Appleyard, S., & Callan, P. (2007). *Chemical safety of drinking water: Assessing priorities for risk management.* WHO.

Turner, M. C., Wigle, D. T., & Krewski, D. (2011). Residential pesticides and childhood leukemia: A systematic review and meta-analysis. *Ciencia & Saude Coletiva, 16*(3), 1915–1931. doi:10.1590/S1413-81232011000300026 PMID:21519680

Vos, J. G., Dybing, E., Greim, H. A., Ladefoged, O., Lambre, C., Tarazona, J. V., & Vethaak, A. D. (2000). Health effects of endocrine-disrupting chemicals on wildlife, with special reference to the European situation. *Critical Reviews in Toxicology, 30*(1), 71–133. doi:10.1080/10408440091159176 PMID:10680769

Weselak, M., Arbuckle, T. E., Wigle, D. T., & Krewski, D. (2007). In utero pesticide exposure and childhood morbidity. *Environmental Research, 103*(1), 79–86. doi:10.1016/j.envres.2006.09.001 PMID:17084836

WHO. (2010). *Water for health. WHO guidelines for drinking water quality.* Retrieved from http://www.who.int/water_sanitation_health/WHS_WWD2010_guidelines_2010_6_en.pdf? ua=1

Windham, G., & Fenster, L. (2008). Environmental contaminants and pregnancy outcomes. *Fertility and Sterility, 89*(2), 111–116. doi:10.1016/j.fertnstert.2007.12.041 PMID:18308050

Wohlfahrt-Veje, C., Andersen, H. R., Jensen, T. K., Grandjean, P., Skakkebaek, N. E., & Main, K. M. (2012a). Smaller genitals at school age in boys whose mothers were exposed to non-persistent pesticides in early pregnancy. *International Journal of Andrology, 35*(3), 265–272. doi:10.1111/j.1365-2605.2012.01252.x PMID:22394112

Wohlfahrt-Veje, C., Andersen, H. R., Schmidt, I. M., Aksglaede, L., Sørensen, K., Juul, A., & Main, K. M. (2012b). Early breast development in girls after prenatal exposure to non-persistent pesticides. *International Journal of Andrology, 35*(3), 273–282. doi:10.1111/j.1365-2605.2011.01244.x PMID:22404257

Xu, W., Wang, X., & Cai, Z. (2013). Analytical chemistry of the persistent organic pollutants identified in the Stockholm Convention: A review. *Analytica Chimica Acta, 790*, 1–13. doi:10.1016/j.aca.2013.04.026 PMID:23870403

Yang, D., Howard, A., Bruun, D., Ajua-Alemanj, M., Pickart, C., & Lein, P. J. (2008). Chlorpyrifos and chlorpyrifos-oxon inhibit axonal growth by interfering with the morphogenic activity of acetylcholinesterase. *Toxicology and Applied Pharmacology, 228*(1), 32–41. doi:10.1016/j.taap.2007.11.005 PMID:18076960

Yang, W., Carmichael, S. L., Roberts, E. M., Kegley, S. E., Padula, A. M., English, P. B., & Shaw, G. M. (2014). Residential agricultural pesticide exposures and risk of neural tube defects and orofacial clefts among offspring in the San Joaquin Valley of California. *American Journal of Epidemiology*, *179*(6), 740–748. doi:10.1093/aje/kwt324 PMID:24553680

This research was previously published in the Handbook of Research on the Adverse Effects of Pesticide Pollution in Aquatic Ecosystems edited by Khursheed Ahmad Wani and Mamta; pages 105-122, copyright year 2019 by Engineering Science Reference (an imprint of IGI Global).

Chapter 13
Environmental Phthalate Exposure in Relation to Reproductive Outcomes and Other Health Endpoints in Humans

Sameena
P. M. B. Gujarati Science College, India

Riyes Un Aziz
Government Holkar College, India

Aubid Bashir
Barkatullah University, India

ABSTRACT

Phthalates are the class of chemicals that exhibit numerous adverse effects to health. These non-persistent chemicals are produced in high volume annually and are used in a wide array of industrial consumer products. The overall exposure of phthalates to humans is via ingestion of contaminated food from wrapped materials or dermally via consumer care products. Pthalates are anti-androgenic compounds, so for this reason, they obtrude with the expression of testosterone by manipulating gene expression of proteins and enzymes involved in production of testosterone. The primarily exposure of Pthalates during fetal development stage results in number of harmful effects in male offspring in humans, like abnormalities of the sperm-producing organs, abnormal development of penile, hypospadias, reduced anogenital distance, as well as a risk for prostate cancer and cryptorchidism. The purpose of this chapter was to review the environmental impact of phthalate exposure in relation to reproductive behavior and other health problems in humans.

DOI: 10.4018/978-1-7998-2351-3.ch013

INTRODUCTION

The advancement of civilization resulted in foundation of new and progressive technologies, consumer products and goods whose manufacture needs new raw materials and chemical compounds. Most of the compounds among them are long-lasting and are not degraded after releasing in to the environment. They get deposited in the food chain and are then migrated across countries or even continents (Ziolkowska and Wyszkowska, 2010). Environmental pollutants affect soil properties (Wyszkowska and Wyszkowski, 2002; Wyszkowski and Sivitskaya, 2012) and exert a generally negative influence on flora, fauna and other forms of life (Ziolkowska and Wyszkowska, 2010; Wyszkowska and Wyszkowski, 2009). They can result in the endocrinological and reproductive problems. Selected chemical substances have androgen synthesis (Adamsson *et al.*, 2009). Phthalates, or esters of phthalic acid, are environmental pollutants (Grynkiewicz, 2011). Those leading plasticizers are added to polyvinyl chloride in order to enhance its hardness and flexibility. Phthalates are used almost in every industry, and they can be found in construction materials, food packaging, pharmaceuticals, varnish, cosmetics, printing inks, latex paint, medical products clothing,, such as intravenous cannulas, and insecticides (Koniecki *et al.*, 2011; Fierens *et al.*, 2012).

The aim of this study was to differentiate phthalates, to find out the sources of phthalate pollution in the environment, and to describe their affect on living organisms.

MODE OF ACTION, MECHANISM OF ACTION AND COMMON ADVERSE OUTCOMES (NATIONAL RESEARCH COUNCIL, 2008)

Mode of action and mechanism of action are terms that are often used in risk assessment and usually used interchangeably. Both these terms refer to the bio-logic pathway to some final health outcome; the difference between the terms is the level of detail used to describe the pathway. Typically, mode of action is used to describe the key events along the pathway and mechanism of action is used to describe the pathway at the molecular level, Although the committee identifies the distinction and does not want to contribute to over confusion regarding the use of the terms, mechanism of action is used in this report to explain the biologic pathway.

Currently, the concentrate in cumulative risk assessment has been on those chemical compounds that have common mechanisms of action. As described below in greater detail, the committee finds that the concentration in cumulative risk assessment must be on the health outcomes and not on the pathways that lead to them, whether defined as modes of action or as mechanisms of action. Several pathways can result to a common outcome, and a focus on only an accurate pathway can lead to limit an approach in conducting a cumulative risk assessment. Accordingly, the chemicals that should be considered for cumulative risk assessment must be ones that cause the same types of health outcomes or the same health outcomes such as specific effects on development of male reproductive system not ones that cause the health issues only by a specific pathway. The committee refers to the health outcomes of interest as common adverse outcomes.

CHARACTERISTICS OF PTHALATES

Phthalates are esters of phthalic acid, also known as esters of benzene-1, 2-dicarboxylic acid are man-made chemicals widely used in industry and commerce. This particular group of manufactured chemicals compounds has a broad spectrum of industrial applications and these chemicals ultimately appear extensively in food processing, consumer products, as well as in medical applications. Phthalates have a benzene ring with two functional (ester) groups. Their solubility in water decreases with an increase in the length of the carbon chain. Phthalates are colorless and odorless oily liquids characterized by limited solubility in water, satisfactory solubility in most organic solvents, high boiling point or molecular weight, low volatility. The esterification reaction to phthalic acid with various alcohols results in the production of the compounds. The amplest use of phthalates in many consumer and personal-care products result in expansive non occupational exposure to humans through several routes (Hauser *et al.*, 2007).

Phthalates are broadly divided into two basic categories; "High molecular-weight phthalates (HMWPs) eg, di2-ethylhexylphthalate (DEHP) and butyl benzyl phthalate (BBzP) include carbon side chains more than 6 (Bradlee and Thomas, 2003), are commonly used in building products, flooring and wall coverings, food packaging and processing materials, and medical devices. Low molecular weight phthalates (LMWPs)" which include carbon chain less than 6, eg, diethyl phthalate (DEP), benzyl butyl phthalate (BBzP), and diisobutyl phthalate (DiBP) are widely used in a variety of cosmetic and personal-hygiene products, toys, childcare products, fragrances as scent stabilizers, varnishes and lacquers (Jurica *et al.*, 2016).

The most widely used phthalates are di(2-ethylhexyl) phthalate (DEHP), diisodecyl phthalate (DIDP), diisononyl phthalate (DINP) and di-n-butyl phthalate (DBP) (Peijnenburg *et al.*, 2008). Di (2-ethylhexyl) phthalate (DEHP): DEHP is also known as dioctyl phthalate (DOP) it is produced by the esterification reaction of 2-ethylhexanol with phthalic anhydride (Ventrice *et al.,* 2013). This is the most common member of the class of phthalates, frequently used in construction materials, consumer goods, and electronics, medical such as infusion fluid containers, surgical drains, intravenous cannulas, blood storage and blood transfusion equipment (Heudorf *et al.,* 2007). According to Lyche, phthalates are ubiquitous contaminants in the environments found in drinking water at the concentration of 0.16-170 μg · dm –3,, in sediments, at 0.0003-218 mg kg –1, indoor air at 20-240 ng · m–3, atmospheric air at <0.4-65 ng · m–3,, dust at 2.38-4.1 g · kg –1, soil at 0.03-1280 mg · kg –1 and wastewater at 0.0004-58.3 g · kg –1. DEHP is characterized by high levels of reproductive toxicity, developmental toxicity and it can also cause reduced fertility, and may damage the neonates.

Diisodecyl Phthalate (DIDP): DIDP is mainly added to polyvinyl chloride (PVC). It can be found in various PVC products, including cable jackets, roofing panels flooring, wall panels, sealants and interior car parts (Risk Assessment Report, (2003) and Kransler *et al.,* (2013).

Diisononyl Phthalate (DINP): DINP is an organic substance. About 95% of globally manufactured DINP is primarily used as PVC plasticizer. It is found in electronics and home appliances footwear, lubricants, paper products inks, pigments flooring, coatings, sealants, varnish and paint (Hays *et al.,* 2011). DINP is a major plasticizer used in children's toys. DINP is obtained by the esterification reaction of phthalic anhydride with isononyl alcohol (Risk Assessment Report, 2003)

Di-n-butyl Phthalate (DBP): DBP is mainly used as a plasticizer for nitrocellulose, polyvinyl chloride and polyvinyl acetate, in coatings, in adhesives and in miscellaneous applications. DBP is obtained by the esterification reaction of phthalic anhydride with n-butanol in the presence of concentrated sulfuric acid. It dissolves easily in most organic solvents, including acetone, diethyl ether, ethanol and benzene (Pałaszewska *et al.,* 2012)

Global assessment of phthalate production in the environment is estimated at 5 million Mg per year, of which more than 60% is used by the processing industries of Japan, North America and Europe (Fierens *et al.,* 2012) When used as plasticizers, phthalates do not bind chemically with the material to which they are added to and are easily released in to the air, water, food and soil. Phthalates are of lipophilic nature, thus are readily dissolved and accumulated in lipids (Fierens *et al.,* 2012 and Heudorf *et al.,* 2007.) The phthalates are not chemically bound in the polymers and hence are leached into the environment from the product and are ubiquitously found in, air, water, soils, and dust. The migration of phthalates occurs during all the stages of life cycle of a product from production, through use, to disposal and the phthalates are thereby ubiquitous in the environment.

Table 1. Phthalate parent compounds and their metabolites

Phthalate name	Abbreviation	Urinary metabolite	Abbreviation
Dimethyl phthalate	DMP	Mono-n-methyl phthalate	MnMP
Diethyl phthalate	DEP	Mono-ethyl phthalate	MEP
Di-isobutyl phthalate	DiBP	Mono-isobutyl phthalate	MiBP
Di-n-butyl phthalate	DnBP	Mono-n-butyl phthalate	MnBP
Di-n-octyl phthalate	DnOP	Mono-(3-carboxypropyl) phthalate	MCPP
Di-isononyl phthalate	DiNP	Mono-carboxyoctyl phthalate	MCOP
Di-isodecyl phthalate	DiDP	Mono-carboxynonyl phthalate	MCNP
Benzylbutyl phthalate	BzBP	Mono-benzyl phthalate	MBzP
Di-2-ethylhexyl phthalate	DEHP	Mono-2-ethylhexyl phthalate	MEHP
		Mono-(2-ethyl-5-hydroxyhexyl) phthalate	MEHHP
		Mono-(2-ethyl-5-oxohexyl) phthalate	MEOHP
		Mono-(2-ethyl-5-carboxypentyl) phthalate	MECPP

STRUCTURE OF PHTHALATES

The viscosity and plasticizer effectiveness of phthalates are because of their chemical structures. Phthalates constitute a broad chemical family comprised of a benzene ring, two carbonyl groups, and two alcohol groups to produce a diester structure. Common branched phthalates such as DINP DBP, DEHP, and BBP feature branched-chain alcohol moieties of 6 to 13 carbons. The linear phthalates contain linear alcohol groups and include short chain phthalates such as DMP and DEP, and other phthalates with chain lengths of 7 to 11 carbons are used to impart increased flexibility at lower temperatures. The benzene ring based structure of phthalates leads to decrease their viscosity level but also makes them harder to degrade. Phthalates move rapidly through the PVC polymer resulting in increased flexibility, softness, and elongation. Since they are not chemically connected to the PVC, and are fairly released in air, water, blood, saliva, since phthalates are highly lipophilic (fat soluble) and get accumulated more readily into lipid-containing solutions. Based on the circumstances of use, 2% - 50% of the phthalate content can emerge from products over their life cycle.

SOURCES OF PHTHALATES IN THE ENVIRONMENT

Phthalates are ubiquitous in household environments in both house dust and indoor air (Rudel *et al.,* 2003). Phthalate levels measured in indoor air are typically many times higher than in outdoor air. People are exposed to phthalates through inhalation and dermal absorption of indoor air. They have also been measured in variety of sources like foodstuff, drinking water and milk. However, the specific share from the various sources and phthalate exposure routes is unknown (Wormuth *et al.,* 2006).

High molecular weight phthalates, such as di(2-ethylhexyl) phthalate [DEHP], di-isononyl phthalate [DiNP], di-n-octyl phthalate [DnoP] are chiefly used as plasticizers to soften polyvinyl chloride (PVC) products which are widely used in personal care products food-containing materials, building materials, cosmetics, medical equipments(ATSDR, 2002). Highest exposure to DEHP can occur in the working environment (e.g. during the manufacture and processing of DEHP or DEHP containing products), during consumer use of these products, or through environmental media (food, air, water, dust). The use of DEHP in consumer products to which children are exposed e.g. toys, bath books, food packaging, and medical devices such as blood, intravenous tubing and nutrient bags are of great concern because of the increased vulnerability of general public

Lower molecular weight phthalates, including di-n-butyl phthalate (DnBP) and diethyl phthalate (DEP), are used personal-care products (e.g. perfumes, lotions, and cosmetics), as solvents and plasticizers for cellulose acetate, in the manufacture of lacquers, varnishes and coatings of drugs (ATSDR, 1995; ATSDR,2001), including those used to make time-release in some pharmaceutical products (Hauser, 2004). DEP (urinary metabolite MEP) levels measured in population samples are found in major quantity than those of DBP and DEHP (CDC, 2003; CDC, 2005). DEP has been found commonly in a large number of cosmetics and personal care products as shampoos, body washes conditioners, shaving gels, hair styling gels, deodorants and lotions and, in adults (Duty, 2005a) and youngsters (Sathyanarayana, 2008) associated with the use of such products

ROUTES OF EXPOSURE TO PHTHALATES

Humans are exposed to phthalates by several routes, and the most likely route varies by phthalate. Exposures can be oral (e.g. DEHP via phthalate-contaminated food, water and other liquids) or dermal (e.g. DEP, via cosmetics and other personal care products) and in infants and toddlers through frequent mouthing of toys) or can also be via inhalational exposure (FDA, 2001).Phthalates exposure to neonates occurs through the placenta or breast-feeding. Breast milk is known to contain detectable amounts of phthalates, particularly the most hydrophobic compounds, DINP and DEHP (Calafat *et al.*, 2004). Parenteral exposure from phthalate containing products and medical devices also lead to higher phthalate exposures mainly Di (2-ethylhexyl) phthalate (DEHP) to hospitalized populations (ATSDR, 2002; Green *et al.*, 2005). Phthalates are readily absorbed into the human blood stream or body fluids and are converted quickly into their respective primary and secondary metabolites. Unlike some other chemicals, they tend to excrete out of the body quickly through fecal matter and urine and. Phthalates can interact and associate with each other and hence enhance the toxicity.

PHTHALATE TOXICITY

Phthalate exposure in human beings is associated with potential disturbance in the development and function of reproductive organs through endocrine disruption, delays in fertility, impairment in fetal development, Sertoli cell dysfunction, and hormonal disruption in Leydig's cells, testicular effects increased risk of allergies, toxicity to kidneys, asthma, and cancer. The current tolerable daily intake (TDI) values for BBP, DBP and DEHP established by the EU Scientific Committee for Toxicity, Ecotoxicity and the Environment (CSTEE) is 37 μg/kg body weight/day based on available studies of reproductive toxicity, since wide spread exposure and reproductive toxicity seem to have greater relevance for humans beings than the proliferation of peroxisome in laboratory animal (rat) liver causing cancer (EFSA, 2003,2005; EU Scientific committee, 2017). One must be fully conscious that phthalate levels determined in the general public are far below the threshold levels at which the first toxic effects were detected in laboratory animals (Koch *et al.*, 2004; Duty *et al.*, 2003). However, because of the multiple contributing sources and routes of human exposure to different chemical classes (e.g. polybrominated diphenyl ethers, polychlorinated biphenyls, currently used pesticides– pyrethroids and organophosphates, bisphenol A, and phthalates) it is of great challenge to recognize which chemical or metabolite is responsible for adverse health outcomes (Robinson and Miller, 2015).

PHTHALATES ARE TOXIC TO MULTIPLE ORGAN SYSTEMS IN HUMANS AND ANIMAL MODELS

Phthalates are a class of chemicals that cause adverse health effects to multiple organ systems in humans and animal models. It is well known that phthalates are anti-androgenic compounds: that is, they alter the expression of the male sex hormone testosterone by reducing the expression or function of genes of enzymes and proteins involved in testosterone secretion. This may result in reduced fertility in males, and the production of non fertile sperm, as well as profound effects on the development of sexual organs during prenatal development. Male sex hormone, testosterone is important during fetal development in mammals, for the development of male reproductive organs. Exposure to phthalates during this critical period results in constellation of effects in male neonates in animal models, including abnormal development penis, abnormalities of the sperm-producing structures, cryptorchidism (undescended testes), reduced anogenital distance (AGD) (a marker of feminization), retained nipples and hypospadias (urethral opening on the underside of the penis instead of the tip) Similar effects have been observed in human studies associated with fetal or infant exposure to phthalates. Decreased anogenital distance and penile size is associated with poor semen quality in young men (Mendiola *et al.,* 2011), as well as higher risk for prostate cancer (Castano-Vinyals *et al.,* 2012). Effects on sexual development in both boys and girls are associated with phthalate exposure during childhood. Reproductive effects such as increased rates of miscarriage and decreased gestational age have also been observed in human studies.

A serious issue is the potential for phthalate exposure to affect intellectual development and other aspects of behavior. Prenatal phthalate exposure in humans is directly correlated with poorer cognitive performance during childhood, poorer psychomotor development during infancy and poorer social behavior. Prenatal exposure to phthalates is associated with a reduced masculine play behavior in boys during childhood. Phthalate exposure during childhood is significantly associated with decreased IQ and vocabulary scores, and learning disabilities and mental disorders, impulsivity, autism spectrum disorder and attention deficit hyperactivity disorder (ADHD) behaviors. Experimental animal studies also documented that phthalate exposure during early life can alter brain neurochemistry and induces abnormal behavioral presentations. Possible mechanisms include maternal thyroid dysfunction during pregnancy; interference with receptors on cells that are involved in various processes during early fetal development; interference with calcium signaling (functionally essential for communication between nerve cells); and interference with normal lipid metabolism, which is crucial for normal functioning and development of brain (Miodovnik *et al.,* 2014). Phthalates also affect normal immune system function by producing and secreting potent inflammatory factors in intact animals in vitro (tissue culture or cell) systems. Prenatal and postnatal exposure to phthalate is strongly linked with an enhancement in allergic responses like increase in asthma, congestion, breathlessness, wheezing, and eczema in children, and an increase in inflammatory response in both children and adults.

Phthalate exposure is strongly correlated with overweight/obesity in both children and adults, as well as an increase in elevated fasting glucose and insulin levels in adults. Phthalate exposure also alters thyroid hormone levels; increased risk of cardiovascular disease increased blood pressure, and increased risk for fibroids and endometriosis.

EVALUATING HUMAN EXPOSURE TO PHTHALATES

Because of the universal nature of environmental phthalate exposure, conventional epidemiological exposure estimation data (questionnaire information, environmental monitoring medical records, etc.) are of confined utility in assessing individual exposure. Instead, biomarkers of exposure are prominent. Urine is the preferred matrix as biomarker for phthalate determination in humans (Calafat and McKee, 2006). As a result of quick metabolism, metabolite levels in urine are typically higher, and are therefore more accurately biomonitored than levels of the total phthalate compound found in other media. Use of metabolites as biomarkers is preferred, because the possibility of accidental contamination during collection, storage and evaluation is greatly reduced. Phthalates or their metabolites have also been detected in many body fluids or secretions, including; urine, plasma, saliva, serum, breast milk, amniotic fluid, me conium and placenta. Phthalate exposures that occur during prenatal development are more likely to result in profound and permanent damaging effects on development than postnatal exposures, conducting such studies in human populations is of great challenge. First, in order to determine exposure precisely during fetal development, it is necessary to carefully monitor the assays by using archived samples from women during pregnancy. Second, such studies need reliable assessment of the offspring of those pregnancies. While this is considerably easy while prenatal stage, in order to examine associated outcomes occurring in postnatal life such as decreased semen quality, impaired fertility- it is essential to follow the pregnancy cohort for decades. The latest availability of various sensitive, specific, and economical assays makes such measures more functional for epidemiological studies (Silva *et al.,* 2007). Moreover, international quality control programs for phthalate metabolite measurements in human samples leads to the enhancement of comparability of results across laboratories worldwide.

Phthalates are quickly metabolized and excreted from the body, with the elimination half-lives less than 24 hours (Koch *et al.,* 2005). Most recent studies have examined the variability of urinary phthalate metabolites within-person (Hoppin *et al.,* 2004) and found that the Pearson correlation coefficient in phthalate or phthalate metabolite concentration in women's samples measured on two consecutive days ranged from 0.5 for mBzP to 0.8 for mBP and concluded that exposure may be adequately stable to assign an exposure level in spite of their short half-lives, based on a single sample. Accordingly,(Hauser, 2004) demonstrated that despite high day-to-day and month-to-month variability in men's individual urinary phthalate metabolite concentrations, a single spot urine sample sufficiently represented average concentration over 3 months period (Teitelbaum *et al.,* 2008) examined that sources of variability in biomarkers of environmental exposures in minority children, including phthalates, and found that a single urine sample is reasonable predictive of exposure over a 6-month interval to authorize its use as an exposure estimate in environmental epidemiology studies The data published on levels of phthalate metabolites in a large population-based sample of the US population over 6 years of age by Centers for Disease Control and Prevention (CDC) (CDC, 2003; CDC, 2005) revealed that widespread nature of phthalate metabolites and variation in measurements by sex ethnicity, age and sex. Wormuth (2006) concluded that phthalate metabolite levels estimated in a European population and estimates of exposure to DEHP and DBP in neonates are about one order of magnitude greater than those in adults. Furthermore, levels of methylbutylphthalate (MBP), monomethylphthalate (MMP) and methylethylphthalate (MEP), in newborns, are directly related to the number of baby care products (creams, powders and lotions) used by their mothers (Sathyanarayana, 2008).

HUMAN FETAL OR INFANT PHTHALATE EXPOSURE AND ASSOCIATED HEALTH OUTCOMES

There were few studies conducted on environmental phthalate exposure associated with human health outcomes prior to 2000.

Evidence for the "Phthalate Syndrome" in Human

Over the past ten years, various experimental studies on rodents reported that several phthalates (most notably, BzBP, DBP and DEHP), disrupt the androgen-signaling pathway in males, causes male reproductive tract abnormalities when administered at the critical window for the development of the reproductive tract (Gray, 2000, Akingbemi, 2004, Foster, 2006). Lee and Koo (2007) the anti-androgenic effects of seven phthalates (DEHP and its metabolite, mono-2-ethyhexyl phthalate (MEHP), BzBP, DBP as well as di-n-heptyl phthalate (DnHP), di-isodecyl phthalate (DIDP), di-isononyl phthalate (DINP), were demonstrated by the Hershberger assay in castrated male SD rats, consequently this anti-androgenic action during prenatal period causes interference with the normal development of reproductive system, most notably results in reduced anogenital distance (AGD). Anogenital distance is the distance between the anus and external genetalia in newborn rodent pups. AGD is used as a sensitive biomarker of prenatal exposure to anti-androgens, including phthalates, flutamide and vinclozilin. Only a single human study had examined AGD in human males (Salazar-Martinez, 2004), although two other studies had examined AGD in female infants prior to 2005 (Callegari, 1987, Phillip *et al.,* 1996). These studies examined the possible sexual dimorphism of AGD in humans, consistent with rodent studies. However, these studies did not address the relationship of AGD to chemical exposure.

Numerous animal studies have reported that DBP, BzBP and DEHP induces marked reductions in testicular testosterone (T) production in neonates and reduces the expression of insulin-like growth factor-3 (Insl-3),exert diverging effects on male reproductive organs which, in addition to shortened AGD, other abnormalities include cryptorchidism, hypospadias, low sperm counts and malformations of the prostate, epididymis,, seminal vesicles, vas deferens and; altered hormone levels together they comprise the "phthalate syndrome" (Foster, 2006; Welsh, 2008).

While a variety of anti-androgens alter anogenital distance AGD in rodents, most are androgen receptor (AR) antagonists. The syndrome induced by the AR-antagonists differs from that induced by the phthalates, which suppress fetal testosterone and Insl-3 synthesis (Wilson *et al.,* 2008, Wilson, 2004). A variety of potentially anti-androgens including linuron (L), procymidone (P), linuron (L), p,p -DDE and flutamide (F) were tested. P, L, and p,p -DDE produced F-like profiles, that include reduced AGD but were different from those produced by DEHP and DBP (Gray, 2000). Thus, detection of male genital defects with reduced anogenital distance (AGD) appears to signal prenatal anti-androgen exposure, but it quiet necessary to broaden up the knowledge of the complete profile of genital dysmorphology and to focus a potential etiologic agent.

Phthalates in Relation to Genital Development in Human Infants

Study population by Shanna and swan (2008)—The SFF (Study for Future Families) is a multi-center pregnancy cohort study in which Shanna and swan (2008) collected and stored serum and urine samples obtained in mid pregnancy. The collection and availability of serum and urine samples, permitted them to link phthalate exposure in prenatal to outcomes in the children born to couples registered in SFF. Hence, Shanna and Swan (2008) started the Study of Phthalates in Pregnant Women and Children (PPWC) in order to observe genital parameters and AGD in human infants in relation to exposure of pthalates to their mother's. Shanna and swan (2008) provided evidence that a human analogue of the "phthalate syndrome" may be observed in male infants.

Infant Measurement (Shanna and Swan, 2008)

Shanna and Swan (2008) carried out the male infant examination included a detailed description of the scrotum and testes, measurement of the penis, AGD and location of testes. All measurements including AGD as well as penile size was done with a precision calipers. AGD (In males) is the distance (mm) from the center of the anus to the cephalad (towards the head) base of the penis, while AGD (female) is the distance (in mm) from the center of the anus to the cephalad base of the clitoris. Examiners studied also testicular descent, which was grouped as "incomplete" if one or both testicles were observed not to be "normal retractile" or "normal". Moreover, penile width and length were observed. Neither the support staff nor the pediatric physicians had any knowledge of level of phthalate concentration in the mother.

Phthalate measurements (Shanna and Swan, 2008) initially as SFF was not, designed to study biomarkers of prenatal exposure, urine collection was begun midway through the assessment only (but rather semen quality across four areas of the US). There were at least 106 pairs of mother-son with both boy's genital measurements and prenatal phthalate concentration. The concentrations of phthalate metabolite were examined in samples of urine provided at the time of pregnancy (mean 28.6 week of pregnancy, as measured from the last menstrual period), by a sensitive method that includes the enzymatic deconjugation of the phthalate metabolites from their glucuronidated form, automated on-line solid-phase extraction, separation with HPLC (high performance liquid chromatography), and observation by isotope-dilution tandem mass spectrometry (Silva, 2007).

Reproductive and Developmental Toxicity (Shanna and Swan, 2008)

Phthalates having a long alkyl side-chain in the ortho position have a strong potential for developmental and reproductive toxic effects in humans. These include (in the order of their toxic potential) DEHP>DBP>BBP as well as diisobutyl phthalate (DiBP), di-n-hexyl phthalate (DnHP), and diisononyl phthalate (DiNP) (Lyche, 2011; Fabjan *et al.*, 2006). Matsumoto *et al.*, (2008) reported a relationship between shorter duration of pregnancy and higher DEHP serum levels. The other reproductive effects such as decreased semen quality and cryptorchidism could be due to the ability of phthalate monoesters to cross the placental barrier and enter the umbilical cord blood of the foetus (Mose *et al.*, 2007).

Most of the studies (Swan *et al.*, 2010; Duty, 2003; Bornehag *et al.*, 2015; Hauser *et al.*, 2007) have provided evidence that changes in male reproductive parameters, such as anogenital distance (AGD, a biomarker of prenatal androgen exposure in male newborns), decreased reproductive hormone levels and DNA sperm damage could be associated with environmental exposure to phthalates. More recent studies with uncertain results suggest for further research of the effects of adult exposure to phthalates on male reproductive endpoints at ambient levels (Sharpe, 2001; Thurston *et al.*, 2016). whereas, studies on animals to the effects of phthalates on female reproductive endpoints (ovary weight, serum oestradiol levels) recommend that exposure to higher levels than ambient ones is essential to induce relevant changes (Kamrin, 2009). Although higher concentration of di-n-octyl phthalate (DOP), DBP, BBP and DEHP levels were observed in the blood of women with endometriosis (Cobellis, 2003; Reddy *et al.*, 2006), the problems in immune system functioning also lead the development of endometriosis (Matsumoto *et al.*, 2008). Several studies report phthalates as hormone disruptors (Lopez carrillo *et al.*, 2010; De coster and Larebeke, 2012), which means that they are able to interfere with the endocrine system responsible for development and growth and ultimately cause feminization of males, called as the "phthalate syndrome" (Wilson, 2008) and typical reduced male behavior in boys (Lovekamp and Davis, 2003; Sharpe *et al.*, 2008). The other syndrome associated to phthalate exposure is the TDS (testicular dysgenesis syndrome), which may involve hypospadias, cryptorchidism, higher incidence of prostate cancer and lower sperm count (Sharpe *et al.*, 2008). Exposure to phthalates in utero may affect production of hormone and formation of testis and later in life cause problems in the reproductive function (Lopez carillo *et al.*, 2010; Latini *et al.*, 2006). Environmental phthalates are able to cross the placental barrier from mother to foetus blood and are excreted in mother's breast milk (Latini, 2003; Calafat *et al.*, 2004; Kavlock *et al.*, 2006). Pthalates metabolites were examined in infants' urine also (Latini *et al.*, 2006). A Danish-Finish cohort study observed that elevated concentrations of DBP metabolites in mother's milk correlated inversely with free serum testosterone levels in three month-old male newborn (Main *et al.*, 2006). Adibi *et al.* (2010) examined intrauterine exposure to phthalates and resulted that urinary levels of phthalate metabolites correlated inversely with trophoblast differentiation gene expression, which is important for development of human placenta. There was no correlation found with the expression of genes characteristic for Steroidogenesis metabolite levels [monoisobutyl phthalate (MiBP), monomethyl phthalate (MMP)and monoethyl phthalate (MEP)] in infants and correlated them with the baby cosmetics that are used in daily basis (shampoo, infant powder and lotions). They recommended that exposure of phthalate can be minimized by lowering the use of childcare products. Most countries for example, European Parliament and the European Commission have set the MAC (maximum allowed concentrations) of phthalates in children's items for relaxation, toys, pacifiers and food, because of these toxic effects, especially on developing organisms like children (Regulations EC, 2017). Stalhnut *et al.* (2007) regarding endocrine disruption studied that least levels of testosterone in adult men exposed to phthalates were related with insulin resistance and obesity. Phthalates may also affect immune functions, thyroid signaling and metabolic homeostasis (Jaakkola and Knight, 2008; Meeker *et al.,* 2007). High concentrations of DEHP metabolite such as mono-(2-ethylhexyl) phthalate (MEHP) in urine are related with lower thyroid stimulating hormone levels and thyroid hormone (Meeker *et al.,* 2007). Urinary DBP metabolite such as monobutyl phthalate (MBP) in some pregnant women correlated inversely with levels of thyroxin (Haung *et al.,* 2009). People especially children who ate food having DEHP had low levels of TSH (thyroid stimulating hormone) in serum (Wu MT *et al.,* 2013). The thyroid hormone is one of the important hormones for the development and growth of the reproductive system. Its deficiency during fetal/ prenatal or postnatal development leads to neurological disorders and brain damage.

Phthalates and Gestational Age at Delivery (Shanna and Swan, 2008)

Latini (2003) measured serum MEHP and DEHP in the cord blood of 84 infants and observed concentrations in relation to gestational age (which was not defined). MEHP and DEHP were present each in 65 of 84 (77.4%) of the examined samples. Infants in which MEHP was observed in cord blood were grouped as "MEHP-positive" (with a definition similar for DEHP). MEHP positive newborn infants showed a lower gestational age significantly when compared with MEHP negative infants (38.16 ± 2.34 vs. 39.35 ± 1.35; $t = -2.163$, $p = 0.033$). There was no relationship found for DEHP and no significant relations were observed between either MEHP or DEHP and birth weight. Colon *et al.* (2000) compared serum levels of phthalates in 35 pediatric controls (median age of 46 months) with forty one Puerto Rican girls (median age of 20 months) with premature thelarche (premature breast development). The highest differences between controls and cases were between serum DEHP concentration in controls and cases; 70 and 450 mg/ml, respectively ($p < 0.05$). There are various concerns involving several aspects of the study design (McKee, 2004) like the fact that exposure was measured concurrent with diagnosis, the large age difference between cases and controls, and potential sample contamination.

Phthalates in Relation to Allergy, Asthma and Respiratory Function

A number of experiments have observed allergy, asthma and respiratory function in children in relation to the use of phthalates in house dust and PVC containing products or articles in the home (Bornehag *et al.,* 2004; Jaakkola, 1999; Jaakkola, 2000) although none has used biomarkers to define exposure. 2 cross-sectional studies had provided relationship between house dust levels of DEHP and BzBP and allergic symptoms (Bornehag *et al.,* 2004; Kolarik *et al.,* 2008).

SUMMARY OF HEALTH OUTCOMES IN ADULTS (SHANNA AND SWAN (2008)

Phthalates in relation to sex hormones in males and semen quality — Most of the researchers published a series of experiments that reported serum reproductive hormones in men attending an infertility clinic, urinary phthalate levels, sperm DNA damage and semen characteristics (Duty, 2005; Duty, 2003a; Duty, 2003b; Hauser *et al.,* 2004). There were dose dependent relationships of low sperm concentration with MBP (smoking status (1.0, 3.1, 2.5, 3.3; P for trend= 0.04), adjusted for age, motility (1.0, 1.5, 1.5, 1.8; P for trend = 0.04), abstinence time, and and odds ratio per quartile. There was higher evidence of an association between the low sperm concentration and highest MBzP quartile (1.0, 1.1, 1.1,1.9; P for trend = 0.13). DEHP, MEP or the MMP metabolites was having no relationship with these semen parameters. These results completely differed from those recorded by Jonsson (2005), who did not recorded any relationship between phthalate exposure and semen quality in a study of young healthy military recruits. A small study in Shanghai (Zhang, 2006) observed concentration of 3 phthalates (DBP, DEP and DEHP) in semen samples. No relationship was seen with sperm concentration. DEHP was correlated significantly to "rate of malformation" (presumably impaired morphology). All three phthalates (DBP, DEP and DEHP) were positively related with sample liquefaction time.

Phthalates in Relation to Metabolism and Thyroid Function in Adults

There are certain human studies of phthalate effects in adults other than studies of male reproduction function.

Only a single study till date has been examined markers of metabolic syndrome in relation to phthalate exposure. Stahlhut *et al.* (2007) examined phthalate exposure and its relation with insulin resistance and abdominal obesity in adult male participants in the National Health and Nutrition Examination Survey (NHANES) 1999–2002. They kept six phthalate metabolites as predictors of HOMA (a measure of insulin resistance) and waist circumference using multiple linear regression, adjusted for urine creatinine, age, fat, race/ethnicity, physical activity level, serum cotinine, and total calorie consumption. Three with elevated HOMA (MBP, MBzP, and MEP) and four metabolites were associated significantly with increased waist circumference (MEHHP, MBzP, MEP and MEOHP).

Meeker *et al.* (2007) recorded urinary concentrations of phthalate monoester metabolites and MEHP in 408 male partners in couples that were sub fertile and resulted that in adult men, Urinary MEHP concentrations may be associated with altered free T3 or/and total T4 levels. Moreover, they saw an inverse association between free T4 and T3 serum levels and MEHP urinary concentrations. The inverse association between free T4 remained and MEHP when adjusting for oxidative metabolite concentrations, which simultaneously reported a positive association with free T4.

RESPIRATORY TOXICITY

Exposure of humans to phthalates during childhood (as well as in the neonatal and foetal period) is often related with impaired lung function, allergies in children, asthma in adults and risk of bronchial obstruction (Jaakkola and Knight, 2008; Hoppin *et al.,* 2004). The lungs of newly born rats exposed to DEHP exhibit histological changes similar to those studied in the lungs of children with a chronic lung disease particularly of preterm infants known as broncho pulmonary dysplasia, (Magliozzi *et al.,* 2003). Asthma, rhinitis and Wheezing in children could be associated with increased concentrations of DEHP and BBP in house dust (Bornehag and Nanberg, 2010; Bornehag *et al.,* 2004; Kolarik *et al.*, 2008). Hoping *et al* (2004) studied the relation between four pulmonary function parameters in the Third National Health and Nutrition Examination Survey (NHANES, 1988–1994) and phthalate exposure. After controlling for smoking, race, height, age and body mass index, there was an inverse relation between three measures of pulmonary function (PEF,FVC, FEV1) and MBP and elevated concentration of MEP was associated with lower FEV1 and FVC values in men. No consistent associations were found with other phthalate metabolites and in females (Hoppin *et al.,* 2004).

DNA DAMAGE AND CARCINOGENESIS

Hauser *et al.*, (2007); Hauser (2008) reported that DEP and DEHP levels are correlated with DNA damage in sperm in exposed humans. Lopez-Carrillo *et al.*, (2010) provided a possible connection between exposure to DEP through a personal care products and cosmetics with an elevated risk of breast cancer, which is related to demethylating DEP the estrogen receptor complex. IARC (The International Agency for Research on Cancer) has provided evidence that DEHP cannot be grouped as human carcinogen because DEHP stimulates liver tumors in rodents by a process activating PPARα that is not found in humans (Klaunig *et al.,* 2003; Guyton *et al.,* 2009). Moreover, as there are no availability of data for DEHP carcinogenicity in humans but there is more evidence of DEHP carcinogenicity in experimental animals, it has been grouped as possibly carcinogenic to humans (Group 2B) (IARC, 2013).

PHTHALATE MIGRATION AND REGULATIONS

Research gives evidence that phthalates are able to migrate to bottled and tap water (Bosnir *et al.*, 2007; Kereszles *et al.*, 2013; IARC, 2013; Khedr, 2013) and alcoholic and soft drinks (Jurica *et al.*, 2016; Bosnir *et al.*, 2007; Chatonnet *et al.*, 2014; March and Cerda, 2015, Wang *et al.*, 2015). Migration of phthalates from plastic packaging to soft drinks is 5 to 40 times more than migration to mineral water (Bosnir *et al.*, 2007). One of the reasons for this higher concentration may be due to the difference in pH: more than 5 in all mineral waters and less than 3 in soft drinks. The MACs of the several common phthalate DEHP in drinking water set by the US EPA and World Health Organization (WHO) are 6 µg L-1 and 8 µg L-1 respectively (US EPA, 2017; WHO, 2017). One of the key acts to mention here is that under the European Regulation (EC) No. 1907/2006 (REACH) and its amendments (until February 2017) (Regulation EC, 2017). It mentions that DIBP, DBP, BBP and DEHP should not be used in any of the childcare products, toys and matrices in specific, from 21 February 2015 (so called "sunset date") due to the evidence of strong toxic effects on reproduction. More particularly, childcare products and toys containing phthalates in a concentration higher than 0.1% of the plasticized material weight must not be marketed. Other phthalates, namely diisodecyl phthalate (DIDP), DOP, and DINP have only been banned in childcare products and toys that children can put in the mouth (Regulation EC, 2017). The tolerable daily intake (TDI) set by the European Food Safety Authority (EFSA) is 500 µg kg-1 bw for BBP (EFSA, 2003-2005), 150 µg kg-1 bw for DINP and DIDP (EFSA, 2003-2005), 50 µg kg-1 bw for DEHP (EFSA, 2003-2005) and 10 µg kg-1 bw for DBP (EFSA, 2003-2005). With EU Regulation No. 10/2011 EC of 14 January 2011 (EU, 2017), the EU has established the so-called SML (specific migration limits) in plastics likely to come into contact with beverages and food. SML (specific migration limits) is the MAC of a given substance released from a article or material into food stimulants or food. For BBP 30.0 mg kg-1 food, for DEHP 1.5 mg kg-1 food and for DBP it is 0.3 mg kg-1 food. DIBP is not permitted in food contact articles. This EU regulation indirectly limits the maximum concentrations of those substances that are undesirable in alcoholic beverages. In some countries, producers of spirits are not required to observe phthalates in alcoholic beverages, but in some MACs are prescribed. Let us take the example of Slovakian Regulations on the General Code for Contaminants and Groceries in Food define the MAC for phthalates as a sum of DBP and DEHP, which is 2 mg kg-1 in alcoholic beverages, fruits, flour, leaved vegetables and 0.7 mg kg-1 in the potatoes and root vegetables (Vinos, 2004).

Magnitude and Time Course

For assessing the overall human exposure to phthalates, two methods have been adopted. One is modeling approach method of exposures based on environmental phthalate behavioral assessments and measurements. The second is biomonitoring of phthalate metabolite or phthalate levels in human fluids especially body fluids like urine and calculating exposures based on these analyses.

Modeling Exposures Using Data From Environmental Analysis and Behaviors

One of the important approaches I.e. modeling approach is examined by combining information on: (1) human behaviors, e.g., the amount of food ingested, the characteristics and duration of toy behavior etc. Based on this information, total exposure through all routes of exposure and the amount of exposure level through each route may be calculated and (2) the levels of phthalates in the environment, e.g., consumer products, food, air, toys, water etc. The accuracy of the resulting value is based upon knowledge of: (1) behaviors, such as frequency of ingestion and amount of food of each type ingested (2) the concentrations of each phthalate in each of the sources and how these levels vary over location and time and (3) all significant sources of each phthalates. Because of the complication in collecting such data on phthalates from the multiplicity of possible sources, uncertainties in level of exposure values derived from this methodology are significant. Moreover, as phthalates are present everywhere, contamination of samples or products from environmental sources may be a serious problem and may lead to large overestimates of exposures. While keeping in mind these difficulties, the modeling approach does have the benefit of giving data for all age groups like infant, children, adults etc. on the apportionment of exposure among sources and on the duration and timing of exposures information that is generally not available from biomonitoring.

Estimating Exposures Based on Biomonitoring Data

The other most important exposure assessment methodology is biomonitoring, which gives direct ways to measure the amount of each phthalate metabolite or phthalate in human body fluids like blood, urine and tissues. These body fluid or tissue levels must be translated then into exposures. This translation needs knowledge of the relation- ship between the amounts of parent metabolites or compounds found in the body fluids or tissues and the magnitude of the phthalate exposure. In the past seven or eight years, several biomonitoring measurements concentrated on phthalate metabolites rather than their parent compounds or metabolite. As there are large significant gaps in knowledge regarding the fate and metabolism of phthalates, it is hard here to mention that which metabolite is the most appropriate or accurate analyte. Since each of metabolite may have a significant impact on the exposure estimate, literature exposure values may significantly vary when they are based on various metabolites (Calafat and McKee, 2006). Another important cause of uncertainty is that the conversion from body fluid concentrations to levels of exposure is based on collected data from adults and it is not even clear how much applicable these data are to other age groups, especially children and infants.

RECOMMENDATIONS FOR EFFECTIVE CONTROL OF PHTHALATE EXPOSURE

As the frequency and quantity of phthalates exposure to human is often unknown, research should concentrate on the routes and sources and try to answer the basic question that at which level the phthalates are hazardous for health of human and other living creatures. It is certainly important to biologically monitor phthalates concentrations by determining their metabolites in body fluids, principally in the urine. Their MACs should be monitored in alcoholic beverages, drinking water and food. In order to avoid economic losses in markets with defined MACs, the producers of food products and alcoholic beverages should introduce phthalate monitoring through product safety systems and internal quality management. Moreover, exposure of phthalates could further be lowered by introducing and finding alternative, plasticizers and phthalate-free materials into the production of consumer products or parts used in beverage and food processing and storage.

CONCLUSION

Phthalates, the esters and salts of phthalic acid, are universal in the environment. They are used as plasticizers during the making of food packaging, adhesives, paint, and cosmetics and PVC. The manufactured compounds are present in every home and they have the ability to easily migrate to the environment and make environment polluted. Phthalates are found everywhere especially in air, soil, treated effluents, water, land filled waste and plants. Moreover, they do not bind themselves permanently with the products to which they are added. Phthalates create a risk of exposure for living organism especially to humans and are rapidly released into the environment. They are represented by reproductive toxicity in animals and humans;

they are able to cause reproductive problems and infertility in males. Phthalates are considered more toxic to young children, which are much more vulnerable to phthalate exposure, including fetal life. Phthalates are very difficult to eliminate from our daily surroundings as they are used in numerous industries.

REFERENCES

Adamsson, A., Salonen, V., Paranko, J., & Toppari, J. (2009). Effects of maternal exposure to di-isononylphthalate (DINP) and 1, 1-dichloro-2, 2-bis (p-chlorophenyl) ethylene (p,p′ -DDE)on steroidogenesis is the fetal rat testis and adrenal gland. *Reproductive Toxicology (Elmsford, N.Y.)*, *28*(1), 66–74. doi:10.1016/j.reprotox.2009.03.002 PMID:19490997

Adibi, J. J., Whyatt, R. M., Hauser, R., Bhat, H. K., Davis, B. J., Calafat, A. M., ... Williams, P. L. (2010). Transcriptional biomarkers of steroidogenesis and trophoblast differentiation in the placenta in relation to prenatal phthalate exposure. *Environmental Health Perspectives*, *118*(2), 291–296. doi:10.1289/ehp.0900788 PMID:20123604

Akingbemi, B. T., Ge, R., Klinefelter, G. R., Zirkin, B. R., & Hardy, M. P. (2004). Phthalate-induced Leydig Cell Hyperplasia is Associated with Multiple Endocrine Disturbances. *Proceedings of the National Academy of Sciences of the United States of America*, *101*(3), 775–780. doi:10.1073/pnas.0305977101 PMID:14715905

ATSDR. (1995) Agency for Toxic Substances and Disease Registry. Atlanta, GA: Division of Toxicology.

ATSDR. (2001). Agency for Toxic Substances and Disease Registry. Atlanta, GA: Division of Toxicology.

ATSDR. (2002) Agency for Toxic Substances and Disease Registry. Atlanta, GA: Division of Toxicology.

ATSDR. (2002). *Toxicological profile for di(2-ethylhexyl)phthalate (DEHP)*. Atlanta, GA: Agency for Toxic Substances and Disease Registry.

Bornehag, C. G., Carlstedt, F., Jönsson, B. A., Lindh, C. H., Jensen, T. K., Bodin, A., ... Swan, S. H. (2015). Prenatal phthalate exposures and anogenital distance in Swedish boys. *Environmental Health Perspectives*, *123*(1), 101–107. doi:10.1289/ehp.1408163 PMID:25353625

Bornehag, C. G., & Nanberg, E. (2010). Phthalate exposure and asthma in children. *International Journal of Andrology*, *33*, 333–345.

Bornehag, C. G., Sundell, J., Weschler, C. J., Sigsgaard, T., Lundgren, B., Hasselgren, M., & Hägerhed-Engman, L. (2004). The association between asthma and allergic symptoms in children and phthalates in house dust: A nested case-control study. *Environmental Health Perspectives*, *112*(14), 1393–1397. doi:10.1289/ehp.7187 PMID:15471731

Bošnir, J., Puntarić, D., Galić, A., Škes, I., Dijanić, T., Klarić, M., ... Šmit, Z. (2007). Migration of phthalates from plastic containers into soft drinks and mineral water. *Food Technology and Biotechnology*, *45*, 91–95.

Calafat, A. M., & McKee, R. H. (2006). Integrating biomonitoring exposure data into the risk assessment process: Phthalates [diethyl phthalate and di(2-ethylhexyl) phthalate] as a case study. *Environmental Health Perspectives*, *114*(11), 1783–1789. doi:10.1289/ehp.9059 PMID:17107868

Calafat, A. M., Slakman, A. R., Silva, M. J., Herbert, A. R., & Needham, L. L. (2004). Automated solid phase extraction and quantitative analysis of human milk for 13 phthalate metabolites. *Journal of Chromatography. B, Analytical Technologies in the Biomedical and Life Sciences*, *805*(1), 49–56. doi:10.1016/j.jchromb.2004.02.006 PMID:15113539

Calafat, A. M., Slakman, A. R., Silva, M. J., Herbert, A. R., & Needham, L. L. (2004). Automated solid phase extraction and quantitative analysis of human milk for 13 phthalate metabolites. *Journal of Chromatography. B, Analytical Technologies in the Biomedical and Life Sciences*, *805*(1), 49–56. doi:10.1016/j.jchromb.2004.02.006 PMID:15113539

Callegari, C., Everett, S., Ross, M., & Brasel, J. A. (1987). Anogenital ratio: Measure of fetal virilization in premature and full-term newborninfants. *The Journal of Pediatrics*, *111*(2), 240–243. doi:10.1016/S0022-3476(87)80075-6 PMID:3612396

Cao, X. L. (2008). Determination of phthalates and adipate in bottled water by headspace solid-phase microextraction and gas chromatography/mass spectrometry. *Journal of Chromatography. A*, *1178*(1-2), 231–238. doi:10.1016/j.chroma.2007.11.095 PMID:18082753

Castaño-Vinyals, G., Carrasco, E., Lorente, J. A., Sabaté, Y., Cirac-Claveras, J., Pollán, M., & Kogevinas, M. (2012). Anogenital distance and the risk of prostate cancer. *BJU International*, *110*(11b), E707–E710. doi:10.1111/j.1464-410X.2012.11516.x PMID:22984847

CDC. (2003). Second national report on human exposure to environmental chemicals. Atlanta, GA: National Center for Environmental Health, Division of Laboratory Sciences.

CDC. (2005). Third national report on human exposure to environmental chemicals. Atlanta, GA: National Center for Environmental Health, Division of Laboratory Sciences.

Chatonnet, P., Boutou, S., & Plana, A. (2014). Contamination of wines andspirits by phthalates: Types of contaminants present, contamination sources and means of prevention. *Food Addit. Contam. Part A*, *31*(9), 1605–1615. doi:10.1080/19440049.2014.941947 PMID:25099435

Cobellis, L. (2003). High plasma concentrations of di-(2-ethylhexyl)-phthalate in women with endometriosis. *Human Reproduction (Oxford, England)*, *18*(7), 1512–1515. doi:10.1093/humrep/deg254 PMID:12832380

Colon, I. (2000). Identification of phthalate esters in the serum of young Puerto Rican girls with premature breast development. *Environmental Health Perspectives*, *108*, 895–900. PMID:11017896

De Coster, S., & van Larebeke, N. (2012). Endocrine-disrupting chemicals: Associated disorders and mechanisms of action. *Journal of Environmental and Public Health*. PMID:22991565

Duty, S. M., Ackerman, R. M., Calafat, A. M., & Hauser, R. (2005a). Personal care product use predicts urinary concentrations of some phthalate monoesters. *Environmental Health Perspectives*, *113*(11), 1530–1535. doi:10.1289/ehp.8083 PMID:16263507

Duty, S. M., Silva, M. J., Barr, D. B., Brock, J. W., Ryan, L., Chen, Z., ... Hauser, R. (2003a). Phthalate exposure and human semen parameters. *Epidemiology (Cambridge, Mass.)*, *14*(3), 269–277. doi:10.1097/01.EDE.0000059950.11836.16 PMID:12859026

Duty, S. M., Singh, N. P., Silva, M. J., Barr, D. B., Brock, J. W., Ryan, L., ... Hauser, R. (2003). The relationship between environmental exposures to phthalates and DNA damage in human sperm using the neutral comet assay. *Environmental Health Perspectives*, *111*(9), 1164–1169. doi:10.1289/ehp.5756 PMID:12842768

Duty, S. M., Singh, N. P., Silva, M. J., Barr, D. B., Brock, J. W., Ryan, L., ... Hauser, R. (2003b). The relationship between environmental exposures to phthalates and DNA damage in human sperm using the neutral comet assay. *Environmental Health Perspectives*, *111*(9), 1164–1169. doi:10.1289/ehp.5756 PMID:12842768

EU Scientific Committee on Toxicity Ecotoxicity and the Environment (CSTEE). (2017). *Opinion on phthalate migration from soft PVC toys and child-care articles*. Brussels: Author.

European Commission. (2011). *Commission Regulation (EU) No 10/2011 of 14 January 2011 on Plastic materials and articles intended to come into contact with food*. Author.

European Food Safety Authority (EFSA). (2003a). *Opinion of the Scientific Panel on food additives, flavourings, processing aids and materials in contact with food (AFC) related to Butylbenzylphthalate (BBP) for use in food contact materials*. Author.

European Food Safety Authority (EFSA). (2003b). *Opinion of the scientific panel on food additives, flavouring, processing aids and material in contact with food on a request from the Commission related to di-isodecylphthalate (DIDP) for use in food contact materials*. Author.

European Food Safety Authority (EFSA). (2005a). *Opinion of the Scientific Panel on food additives, flavourings, processing aids and material in contact with food (AFC) related to di-Butylphthalate (DBP) for use in food contact materials*. Author.

European Food Safety Authority (EFSA). (2005b). *Opinion of the Scientific Panel on food additives, flavourings, processing aids and materials in contact with food (AFC) related to Bis(2-ethylhexyl)phthalate (DEHP) for use in food contact materials*. Author.

European Food Safety Authority (EFSA). (2005c). *Opinion of the scientific panel on food additives, flavouring, processing aids and material in contact with food on a request from the Commission related to di-isononylphthalate (DINP) for use in food contact materials*. Author.

Fabjan, E., Hulzebos, E., Mennes, W., & Piersma, A. H. (2006). A category approach for reproductive effects of phthalates. *Critical Reviews in Toxicology*, *36*(9), 695–726. doi:10.1080/10408440600894914 PMID:17050082

FDA. (2001). Food and Drug Administration Total Diet Study; summary of residues found ordered by pesticide market baskets 91-3--99-1. Rockville, MD: Office of Plant and Dairy Foods and Beverages.

Fierens, T., Servaes, K., Van Holderbeke, M., Geerts, L., De Henauw, S., Sioen, I., & Vanermen, G. (2012). Analysis of phthalates in food products and packaging materials sold on the Belgian market. *Food and Chemical Toxicology*, *50*(7), 2575–2583. doi:10.1016/j.fct.2012.04.029 PMID:22554646

Fierens, T., Van Holderbeke, M., Willems, H., De Henauw, S., & Sioen, I. (2012). Transfer of eight phthalates through the milk chain - A case study. *Environment International*, *2013*(51), 1–7. PMID:23138015

Foster, P. M. (2006). Disruption of Reproductive Development in Male Rat Offspring Following in Utero Exposure to Phthalate Esters. *International Journal of Andrology, 29*(1), 140–147. doi:10.1111/j.1365-2605.2005.00563.x PMID:16102138

Gray, L. E. J. R. (2000). Perinatal exposure to the phthalates DEHP, BBP, and DINP, but not DEP, DMP, or DOTP, alters sexual differentiation of the male rat. *Toxicological Sciences, 58*(2), 350–365. doi:10.1093/toxsci/58.2.350 PMID:11099647

Green, R., Hauser, R., Calafat, A. M., Weuve, J., Schettler, T., Ringer, S., ... Hu, H. (2005). Use of di(2-ethylhexyl) phthalate-containing medical products and urinary levels of mono(2-ethylhexyl) phthalate in neonatal intensive care unit infants. *Environmental Health Perspectives, 113*(9), 1222–1225. doi:10.1289/ehp.7932 PMID:16140631

Grynkiewicz-Bylina, B. (2011). Dangerous phthalates in children's environment. *Ecological Chemistry and Engineering. S, 18*(4), 455–463.

Guyton, K. Z., Chiu, W. A., Bateson, T. F., Jinot, J., Siegel Scott, C., Brown, R. C., & Caldwell, J. C. (2009). A reexamination of the PPAR-alpha activation mode of action as a basis for assessing human cancer risks of environmental contaminants. *Environmental Health Perspectives, 117*(11), 1664–1672. doi:10.1289/ehp.0900758 PMID:20049115

Hauser, R. (2008). *Urinary phthalate metabolites and semen quality:a review of a potential biomarker of susceptibility*. Academic Press.

Hauser, R., Duty, S., Godfrey-Bailey, L., & Calafat, A. M. (2004a). Medications as a source of human exposure tophthalates. *Environmental Health Perspectives, 112*(6), 751–753. doi:10.1289/ehp.6804 PMID:15121520

Hauser, R., Meeker, J. D., Park, S., Silva, M. J., & Calafat, A. M. (2004b). Temporal variability of urinary phthalate metabolite levels in men of reproductive age. *Environmental Health Perspectives, 112*(17), 1734–0. doi:10.1289/ehp.7212 PMID:15579421

Hauser, R., Meeker, J. D., Singh, N. P., Silva, M. J., Ryan, L., Duty, S., & Calafat, A. M. (2007). DNA damage in human sperm is related to urinary levels of phthalate monoester and oxidative metabolites. *Human Reproduction (Oxford, England), 22*(3), 688–695. doi:10.1093/humrep/del428 PMID:17090632

Hays, S. M., Aylward, L. L., Kirman, C. R., Krishnan, K., & Nong, A. (2011). Biomonitoring equivalents for di-isononyl phthalate (DINP). *Regulatory Toxicology and Pharmacology, 60*(2), 181–188. doi:10.1016/j.yrtph.2011.03.013 PMID:21466828

Heudorf, U., Mersch-Sundermann, V., & Angerer, J. (2007). Phthalates: Toxicology and exposure. *International Journal of Hygiene and Environmental Health, 210*(5), 623–634. doi:10.1016/j.ijheh.2007.07.011 PMID:17889607

Hoppin, J. A., Ulmer, R., & London, S. J. (2004). Phthalate exposure and pulmonary function. *Environmental Health Perspectives, 112*(5), 571–574. doi:10.1289/ehp.6564 PMID:15064163

Huang, P. C., Kuo, P. L., Chou, Y. Y., Lin, S. J., & Lee, C. C. (2009). Association between prenatal exposure to phthalates and the health of newborns. *Environment International, 35*(1), 14–20. doi:10.1016/j.envint.2008.05.012 PMID:18640725

IARC. (2013). Working Group on the Evaluation of Carcinogenic Risks to Humans. Some chemicals present in industrial and consumer products, food and drinking-water. *IARC Monographs on the Evaluation of Carcinogenic Risks to Humans, 101*, 9–549. PMID:24772663

Jaakkola, J. J. (2000). Plastic wall materials in the home and respiratory health in young children. *American Journal of Public Health, 90*(5), 797–799. doi:10.2105/AJPH.90.5.797 PMID:10800434

Jaakkola, J. J., Oie, L., Nafstad, P., Botten, G., Samuelsen, S. O., & Magnus, P. (1999). Interior surface materials in the home and the development of bronchial obstruction inyoung children in Oslo, Norway. *American Journal of Public Health, 89*(2), 188–192. doi:10.2105/AJPH.89.2.188 PMID:9949747

Jaakkola, J. J. K., & Knight, T. L. (2008). The role of exposure to phthalates from polyvinyl chloride products in the development of asthma and allergies: A systematic review and meta-analysis. *Environmental Health Perspectives, 116*(7), 845–853. doi:10.1289/ehp.10846 PMID:18629304

Jonsson, B. A. (2005). Urinary phthalate metabolites and biomarkers of reproductive function in young men. *Epidemiology (Cambridge, Mass.), 16*, 487–493. doi:10.1097/01.ede.0000164555.19041.01 PMID:15951666

Jurica, K., Brčić Karačonji, I., Lasić, D., Vukić Lušić, D., Anić Jurica, S., & Lušić, D. (2016). Determination of phthalates in plum spirit and their occurrence during plum spirit production. *Acta Alimentaria, 45*(1), 141–148. doi:10.1556/066.2016.45.1.17

Kamrin, M. A. (2009). Phthalate risks, phthalate regulation, and public health: A review. *Journal of Toxicology and Environmental Health. Part B, Critical Reviews, 12*(2), 157–174. doi:10.1080/10937400902729226 PMID:19235623

Kavlock, R., Barr, D., Boekelheide, K., Breslin, W., Breysse, P., Chapin, R., ... Williams, P. (2006). NTP-CERHR Expert Panel update on the reproductive and developmental toxicity of di(2-ethylhexyl) phthalate. *Reproductive Toxicology (Elmsford, N.Y.)*, *22*(3), 291–399. doi:10.1016/j.reprotox.2006.04.007 PMID:17068859

Keresztes, S., Tatár, E., Czégény, Z., Záray, G., & Mihucz, V. G. (2013). Study on the leaching of phthalates from polyethylene terephthalate bottles into mineral water. *The Science of the Total Environment*, *458-460*, 451–458. doi:10.1016/j.scitotenv.2013.04.056 PMID:23688967

Khedr, A. (2013). Optimized extraction method for LC-MS determination of bisphenol A, melamine and di(2-ethylhexyl) phthalate in selected soft drinks, syringes, and milk powder. *Journal of Chromatography. B, Analytical Technologies in the Biomedical and Life Sciences*, *930*, 98–103. doi:10.1016/j.jchromb.2013.04.040 PMID:23727873

Klaunig, J. E., Babich, M. A., Baetcke, K. P., Cook, J. C., Corton, J. C., David, R. M., ... Fenner-Crisp, P. A. (2003). PPARalpha agonist-induced rodent tumors: Modes of action and human relevance. *Critical Reviews in Toxicology*, *33*(6), 655–780. doi:10.1080/713608372 PMID:14727734

Koch, H. M., Drexler, H., & Angerer, J. (2004). Internal exposure of nursery-school children and their parents and teachers to di(2-ethylhexyl)phthalate (DEHP). *International Journal of Hygiene and Environmental Health*, *207*(1), 15–22. doi:10.1078/1438-4639-00270 PMID:14762970

Kolarik, B., Naydenov, K., Larsson, M., Bornehag, C. G., & Sundell, J. (2008). The association between phthalates in dust and allergic diseases among Bulgarian children. *Environmental Health Perspectives*, *116*(1), 98–103. doi:10.1289/ehp.10498 PMID:18197306

Kransler, K. M., Bachman, A. N., & McKee, R. H. (2013). Estimates of daily di-isodecyl phthalate (DIDP) intake calculated from urinary biomonitoring data. *Regulatory Toxicology and Pharmacology*, *65*(1), 29–33. doi:10.1016/j.yrtph.2012.11.004 PMID:23174424

Latini, G., De Felice, C., Presta, G., Del Vecchio, A., Paris, I., Ruggieri, F., & Mazzeo, P. (2003). In utero exposure to di-(2-ethylhexyl)phthalate and duration of human pregnancy. *Environmental Health Perspectives*, *111*(14), 1783–1785. doi:10.1289/ehp.6202 PMID:14594632

Latini, G., Del Vecchio, A., Massaro, M., Verrotti, A., & De Felice, C. (2006). *In utero exposure to phthalates and fetal development*. Academic Press.

Lee, B. M., & Koo, H. J. (2005). (DEHP) in human urine and serum after single oral doses of deuterium-labeled DEHP. *Archives of Toxicology*, *79*, 367–376. doi:10.100700204-004-0642-4 PMID:15700144

López-Carrillo, L., Hernández-Ramírez, R. U., Calafat, A. M., Torres-Sánchez, L., Galván-Portillo, M., Needham, L. L., ... Cebrián, M. E. (2010). Exposure to phthalates and breast cancer risk in northern Mexico. *Environmental Health Perspectives*, *118*(4), 539–544. doi:10.1289/ehp.0901091 PMID:20368132

Lovekamp-Swan, T., & Davis, B. J. (2003). Mechanisms of phthalate ester toxicity in the female reproductive system. *Environmental Health Perspectives*, *111*(2), 139–145. doi:10.1289/ehp.5658 PMID:12573895

Lyche, J. L. (2011). Phthalates. In R. C. Gupta (Ed.), *Reproductive andDevelopmental Toxicology* (1st ed.; pp. 637–655). Amsterdam: Academic Press. doi:10.1016/B978-0-12-382032-7.10048-7

Magliozzi, R., Nardacci, R., Scarsella, G., Di Carlo, V., & Stefanini, S. (2013). Effects of the plasticiser DEHP on lung of newborn rats: Catalase immunocytochemistry and morphometric analysis. *Histochemistry and Cell Biology*, *120*(1), 41–49. doi:10.100700418-003-0543-2 PMID:12802597

Main, K. M., Mortensen, G. K., Kaleva, M. M., Boisen, K. A., Damgaard, I. N., Chellakooty, M., ... Skakkebæk, N. E. (2006). Human breast milk contamination with phthalates and alterations of endogenous reproductive hormones in infants three months of age. *Environmental Health Perspectives*, *114*(2), 270–276. doi:10.1289/ehp.8075 PMID:16451866

March, J. G., & Cerdà, V. (2015). An innovative arrangement for in-vial membrane-assisted liquid-liquid microextraction: Application to the determination of esters of phthalic acid in alcoholic beverages by gas chromatography-mass spectrometry. *Analytical and Bioanalytical Chemistry*, *407*(14), 4213–4217. doi:10.100700216-015-8646-x PMID:25876533

Matsumoto, M., Hirata-Koizumi, M., & Ema, M. (2008). Potential adverse effects of phthalic acid esters on human health: A review of recent studies on reproduction. *Regulatory Toxicology and Pharmacology*, *50*(1), 37–49. doi:10.1016/j.yrtph.2007.09.004 PMID:17983696

McKee, R. H. (2004). Toxicology Research Task G. Phthalate exposure and early thelarche. *Environmental Health Perspectives*, *112*(10), A541–A543. doi:10.1289/ehp.112-a541b PMID:15238295

Meeker, J. D., Calafat, A. M., & Hauser, R. (2007). Di(2-ethylhexyl) phthalate metabolites may alter thyroid hormone levels in men. *Environmental Health Perspectives, 115*(7), 1029–1034. doi:10.1289/ehp.9852 PMID:17637918

Meeker, J. D., Calafat, A. M., & Hauser, R. (2007). Di(2-ethylhexyl) phthalate metabolites may alter thyroid hormone levels in men. *Environmental Health Perspectives, 115*(7), 1029–1034. doi:10.1289/ehp.9852 PMID:17637918

Mendiola, J., Stahlhut, R. W., Jørgensen, N., Liu, F., & Swan, S. H. (2011). Shorter anogenital distance predicts poorer semen quality in young men in Rochester, New York. *Environmental Health Perspectives, 119*(7), 958–963. doi:10.1289/ehp.1103421 PMID:21377950

Miodovnik, A., Edwards, A., Bellinger, D. C., & Hauser, R. (2014). Developmental neurotoxicity of ortho-phthalate diesters: Review of human and experimental evidence. *Neurotoxicol., 41*, 112–122. doi:10.1016/j.neuro.2014.01.007 PMID:24486776

Mose, T., Mortensen, G. K., Hedegaard, M., & Knudsen, L. E. (2007). Phthalate monoesters in perfusate from a dual placenta perfusion system, the placenta tissue and umbilical cord blood. *Reproductive Toxicology (Elmsford, N.Y.), 23*(1), 83–91. doi:10.1016/j.reprotox.2006.08.006 PMID:17049806

National Research Council. (2008). *Pthalates and cumulative risk assessment the task ahead. Committee on the health risk of pthalates*. National research council.

Pałaszewska-Tkacz, A., & Czerczak, S., & Dibutylu, F. (2012). (Di-n-butyl phthalate - inhaled fraction. Occupational exposure limits for phthalates). *Podstawy i Metody Oceny Środ Pracy., 73*(3), 37–70.

Peijnenburg, W. J. G. M., Sven, E. J., & Brian, F. (2008). Phthalates. In S. E. Jørgensen & B. D. Fath (Eds.), *Encyclopedia of Ecology*. Oxford, UK: Academic Press. doi:10.1016/B978-008045405-4.00419-5

Phillip, M. (1996). Clitoral and penile sizes of full term newborns in two different ethnic groups. *Journal of Pediatric Endocrinology & Metabolism, 9*, 175–179. PMID:8887140

Reddy, B. S., Rozati, R., Reddy, B. V. R., & Raman, N. V. V. S. S. (2006). Association of phthalate esters with endometriosis in Indian women. *BJOG Int J Obstet Gynaecol, 113*(5), 515–520. doi:10.1111/j.1471-0528.2006.00925.x PMID:16637895

Regulation (EC) No 1907/2006 of the European Parliament and of the Council of 18 December 2006 concerning the Registration, Evaluation, Authorisation and Restriction of Chemicals (REACH), establishing a European Chemicals Agency, amending Directive 1999/45/EC and repealing Council Regulation (EEC) No 793/93 and Commission Regulation (EC) No 1488/94 as well as Council Directive 76/769/EEC and Commission Directives 91/155/EEC, 93/67/ EEC, 93/105/EC and 2000/21/EC [displayed 8 May 2017].

Report, R. A. (2003a). 1,2-benzenedicarboxylic acid, di-C9-11-branched alkyl esters, C10-rich and di-"isodecyl" phthalate (DIDP). Institute for Health and Consumer Protection. *European Chemicals Bureau, 36*, 234.

Report, R. A. (2003b). 1,2-benzenedicarboxylic acid, di-C8-10-branched alkyl esters, C9-rich and di-"isononyl" phthalate (DINP). Institute for Health and Consumer Protection. *European Chemicals Bureau, 35*, 290.

Robinson, L., & Miller, R. (2015). The impact of bisphenol A and phthalates on allergy, asthma, and immune function: A review of latest findings. *Current Environmental Health Reports, 2*(4), 379–387. doi:10.100740572-015-0066-8 PMID:26337065

Rudel, R. A., Camann, D. E., Spengler, J. D., Korn, L. R., & Brody, J. G. (2003). Phthalates, alkylphenols, pesticides, polybrominated diphenyl ethers, and other endocrine-disrupting compounds in indoor air and dust. *Environmental Science & Technology, 37*(20), 4543–4553. doi:10.1021/es0264596 PMID:14594359

Salazar-Martinez, E., Romano-Riquer, P., Yanez-Marquez, E., Longnecker, M. P., & Hernandez-Avila, M. (2004). Anogenital distance in human male and female newborns: A descriptive, cross-sectional study. *Environmental Health, 3*(1), 8–8. doi:10.1186/1476-069X-3-8 PMID:15363098

Sathyanarayana, S. (2008) Baby care products: possible sources of infant phthalate exposure. *Pediatrics, 121.*

Shanna, H. (2008). Environment pthalate exposure in relation to reproductive outcomes and other health endpoints in humans. *Environmental Research, 108*(2), 177–184. doi:10.1016/j.envres.2008.08.007 PMID:18949837

Sharpe, R. M. (2001). Hormones and testis development and the possible adverse effects of environmental chemicals. *Toxicology Letters, 120*(1-3), 221–232. doi:10.1016/S0378-4274(01)00298-3 PMID:11323180

Sharpe, R. M., & Skakkebaek, N. E. (2008). Testicular dysgenesis syndrome: Mechanistic insights and potential new downstream effects. *Fertility and Sterility, 89*(Suppl 2), e33–e38. doi:10.1016/j.fertnstert.2007.12.026 PMID:18308057

Silva, M. J. (2007). Quantification of 22 phthalate metabolites in human urine. *Journal of Chromatography. A, 860*, 106–112. PMID:17997365

Stahlhut, R. W., van Wijngaarden, E., Dye, T. D., Cook, S., & Swan, S. H. (2007). Concentrations of urinary phthalate metabolites are associated with increased waist circumference and insulin resistance in adult U.S. males. *Environmental Health Perspectives, 115*(6), 876–882. doi:10.1289/ehp.9882 PMID:17589594

Swan, S., Liu, F., Hines, M., Kruse, R. L., Wang, C., Redmon, J. B., ... Weiss, B. (2010). Prenatal phthalate exposure and reduced masculine play in boys. *International Journal of Andrology, 33*(2), 259–269. doi:10.1111/j.1365-2605.2009.01019.x PMID:19919614

Teitelbaum, S. L., Britton, J. A., Calafat, A. M., Ye, X., Silva, M. J., Reidy, J. A., ... Wolff, M. S. (2008). Temporal variability in urinary concentrations of phthalate metabolites, phytoestrogens and phenols among minority children in the United States. *Environmental Research, 106*(2), 257–269. doi:10.1016/j.envres.2007.09.010 PMID:17976571

Thurston, S. W., Mendiola, J., Bellamy, A. R., Levine, H., Wang, C., Sparks, A., ... Swan, S. H. (2016). Phthalate exposure and semen quality in fertile US men. *Andrology, 4*(4), 632–638. doi:10.1111/andr.12124 PMID:26601918

US Environmental Protection Agency (2012). Phthalates Action Plan, Revised 03/14/2012.

Ventrice, P., Ventrice, D., Russo, E., & De Sarro, G. (2013). Phthalates: European regulation, chemistry, pharmacokinetic and related toxicity. *Environmental Toxicology and Pharmacology, 36*(1), 88–96. doi:10.1016/j.etap.2013.03.014 PMID:23603460

Výnos Ministerstva Pôdohospodárstva Slovenskej republiky a Ministerstva Zdravotníctva Slovenskej republiky z 15. marca 2004 No. 608/3/2004 - 100, ktorým sa vydáva hlava Potravinového Kódexu Slovenskej republiky upravujúca kontaminanty v potravinách [Slovak decree of the Ministry of Agriculture of the Slovak Republic and the Slovak Ministry of Health of 15 March 2004 No. 608/3/2004 - 100, issuing the chapter Slovak Republic Foodstuffs Code governing contaminants in food, in Slovak]. Ministerstva Pôdohospodárstva Slovenskej republiky 2004.

Wang, J., Li, X., Zhang, Q., Xiong, J., & Li, H. (2015). Determination of phthalate esters in Chinese spirits using isotope dilution gaschromatography with tandem mass spectrometry. *Journal of Separation Science, 38*(10), 1700–1710. doi:10.1002/jssc.201401001 PMID:25755215

Welsh, M., Saunders, P. T. K., Fisken, M., Scott, H. M., Hutchison, G. R., Smith, L. B., & Sharpe, R. M. (2008). Identification in rats of a programming window for reproductive tract masculinization, disruption of which leads to hypospadias and cryptorchidism. *The Journal of Clinical Investigation*, *118*(4), 1479–1490. doi:10.1172/JCI34241 PMID:18340380

Wilson, V. S., Blystone, C. R., Hotchkiss, A. K., Rider, C. V., & Gray, L. E. (2008). Diverse mechanisms of anti-androgen action: Impact on male rat reproductive tractdevelopment. *International Journal of Andrology*, *31*(2), 178–187. doi:10.1111/j.1365-2605.2007.00861.x PMID:18315717

Wilson, V. S., Blystone, C. R., Hotchkiss, A. K., Rider, C. V., & Gray, L. E. (2008). Diverse mechanisms of anti-androgen action: Impact on male rat reproductive tract development. *International Journal of Andrology*, *31*(2), 178–187. doi:10.1111/j.1365-2605.2007.00861.x PMID:18315717

Wilson, V. S., Lambright, C., Furr, J., Ostby, J., Wood, C., Held, G., & Gray, L. E. Jr. (2004). Phthalate ester-induced gubernacular lesions are associatedwith reduced insl3 gene expression in the fetal rat testis. *Toxicology Letters*, *146*(3), 207–215. doi:10.1016/j.toxlet.2003.09.012 PMID:14687758

World Health Organization (WHO). (2017). *Guidelines for Drinking-Water Quality*. WHO.

Wormuth, M., Scheringer, M., Vollenweider, M., & Hungerbuhler, K. (2006). What are the sources of exposure to eight frequently used pthalic acid esters in Europeans. *Risk Analysis*, *26*(3), 803–824. doi:10.1111/j.1539-6924.2006.00770.x PMID:16834635

Wu, M. T., Wu, C. F., Chen, B. H., Chen, E. K., Chen, Y. L., Shiea, J., ... Wu, J. R. (2013). Intake of phthalate-tainted foods alters thyroid functions in Taiwanese children. *PLoS One*, *8*(1), e55005. doi:10.1371/journal.pone.0055005 PMID:23383031

Wyszkowska, J., & Wyszkowski, M. (2002). Effect of cadmium and magnesium on microbiological activity in soil. *Polish Journal of Environmental Studies*, *11*(5), 585–591.

Wyszkowski, M., & Sivitskaya, V. (2012). Changes in the content of organic carbon and available forms of macronutrients in soil under the influence of soil contamination with fuel oil and application of different substances. *Journal of Elementology*, *17*(1), 139–148.

Wyszkowski, M., & Wyszkowska, J. (2009). The effect of contamination with cadmium on spring barley (Hordeum vulgare L.) and its relationship with the enzymatic activity of soil. *Fresenius Environmental Bulletin, 18*(7), 1046–1053.

Zhang, Y. H. (2006). Phthalate exposure and human semen quality in Shanghai: a cross-sectional study. *Biomedical and Environmental Sciences, 19*, 205–209. PMID:16944777

Ziółkowska, A., & Wyszkowski, M. (2010). Toxicity of petroleum s ubstances to microorganisms and plants. *Ecological Chemistry and Engineering. S, 17*(1), 73–82.

ADDITIONAL READING

Swan, S. H., Main, K. M., Liu, F., Stewart, S. L., Kruse, R. L., Calafat, A. M., ... Teague, J. L. (2005). the Study for Future Families Research Team. Decrease in anogenital distance among male infants with prenatal phthalate exposure. *Environmental Health Perspectives, 113*(8), 1056–1061. doi:10.1289/ehp.8100 PMID:16079079

Talsness, C. E., Andrade, A. J. M., Kuriyama, S. N., Taylor, J. A., & vom Saal, F. S. (2009). Components of plastic: Experimental studies in animals and relevance for human health. *Philosophical Transactions of the Royal Society of London. Series B, Biological Sciences, 364*(1526), 2079–2096. doi:10.1098/rstb.2008.0281 PMID:19528057

Wang, Y. C., Chen, H. S., Long, C. Y., Tsai, C. F., Hsieh, T. H., Hsu, C. Y., & Tsai, E. M. (2012). Possible mechanism of phthalates-induced tumorigenesis. *The Kaohsiung Journal of Medical Sciences, 28*(7), S22–S27. doi:10.1016/j.kjms.2012.05.006 PMID:22871597

Whyatt, R. M., Liu, X., Rauh, V. A., Calafat, A. M., Just, A. C., Hoepner, L., ... Factor-Litvak, P. (2012). Maternal prenatal urinary phthalate metabolite concentrations and child mental, psychomotor,and behavioral development at 3 years of age. *Environmental Health Perspectives, 120*(2), 290–295. doi:10.1289/ehp.1103705 PMID:21893441

KEY TERMS AND DEFINITIONS

Asthma: A condition in which a person's airways become inflamed, narrow and swell, and produce extra mucus, which makes it difficult to breathe.

Biomonitoring: It is the measurement of the body burden of toxic chemical compounds, elements, or their metabolites, in biological substances. Often, these measurements are done in blood and urine.

Cryptorchidism: It is the absence of one or both testes from the scrotum.

Pthalates: Phthalates, or phthalate esters, are esters of phthalic acid. They are mainly used as plasticizers (i.e., substances added to plastics to increase their flexibility, transparency, durability, and longevity). They are used primarily to soften polyvinyl chloride.

Steroidogenesis: It is a synthetic process that begins with cholesterol as a substrate and, through a series of enzymatic reactions, produces a wide array of bioactive interrelated signaling molecules.

This research was previously published in the Handbook of Research on Environmental and Human Health Impacts of Plastic Pollution edited by Khursheed Ahmad Wani, Lutfah Ariana, and S.M. Zuber; pages 314-339, copyright year 2020 by Engineering Science Reference (an imprint of IGI Global).

Section 3
Postpartum Care

Chapter 14
An Analysis of Factors Affecting Postnatal Depression Intervention Adherence

Omobolanle Omisade
University of Portsmouth, UK

Alice Good
University of Portsmouth, UK

Tineke Fitch
University of Portsmouth, UK

Jim Briggs
University of Portsmouth, UK

ABSTRACT

Adjunct mobile support for postnatal depression could promote treatment adherence and long-term maintenance of behavioural change. The aim of this article is to establish the factors that determine adherence to postnatal depression intervention and support. Also, this article is intended to establish attitudes that women have towards postnatal depression intervention and support. Eighty-four women with a previous diagnosis of postnatal depression completed an online questionnaire on their previous use of postnatal depression intervention and factors inhibiting adherence, as well as attitudes towards the intervention. Results showed that adjunct support and combining multiple interventions would improve adherence. The provision of treatment guidance will also positively enhance treatment uptake and retention. Therefore, these factors should be considered for the development of theory-based adjunct mobile application for postnatal depression.

DOI: 10.4018/978-1-7998-2351-3.ch014

INTRODUCTION

Women are vulnerable to the affective mood disorder postnatal depression (PND), which can occur in the first three months after childbirth (Culjak & Spranca, 2006; O'Mahen et al., 2013). From the literature, PND represents the most frequent form of maternal morbidity following delivery (Cuijper, Brannmark, & Van Straten, 2008; Gibson, McKenzie-McHarg, Shakespeare, Price, Gray, 2009). A meta-analysis of 59 studies reports that 13% of women having babies suffer from PND with about 70,000 women experiencing PND in the United Kingdom every year (Caramlau, Barlow, Sembi, McKenzie-McHarg, & McCabe, 2011; Dennis, 2003; Evans, Donelle, Hume-Loveland, 2011; Glover, Onozawa, & Hodgkinson, 2002; Morrell, 2006). Like other episodes of depression, PND affects a postnatal woman's feelings about herself and her interpersonal relationships; and she may be functioning only minimally in her role as a mother (Beck, 2001). Additionally, PND can have serious consequences for the infant, which can include lower weight; impaired mental and emotional development; difficult temperament; poor self-regulation; low self-esteem; sudden infant death syndrome; or an overall higher frequency of hospital admissions and long-term behavioural problems (Forman, Videbech, Hedegaard, Salvig, & Secher, 2000; Glover et al., 2002; Grace, Evindar, & Stewart, 2003 Morrell, 2006; O'Mahen, 2013).

Antidepressant medication is usually the first treatment offered to treat the symptoms of PND. There is evidence to support its efficacy when used as prescribed, but it is often associated with side effects (Hou et al., 2013; Kaltenthaler et al., 2002). A study compared the effectiveness of antidepressants with placebo for the treatment of PND in an 8-week study (Yonkers, Lin, Howell, Heath, & Cohen, 2008). Women were randomised to either a placebo group or to take paroxetine antidepressant. Seventy women qualified for the study and only 31 completed between 7 and 8 weeks of treatment. While results indicated that there was a great improvement in the overall clinical severity for the paroxetine group compared with the controlled group, the study was restricted by high attrition rate and this complicated the interpretation of the findings. The high attrition rate in PND interventions remains a major problem that needs to be solved. One possible reason for high attrition for the use of antidepressants might be related to the fact that postnatal depressed mothers consistently indicate that they prefer therapy to antidepressants because of the concern over safety when breastfeeding (Hou et al., 2013; Ruaro, 2013). However, the authors cannot make a general conclusion.

Alternatively, psychotherapy is an effective treatment and support for PND. Milgrom et al. (2006) suggested that counselling informed by the principles of Cognitive Behavioural Therapy (CBT) (a form of psychotherapy) is effective when delivered by maternal and child health nurses. Interpersonal Therapy (IPT) has also been found to be effective for this population (Klier, Muzik, Rosenblum, & Lenz, 2001). However, the postnatal period still presents specific barriers to adequate improvement in depression, and a large number of women remain without treatment, do not adhere to the prescribed intervention or show only moderate improvement in depression (Boath, Bradley, Anthony, 2004; O'Mahen, 2013). More recently, computerised self-help approaches using the Internet have been developed to provide greater access and flexibility of receiving psychotherapy while requiring minimal input from a therapist (O'Mahen, 2013). The National Institute for Health and Care Excellence (NICE) has recommended the use of Computerized Cognitive Behavioural Therapy (CCBT) software for depression (NICE, 2006). CCBT has shown to be effective, with less time required in usual care and shorter therapist time needed while providing engagement and quality support (Churchill, et al., 2001; Gerhards, et al., 2010; Giridher, Wasilewska, Wong, & Rekhi, 2010; Graham, Franses, Kenwright, & Marks, 2000; Ingram, 2013; Kaltenthaler, Parry, Beverley, & Ferriter, 2008; Kaltenthaler et al., 2002; Marks, Shaw, & Parkin, 1998; Merry et al., 2012). However, in clinical settings where women are only able to access CCBT from health centres, there is still the problem of long waiting lists for assessments and support (Andersson et al., 2005; Henshaw, 2004; Marks, Cavanagh, & Gega, 2007; O'Mahen et al., 2013; Proudfoot et al., 2004). The number of sessions of CCBT ranges from four to a maximum of 12 sessions and, in some cases, these sessions do not fit into a baby's variable and demanding schedule, resulting in poor adherence and inequality in access to appropriate treatment (Kaltenthaler et al., 2002; O'Mahen et al., 2013; Wan, Hu, Moore, & Ashford, 2008).

Research suggests that, despite effective treatment options, a large number of depressed women comply poorly with treatment or show only moderate improvement in depression (McCarthy & McMahon, 2008). In some cases, depressed women with other young children attributed poor adherence to struggles and cost associated with transportation or overwhelming responsibilities that can interfere with the ability to attend regularly scheduled appointments (De Graaf et al., 2009; Kaltenthaler et al., 2008; McCarthy & McMahon, 2008; Merry et al., 2012; Wan et al., 2008). Other barriers include stigma, long treatment sessions, sleep difficulties associated with infant sleep schedules and problems adjusting to and managing busy schedules of an infant balanced against other valued tasks (Kaltenthaler et al., 2008; O'Mahen et al., 2013).

The increase in the use of mobile phones and mobile applications may offer additional opportunities to provide support and may circumvent many of the difficulties that lead to poor adherence in PND. An adjunct mobile application could potentially be used to motivate postnatal depressed women to adhere to treatment and sustain treatment outcome in the long-term by providing guided support (Cuijpers, Donker, van Straten, Li, & Andersson, 2010; O'Mahen et al., 2013). It could offer the opportunity to provide just-in-time support and resources to those that have particular needs for flexibility (Kaltenthaler et al., 2008). A mobile application for PND would enable personalised interaction in a more practical and nonintrusive fashion as well as specialised treatment adaptation (O'Mahen et al., 2013). However, to develop an intervention that will increase adherence, there is a need to identify the factors that determine positive intentions to adhere to PND treatment. Furthermore, if you want to change the attitude towards a behaviour, you need to find out the beliefs people hold and the consequences of their attitude. A knowledge of these will also help to adapt the right kinds of beliefs, and, thus, a change in behaviour (Ajzen, 2002).

Studies have shown that, for optimum effectiveness, an intervention should have a sound theoretical basis. According to the Theory of Planned Behaviour (TPB), human action is influenced by three major constructs: behavioural beliefs/attitude (favourable or unfavourable), subjective norm (pressure to perform or not perform the behaviour) and control belief (perceived capacity to perform the behaviour) (Ajzen, 2002). They are all conceptualised as directly related to intentions towards behaviour. The targets of this paper are the behavioural beliefs and attitudes women have towards adhering to PND treatments as well as the control beliefs. Attitude towards a behaviour is assumed to be a function of beliefs about the behaviour's likely consequences, together with the valence attached to those consequences (Ajzen, 2011). It is assumed that a knowledge of women's beliefs and attitudes towards intervention outcome could predict their behaviour towards treatment adherence and their intention to use a support application. Fishbein advocates identifying salient beliefs from the intended population and developing suitable and appropriate materials based on the elicited beliefs (Fishbein, von Haeften, & Appleyard, 2001). Furthermore, a person may hold a positive attitude concerning a behaviour, but not always carry out their intentions towards it (Ajzen, 2011). In this context, a postnatal depressed woman might have positive intentions towards treatment, but there are many reasons as to why she does not adhere to it, and this can be classified as the degree of control that the woman has over behavioural performance. If a depressed woman has the capacity, skills, time, resources or whatever it takes to perform the adherence behaviour, then she will be able to carry out her intention, but not if some of these are lacking. However, women with PND are faced with overwhelming responsibilities and undergo some changes after childbirth that could affect their adherence behaviour (De Graaf et al., 2009; Kaltenthaler et al., 2002). There is, therefore, need to understand women's beliefs and attitudes toward interventions, control beliefs and how they form their intentions to engage, perform or not the adherence behaviour.

Identifying women's beliefs and attitudes towards PND interventions could potentially benefit practitioners who intend to change or motivate the adherence behaviour. In this context, this knowledge will inform the development of a theory-based adjunct mobile application to support the wellbeing of women with PND. It will also help to decide on the factors and beliefs that should be supported or discouraged by a mobile application for PND. The authors envisage that an adjunct mobile application would promote the self-monitoring and social support needed to motivate treatment adherence and long-term maintenance and control over adherence behaviour.

Study Aims and Objectives

This study aims to investigate the TPB constructs, behavioural and control beliefs to establish some of the factors that lead to treatment adherence and sustained outcome. The objectives are to identify the obstacles to the performance of adherence behaviour that should be discouraged within the mobile application. For women who are already motivated, the authors will also identify factors that could facilitate them to implement their intentions to adhere to treatment. This study will be more related to the type of treatment used and its effectiveness, as opposed to relaying past experiences of PND specifically.

METHOD

Design

The study used an online survey to collect data from participants. Ethical approval was obtained from the author's University Ethics Committee (ID number - BO1/OM1)

Recruitment

Participants were recruited by advertising on UK-based social media platforms, sending email invitations to women who are members of parenting support groups and fertility forums. This took place from February to May 2016. Moderators of the groups were consulted concerning the research, prior to actively targeting potential participants. Once approval had been granted, recruitment involved voluntary participation of women with previous diagnosis of PND.

Interested participants provided informed consent prior to participating and then accessed information describing the aims and objectives of the study and eligibility. It was recognised there may be a possibility that participants might have found that some of the study questions triggered distressing memories; therefore, the authors designed the questionnaire to ensure that questions related more to the type of therapy used and its effectiveness, as opposed to relaying past experiences of PND specifically. In the event they became distressed, the study also provided a set of resources that could support women. The authors did not ask any questions relating to children being at risk or other likely distressing memories.

Participants were provided with sufficient details of the study at an appropriate level of understanding and were informed that they had the right to withdraw at any time during the course of completing the questionnaire. Given the possibility, albeit minimal, that participants may incur psychological stress in relation to carrying out the survey, information was provided at the end of the survey advising women where they could seek support. The survey was designed to exclude any women who had a current or recent diagnosis of PND.

Instrument

Ajzen's (2002) instructions for constructing a TPB questionnaire were adopted to develop items used to collect data on treatment adherence behaviour. This study is simply measuring the attitude towards PND treatment adherence and the perceived control beliefs; therefore, this was measured by eight items with possible responses ranging from strongly disagree to strongly agree. See Figure 1 for how the construct was operationalised in the current study. The questionnaire included questions about the types of intervention participants have used in the past, the effectiveness of intervention on wellbeing, the effect of intervention on symptoms, factors that might cause non-adherence and demographics. See appendices for questionnaire items.

For the purpose of this study, eight PND interventions are considered in order to identify participant's attitude towards treatment adherence:

- Cognitive Behavioural Therapy (CBT)
- Medication (Med)
- Monitoring and Assistance (MA)
- Self-Help from peer group (SHP)
- Psycho-education
- Wellbeing therapy
- Interpersonal therapy
- Problem solving therapy

The natures of these interventions are described in the following studies: Klier et al. (2001), Cooper (2003), Milgrom, Ericksen, McCarthy, & Gemmill (2006), Pampallona et al. (2002 and Yonker et al. (2008). This study classified symptoms as:

Figure 1. Adapted Theory of Planned Behaviour Construct for predicting treatment adherence behavior (Ajzen, 2002)

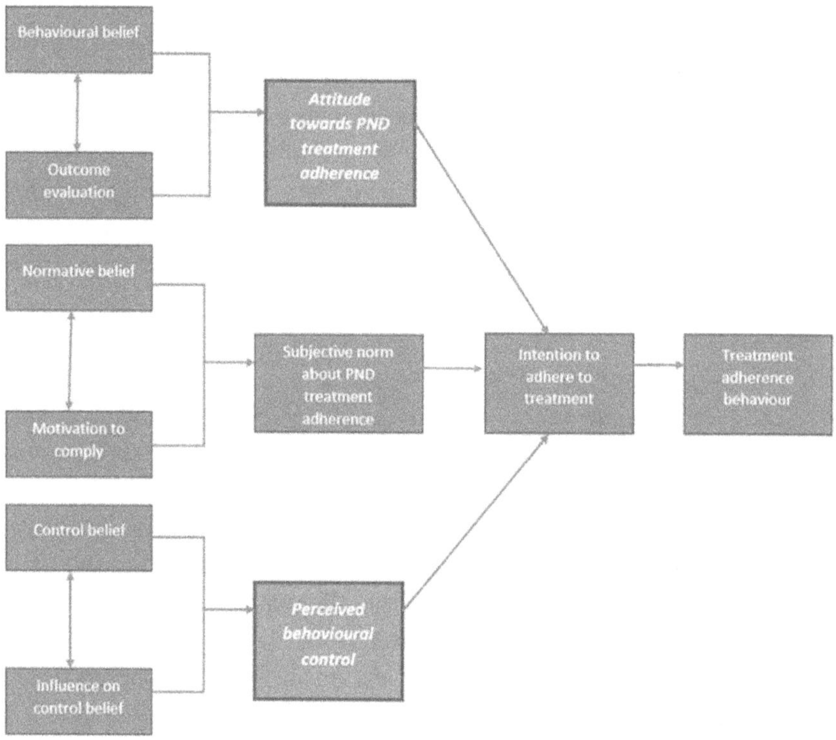

- Isolation
- Poor communication
- Prioritising demand
- Relationships
- Stress management
- Negative thoughts
- Self-confidence

Participants

Potential participants were screened for eligibility using multiple questions in the questionnaire. In order to determine whether a participant is currently ill or well, the authors asked the question “Do you presently suffer from postnatal depression”. Eligible participants were women with previous diagnosis of PND, yet who had not suffered any symptoms of PND in the last two years prior to recruitment. This study group was used because it places us in a position to explore women's view about the short and long-term effectiveness of the intervention on their recovery from PND. Men, women who currently suffer from PND, have experienced PND in the last two years, or have not received treatment in the past were excluded from the study.

Sample

This study estimated a sample size of 382 postnatal mothers to achieve effect size. This is based on a population of about 70,000 women suffering from PND in the UK (Caramlau et al., 2011; Dennis, 2003; Evans et al., 2011; Glover et al., 2002), with 5% margin of error and confidence level of 95%. 460 women were invited and, in total, 181 participants started the survey. After screening for depression, 97 were not eligible for the study. Of those, 55 (30.4%) were excluded because they were current sufferers of PND, 11 because they had never suffered from PND and 23 (12.7%) because they had not received any treatment for PND. A further eight respondents that did not complete any further questions had to be excluded due to the lack of further responses to analyse. The final group of participants comprised 84 (46.4%) postnatal women (mean age = 32 years, range 27-41). It is important to note that not all participants responded to all questions asked. Table 1 presents further details on the number of included and excluded participants.

Data Analysis

Throughout this study, the widely used IBM SPSS statistics package was used to analyse quantitative data (Brace, Kemp, & Snelgar, 2012). For this study, an outcome is statistically significant if the significance level "p" is less than 0.05. This study explored the differences in scores of a non-parametric dependent variable between three or more groups of a single independent variable. Therefore, the Kruskal-Wallis

Table 1. Number of included and excluded women

	Excluded women	Included women	Percentage (%)
Women not suffering from PND	11		6.1
Women not treated for PND	23		12.7
Women excluded due to the lack of further responses to analyse	8		4.4
Current sufferers	55		30.4
Treated and not currently suffering		84	46.4
Total	97	84	100.0

test, which is a non-parametric equivalent of the between subject analysis of variance (ANOVA) test, was employed to evaluate significant differences. The Kruskal-Wallis test only tells us that there is a difference, but does not tell us where the differences are according to each pair of analyses (Brace, et al., 2012). Therefore, an additional Mann-Whitney U test was used to locate the differences, one for each pair of groups.

Furthermore, this study measured the degree of relationship and association between symptoms and adherence variables. However, it is important to note that correlation does not imply causation, but will provide a measure of strength and direction of relationship. The Pearson correlation was used for normal data. For non-parametric data, Kendall's Tau-b test of correlation was used to predict the relationship between variables. The study assessed relationships in terms of the positive or negative correlation coefficient (r). The correlation coefficient describes the strength of the association between two variables. It provides a direct representation of effect size. Using Cohen's (1988) conventions for categorising effects sizes, the study described the strength and size of the relationship for particular values of correlation coefficient.

RESULTS

Depressed Women Without Treatment

Our survey revealed that, despite effective treatment options, some women remain without treatment. Although those women who had PND and remained without treatment were excluded from the main part of this study (see Table 1), our sample showed that 12.7% (23/181) of respondents fell into this category. Our findings agree with the literature that suggests that, despite effective intervention options, postnatal depressed women remain without treatment (Kaltenthaler et al., 2002; O'Mahen, 2013; Wan et al., 2008).

The Use of Multiple Interventions

Our results showed that 81% of depressed women rely on combinations of treatment strategies, with medication being the most common intervention that was combined. Figure 2 presents the frequency of the number of women who used multiple interventions. Table 2 shows that women found one intervention more effective than the other.

Figure 2. Frequency of number women who used multiple interventions

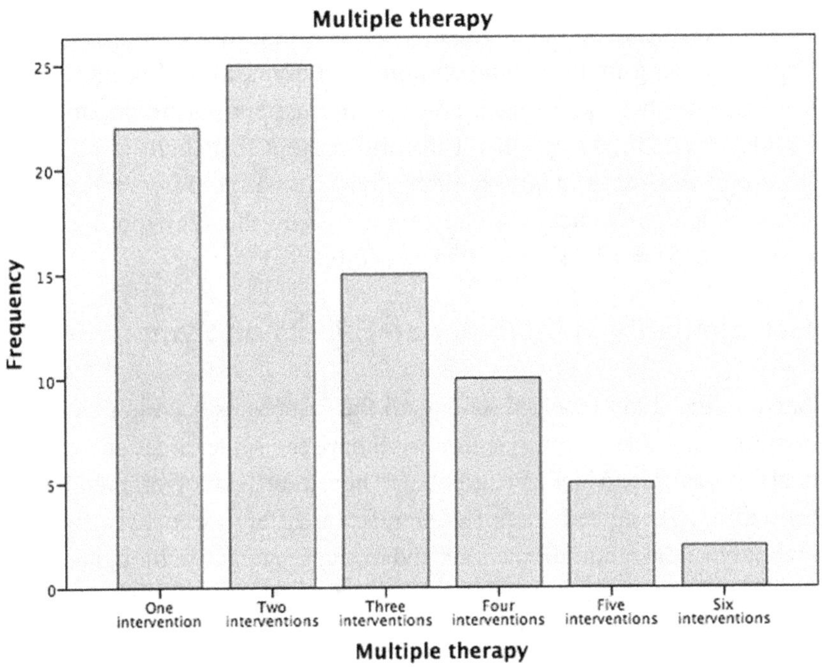

Table 2. Frequency of participants' most effective intervention and percentage score of women that have used multiple interventions

Intervention	Number of women who used intervention	Number of women for whom this was the most effective intervention	Number of women for whom this was one of a set of multiple interventions
Cognitive Behavioural Therapy	29	12	12
Monitoring and assistance (GP, Nurse or Therapist)	37	6	6
Medication	67	40	27
Psycho-education and information	3	1	
Self-help from peer group	26	10	7
Interpersonal Therapy	7	3	5
Wellbeing Therapy	5	5	5
Problem Solving Therapy	2	2	2
Total	176	79	64

Can Combine Multiple Intervention Aid Symptoms

Further tests were carried out to identify women's attitudes towards the benefits and purpose of using multiple interventions. The Kruskal-Wallis test was used to identify differences between using one intervention as opposed to combining multiple interventions for PND symptoms. The results show that there is no significant difference between using one, two, three, four, five or six interventions on PND symptoms. Non-significance was apparent across all the symptom factors except relationship: $\chi 2$ (5) = 12.942, p = .024, see Table 3.

Is There Similarity in Intervention Effects on Symptoms

All women in the study reported having all the symptoms used in this study. This study assumes that several interventions will have the same effect on symptoms. A statistical test was used to identify the belief of how the effects of intervention on PND symptoms differ. The authors identified significant differences between intervention groups about isolation, communication and managing negative thoughts. The result for prioritising demands, relationship, self-confidence, and stress management that were not statistically significant. A subsequent Mann-Witney U-test showed that these differences were particularly apparent between CBT and SHP (z = -2.318, p = 0.02), MED and SHP (z = -2.540, p = 0.01). Concerning scores on isolation and for communication, differences were found between the MED and SHP categories (z = -2.863, $p < 0.05$) and between managing negative thought CBT and SHP (z = -2.451, p = 0.02). Although, the results were apparently between neutral and disagree, it shows that various interventions have different effects on symptoms.

Table 3. Effects of using multiple interventions to aid symptoms

Symptoms factors	**Kruskal-Wallis test**		
	H	**df**	**P-value**
Isolation	2.794	0.73	0.73
Communication	2.042	0.84	0.84
Prioritise demands	2.995	0.71	0.71
Relationship	12.942	5.00	0.02
Stress management	6.392	5.00	0.27
Manage negative thoughts	2.626	5.00	0.76
Self confidence	6.399	5.00	0.27

Association Between Non- Adherence and PND Symptoms

This study assumes that there is a relationship between non-adherence factors and the effect of PND intervention on symptoms. To evaluate this assumption, the authors considered poor adherence control factors available from the literature to be the cost of receiving intervention; the duration of appointments; waiting times; and location convenience. All women in the study reported facing the control factors used in this study. The results in Table 4 show that there was a weak and non-significant correlation between most of these. Although the correlation between the location and stress management was significant, it is a small effect (r= 249, p= .01).

Furthermore, we identified how women followed treatment instructions as prescribed by their practitioners. Research suggests that half of those women for whom treatment regimens were prescribed do not follow them as directed - this is termed as non-adherence (World Health Organisation, 2003). The researchers asked women how often they followed their treatment instructions. Table 5 shows that 63% (mean = 3.77; sd = .89) of the final group of the women followed the instructions as directed by their practitioners. However, there was a weak and non-significant relationship between the frequency of following instructions and the effect on symptoms (see Table 6).

Table 4. Association between PND symptoms and factors that might affect adherence to PND treatment (control factors)

Symptoms factors	Kendall's Tau_b correlation							
	Cost factor		Duration factors		Waiting times factor		Location factor	
	r	p	r	p	r	p	r	p
Isolation	.151	.12	.068	.49	.013	.90	.019	.85
Communication	-.070	.45	.004	.97	.108	.27	.011	.91
Prioritise demands	.059	.54	.172	.08	.057	.57	.010	.91
Relationship	.015	.88	-.096	.32	.031	.76	.124	.20
Stress management	.023	.81	-.047	.63	-.113	.26	.249	.01
Manage negative thoughts	.006	.95	-.169	.09	-.088	.39	.109	.27
Self confidence	.068	.48	.050	.61	.001	.99	.059	.54

Table 5. Number of women that follow instructions as directed by practitioner

	Frequency	Percentage (%)
Never	4	6.1
Sometimes	20	30.3
Regularly	42	63.6
Total	66	100.0

Table 6. Summary of relationship between following instructions and symptom control factors

Symptoms factors	Kendall's tau_b correlation		
	r	P-value	Variance
Isolation	-.033	0.76	.729
Communication	.096	0.37	.921
Prioritise demands	-.113	0.29	.127
Relationship	-.021	0.85	.289
Stress management	.005	0.96	.25
Manage negative thoughts	-.066	0.55	.291
Self confidence	.081	0.45	.656

The Soothing of One PND Symptom Might Alleviate the Effect of Other Symptoms

The Pearson correlation coefficient was used to examine the degree of association between symptom factors. This test was used because there was a normal distribution of data. Prioritising demands was found to be significantly and positively correlated with communication ($r(n=79) = 0.464$, $p < 0.001$); relationship ($r(n=79) = 0.434$, $p < 0.001$); stress management ($r(n=79) = 0.408$, $p < 0.001$); managing negative thoughts ($r(n=79) = 0.329$, $p < 0.001$) and self-confidence ($r(n=79) = 0.474$, $p < 0.001$). These indicate that depressed women with a higher level of prioritising their demands tended to have a good relationship with people, have reduced stress, are able to manage negative thoughts and have faith in themselves. However, isolation was found to have a very weak relationship with prioritising demands ($r(n=79) = 0.164$, $p = 0.148$), communication ($r(n=79) = 0.208$, $p = 0.065$), and relationship ($r(n=79) = 0.177$, $p = 0.119$) (see Table 7).

Table 7. Association between symptoms considered in this study

Symptom	2	3	4	5	6	7
1. Communication	.208	.464**	.438**	.335**	.301**	.493**
2. Isolation	-	.164	.177	.252*	.325**	.308**
3. Prioritising demands		-	.434**	.408**	.329**	.474**
4. Relationships			-	.520**	.390**	.550**
5. Managing stress				-	.777**	.557**
6. Managing negative thoughts					-	.512**
7. Self confidence						-

DISCUSSION

This study documents the beliefs and factors that might determine adherence to PND treatment, and ensure increased sustained outcome. Firstly, a favourable attitude towards combining multiple interventions influences the actual adherence behaviour. There are several possible reasons why depressed women combine interventions, one being seeking support for normalisation of their mothering (O'Mahen et al., 2013). Previous research has shown that many women begin to incorporate alternate plans after the initial core sessions of their initial intervention (Christensen, Griffiths, & Farrer, 2009; O'Mahen et al., 2013). A poor patient-doctor relationship might cause some women to be inconsistent in attending treatment sessions, thus finding themselves using alternative treatments. In previous research, women have expressed negative experiences of seeking help, and this is particularly likely to cause them to seek additional treatments. Long waiting lists for treatments might be a barrier; therefore, they then seek additional support during waiting times. In some cases, treatments are not equivalently distributed geographically (Goodman 2009; Payne & Myhr, 2010). Finally, perceived stigma can also lead to women seeking additional support that will provide the level of anonymity they require (Dennis & Chung-Lee, 2006; Goodman, 2009; O'Mahen, et al., 2013). Although our results show that combining multiple interventions does not have any significant effect on symptoms, the authors identified, however, that different interventions have different levels of effect on PND symptoms, therefore combining multiple interventions should be increased. This is further supported by research that suggested that to improve adherence, medication should be combined with other support strategies such automatic reminders, reminder packaging, medication boxes, device aids, counselling, telephone support, patient education etc., (Desteghe et al., 2017).

In this present study, women's belief is that the soothing of one symptom factor alleviates the effects of other symptoms. The authors identified a weak relationship between symptoms; this could mean that women are encouraged to adhere or not when the effect of treatment on one or more symptoms is obvious. This is similar to a study that revealed that it was only after women got into a supportive treatment relationship and improved their communication that they felt able to disclose their distress to others (McCarthy & McMahon, 2008). However, further study may be needed to highlight the factors that suggest the relationship between PND symptoms and the effect they have on each other.

Another strength of this study is that treatment cost, duration, location and waiting time, identified as control factors that inhibit adherence to PND treatment, are not related to increased adherence, but not in all cases. One possible explanation is that these factors should not totally hinder women from adhering to prescribed treatments. However, the location where intervention is received is seen to have a relationship with stress management; therefore, it should be recognised that there may be a possibility that depressed women become distressed by the location of receiving treatment. This could be due to transportation difficulties faced by some women. In regard to location, studies have documented the inability of women to attend regularly scheduled appointments (Goodman, 2009; O'Mahen et al., 2014). Additionally, this might mean that an adjunct support should be provided as a control measure in the event they should become distressed by the treatment location. It is also useful to provide guidance as moderator of intention-behaviour and, thus, this might enhance treatment uptake and retention (Cuijpers et al., 2010; O'Mahen et al., 2013). This compares favourably with other research suggestions that only women who get a supportive treatment are able to show sustained outcome (Cuijpers et al., 2008; O'Mahen et al., 2013; McCarthy & McMahon, 2008). Furthermore, following instructions as prescribed by practitioners did not have an effect on PND symptoms. The underlying causes as to why following instructions did not have effect on symptom are still unclear. Therefore, the authors are careful in making their conclusions on this finding.

Implications

This study identified women's attitudes towards postnatal depression interventions and the factors that could motivate improved adherence. A knowledge of these factors will allow the development of a set of guidelines which can inform the development of an adjunct mobile application for postnatal depression and future improvement research. This will also facilitate the development of a mobile application that is tailored towards positive treatment adherence attitudes. Furthermore, it will potentially support future applications for a larger study to undertake a full trial of mobile applications for PND.

Limitations

Limitations of the current study are largely related to the fact that not all participants provided us with a complete data set. Although all participants satisfied the eligibility criteria, the women who completed the study are best considered a convenient sample that may not be generalised to all postnatal depressed mothers. Finally, it is possible that the use of only two TPB constructs (behavioural and control beliefs) might have influenced the ability to identify more factors that facilitate or inhibit adherence behaviour.

CONCLUSION

This study has identified the TPB variables that might predict the intention to adherence to PND treatments. Firstly, increasing access to adjunct support for PND has the potential to influence adherence positively, and long-term sustained treatment outcome. In particular, providing an intervention that combines support features of several interventions is recommended for increased adherence. This intervention could also provide the flexibility of treatment adaptation. Additionally, it may circumvent many of the barriers to treatment delivery and motivate women to self-manage their wellbeing as well as give them access to supplementary wellbeing support.

It is essential that the option to combine multiple interventions should also be balanced, this could mean that it should not be encouraged or discouraged. This is because combining multiple interventions does not have any significant effect on symptoms; however, different interventions have different levels of effect on PND symptoms. Therefore, the authors recommend a platform that will facilitate using additional support to prescribed treatments for PND. This is in line with a growing body of research demonstrating that the provision of additional support to prescribed treatment could enhance achieving the desired outcome and sustained effect (Broom, Ladley, Rhyne, & Halloran, 2015). Adjunct treatment needs to remain available to women receiving intervention, both during and after the intervention has ended (Turner, Chew-Graham, & Folkes, 2010). The effect of adjunct support was revealed in a study that recorded high compliance (Rojas et al., 2007). The multicomponent intervention used in that study was supported by regular phone calls from trained mental health workers, and depressed women were constantly reminded in sessions about the need to take medications as prescribed (Rojas, et al., 2007). The authors also recommend that, rather than providing women with a single intervention for all PND symptoms, there should be a multiple-choice option that is open to adapting support to depressed women's specific needs. This should hopefully give them the opportunity to have control over their desired intervention outcome.

Furthermore, this study demonstrated that a greater guidance tool designed to make treatment effect on symptoms noticeable could be beneficial and help control adherence behaviour. A structured support plan is viewed as a behavioural control tool, critical for achieving increased treatment understanding, self-management and adherence.

Given these promising findings, there is a need to develop and evaluate methods of promoting adherence and sustained treatment outcome in the PND population. Mobile Health is growing as a method to improve adherence and health outcomes. An adjunct mobile application is one method that may hold the promise of doing such. Developing a suitable and appropriate mobile application is desirable, given its potential to increase adherence to the behaviour being promoted (Desteghe et al., 2017). This tool could support individuals with treatment/work already offered by practitioners, thus allowing sessions to be offered at a reduced frequency, duration and at a cheaper cost and convenient location. In order to develop a mobile health intervention that will increase adherence, using a theory based approach, this study sought to understand women's perspective on obstacles to the performance of adherence behaviour that should be discouraged within the mobile application as well as factors that could facilitate them to implement their intentions to adhere to treatment. Based on our findings, we recommend that the development of a PND adherence mobile application should include features designed to:

- Help manage and monitor the use of multiple interventions.
- Keep a record and manage the impact of symptoms so that changes are noticeable.
- Keep records of prescription instructions and provide positive prompts to users for better communication.
- Include prompts and reminders as a means of self-guidance.
- Help users stay in contact with healthcare providers, family and friends when further guidance or help is needed.

Additionally, research has shown that self-incentives are key motivators and successful in changing health behaviours, adherence to daily care and improve health outcome. As a result of this insight we recommend that the mobile app should also include a feature that is:

- Related to self-incentives and will make the environment enjoyable and stimulating for users.

The current findings highlight beliefs about PND interventions that are necessary for developing adherence behaviour change intervention for this population. These findings will inform the design of an adjunct mobile application for PND. However, there is a need to establish the suitability and appropriateness of a mobile application. The mobile application should be evaluated for suitability and appropriateness to enhance the likelihood that the tool can effectively change behaviour. Further research is also needed to determine the acceptance of such a mobile application by both women with PND and practitioners. Such research should allow us to establish the requirements under which a mobile application for PND may be offered as effective and accessible support.

REFERENCES

Ajzen, I. (2002). Perceived behavioural control, self-efficacy, locus of control and the theory of planned behaviour. *Journal of Applied Social Psychology*, *32*(4), 665–683. doi:10.1111/j.1559-1816.2002.tb00236.x

Ajzen, I. (2011). Behavioral interventions: Design and evaluation guided by the theory of planned behavior. In M. M. Mark, S. I. Donaldson, & B. C. Campbell (Eds.), *Social psychology for program and policy evaluation New York* (pp. 74–100). Guilford.

Andersson, G., Bergstrom, J., Hollandare, F., Carbring, P., Viktor, K., & Ekselius, L. (2005). Internet-based self help for depression. *The British Journal of Psychiatry*, *187*(5), 456–461. doi:10.1192/bjp.187.5.456 PMID:16260822

Beck, C. T. (2001). Revision of the Postpartum Depression Predictors Inventory. *JOGNN principles and practice*, *31*(4), 394-402.

Boath, E., Bradley, E., Anthony, P. (2004) Users' views of two alternative approaches to the treatment of postnatal depression. *Journal of Reproductive and Infant Psychology*, *22*(1), 13-24.

Brace, N., Kemp, R. and Snelgar, R.(2012). *SPSS for Psychologist* (5th ed.). Basingstoke, UK: Macmillan Publishers.

Broom, M. A., Ladley, A. S., Rhyne, E. A., & Halloran, D. A. (2015). Feasibility and perception of using text messages as an adjunct therapy for low-income, minority mothers with postnatal depression. *JMIR Mental Health*, *2*(1), e4. doi:10.2196/mental.4074 PMID:26543910

Caramlau, I., Barlow, J., Sembi, S., McKenzie-McHarg, K., & McCabe, C. (2011). Mums 4 Mums: Structured telephone peer-support for women experiencing PND. Pilot and exploratory RCT of its clinical and cost effectiveness. *Trials*, *12*, 88. doi:10.1186/1745-6215-12-88 PMID:21439042

Christensen, H., Griffiths, K. M., & Farrer, L. (2009). Adherence in internet interventions for anxiety and depression. *Journal of Medical Internet Research*, *11*(2), e13. doi:10.2196/jmir.1194 PMID:19403466

Churchill, R., Hunot, V., Corney, R., Knapp, M., McGuire, H., Tyleem, A., & Wessely, S. (2001). A systematic review of controlled trials of the effectiveness and cost-effectiveness of brief psychological treatments for depression. *Health Technology Assessment*, *5*, 1–173. PMID:12387733

Cooper, J. E. (2003). Detection and Management of Psychiatric Disorders in Primary Care. *The British Journal of Psychiatry*, *182*(1), 1–4. doi:10.1192/bjp.182.1.1 PMID:12509308

Cuijper, P., Brannmark, J. G., & Van Straten, A. (2008). Psychological Treatment of Postpartum Depression: A meta-analysis. *Journal of Clinical Psychology*, *64*(1), 113–118. PMID:18161036

Cuijpers, P., Donker, T., van Straten, A., Li, J., & Andersson, G. (2010). Is guided self-help as effective as face-to-face psychotherapy for depression and anxiety disorders? A systematic review and meta-analysis of comparative outcome studies. *Psychological Medicine*, *40*(12), 1943–1957. doi:10.1017/S0033291710000772 PMID:20406528

Culjak, G., & Spranca, M. (2006). Internet Improves Health Outcome in Depression. In *Proceedings of the Hawaii International Conference on System Sciences*.

De Graaf, L. E., Gerhards, S. A. H., Arntz, A., Riper, H., Metsemakers, J. F. M., Evers, S. M., ... Huibers, M. J. (2009). Clinical effectiveness of online computerised cognitive–behavioural therapy without support for depression in primary care: Randomised trial. *The British Journal of Psychiatry*, *195*(1), 73–80. doi:10.1192/bjp.bp.108.054429 PMID:19567900

Dennis, C. (2003). The effect of peer support on postpartum depression: A pilot randomized controlled trial. *Canadian Journal of Psychiatry*, *48*(2), 115–125. doi:10.1177/070674370304800209 PMID:12655910

Dennis, C.-L., & Chung-Lee, L. (2006). Postpartum depression help-seeking barriers and maternal treatment preferences: A qualitative systematic review. *Birth (Berkeley, Calif.)*, *33*(4), 323–331. doi:10.1111/j.1523-536X.2006.00130.x PMID:17150072

Desteghe, L., Vijgen, J., Koopman, P., Dilling-Boer, D., Schurmans, J., Dendale, P., & Heidbuchel, H. (2017). The Health Buddies App as a Novel Tool to Improve Adherence and Knowledge in Atrial Fibrillation Patients: A Pilot Study. *JMIR mHealth and uHealth*, *5*(7), e98. doi:10.2196/mhealth.7420 PMID:28724512

Evans, M., Donelle, L., & Hume-Loveland, L. (2011). Social support and online postpartum depression discussion groups: A content analysis. *Patient Education and Counseling*, *87*(3), 405–410. doi:10.1016/j.pec.2011.09.011 PMID:22019021

Fishbein, M., von Haeften, I., & Appleyard, J. (2001). The role of theory in developing effective interventions: Implications from Project SAFER. *Psychology Health and Medicine*, *6*(2), 223–238. doi:10.1080/13548500123176

Forman, N. D. (2000). Postpartum Depression: Identification of women at risk. *British Journal of Obstetrics and Gynaecology*, *107*(10), 1210–1217. doi:10.1111/j.1471-0528.2000.tb11609.x PMID:11028570

Gerhards, S. A. H., de Graaf, L. E., Jacobs, L. E., Severens, L. J., Huibers, M. J. H., Arntz, A., ... Evers, S. M. (2010). Economic evaluation of online computerised cognitive-behavioural therapy without support for depression in primary care: Randomised trial. *The British Journal of Psychiatry*, *196*(4), 310–318. doi:10.1192/bjp.bp.109.065748 PMID:20357309

Gibson, J., McKenzie-McHarg, K., Shakespeare, J., Price, J., & Gray, R. (2009). A systematic review of studies validating the Edinburgh PND Scale in antepartum and postpartum women. *Acta Psychiatrica Scandinavica*, *119*, 350–364. doi:10.1111/j.1600-0447.2009.01363.x PMID:19298573

Giridher, I., Wasilewska, A., Wong, J. L., & Rekhi, K. S. (2010). Global mobile application for monitoring health. In *Proceedings of the 2010 International Multiconference on Computer Science and Information Technology* (pp. 855-859).

Glover, V., Onozawa, K., & Hodgkinson, A. (2002). Benefits of infant massage for mothers with PND. *Seminars in Neonatology*, *7*, 495–500. doi:10.1053iny.2002.0154 PMID:12614602

Goodman, J. H. (2009). Women's attitudes, preferences and perceived barriers to treatment for perinatal depression. *Birth (Berkeley, Calif.)*, *36*(1), 60–69. doi:10.1111/j.1523-536X.2008.00296.x PMID:19278385

Grace, S. L., Evindar, A., & Stewart, D. E. (2003). The effect of postpartum depression on child cognitive development and behavior: A review and critical analysis of the literature. *Archives of Women's Mental Health*, *6*(4), 263–274. doi:10.100700737-003-0024-6 PMID:14628179

Graham, C., Franses, A., Kenwright, M., & Marks, I. (2000). Psychotherapy by Computer: A postal survey of responders to a teletext article. *Psychiatric Bulletin*, *24*(9), 331–332. doi:10.1192/pb.24.9.331

Henshaw, C. A. (2004). What do women think about treatments for PND. *Clinical Effectiveness in Nursing*, *8*, 170–175. doi:10.1016/j.cein.2005.03.003

Hou, Y., Hu, P., Zhang, Y., Lu, Q., Wang, D., Yin, L., ... Zou, X. (2013). Cognitive behavioral therapy in combination with systemic family therapy improves mild to moderate postpartum depression. *Revista Brasileira de Psiquiatria (Sao Paulo, Brazil)*, *36*(1), 47–52. doi:10.1590/1516-4446-2013-1170 PMID:24604461

Ingram, D., & Moreno, M. (2013). A computerized self-help intervention is as effective as face-face counselling for adolescents seeking help for depression. *The Journal of Pediatrics*, *161*(5), 967–968. doi:10.1016/j.jpeds.2012.08.050 PMID:23095695

Kaltenthaler, E., Parry, G., Beverley, C., & Ferriter, M. (2008). Computerised cognitive-behavioural therapy for depression: Systematic review. *The British Journal of Psychiatry*, *193*(3), 181–184. doi:10.1192/bjp.bp.106.025981 PMID:18757972

Kaltenthaler, E., Shackley, K., Stevens, K., Beverly, C., & Parry, G. (2002). A systematic review and economic evaluation of computerized cognitive behaviour therapy for depression and anxiety. *Health Technology Assessment*, *6*(22). doi:10.3310/hta6220 PMID:12433315

Klier, C. M., Muzik, M., Rosenblum, K. L., & Lenz, G. (2001). Interpersonal Psychotherapy adapted for group setting in the treatment of postnatal depression. *The Journal of Psychotherapy Practice and Research*, *10*, 124–131. PMID:11264336

Marks, I. M., Cavanagh, K., & Gega, L. (2007). *Hands-on Help: Computer-aided Psychotherapy*. Psychology Press Ltd.

Marks, I. M., Shaw, S. C., & Parkin, R. (1998). Computer-aided treatments of mental health problems. *Clinical Psychology: Science and Practice*, *5*(2), 151–170. doi:10.1111/j.1468-2850.1998.tb00141.x

McCarthy, M., & McMahon, C. (2008). Acceptance and Experience of Treatment for PND in a Community Mental Health Setting. *Health Care for Women International*, *29*, 618–637. doi:10.1080/07399330802089172 PMID:18569047

Merry, S. N., Stasiak, K., Shepheard, M., Frampton, C., Fleming, T., & Lucassen, M. F. G. (2012). The effectiveness of SPARX, a computerised self help intervention for adolescents seeking help for depression: Randomised controlled non-inferiority trial. *BMJ (Clinical Research Ed.)*, *344*, 1–16. PMID:22517917

Milgrom, J., Ericksen, J., McCarthy, R., & Gemmill, A. W. (2006). Stressful impact of depression on early mother–infant relations. *Stress and Health*, *22*(4), 229–238. doi:10.1002mi.1101

Morrell, J. C. (2006). Review of interventions to prevent or treat PND. *Clinical Effectiveness in Nursing*, 9(Suppl. 2), e135–e161. doi:10.1016/j.cein.2006.11.006

NICE. (2006). Computerised cognitive behavioural therapy for depression and anxiety. Retrieved December. 2015. Technology appraisal guidance. http://www.nice.org.uk/nicemedia/pdf/ccbtassessmentreport.pdf

O'Mahen, H. A., Richards, D. A., Woodford, J., & Wilkinson, E., McGinley. J., Taylor, R. S., Warren. (2013). Netmum, a phase II randomized controlled trial of guide Internet behavioural activation treatment for postpartum depression. *Psychological Medicine*. PMID:24148703

Pampallona, S., Bollini, P., Tibaldi, G., Kupelnick, B., & Munizza, C. (2002). Patient adherence in the treatment of depression. *The British Journal of Psychiatry*, *180*(2), 104–109. doi:10.1192/bjp.180.2.104 PMID:11823317

Payne, K. A., & Myhr, G. (2010). Increasing access to cognitive–behavioral therapy (CBT) for the treatment of mental illness in Canada: A research framework and call for action. *Healthcare Policy*, *5*, e173–e175. PMID:21286263

Proudfoot, J., Ryen, C., Everitt, B., Sharpio, D., Goldberg, D., Mnn, A., ... Gray, J. A. (2004). Clinical efficacy of computerized cognitive-behavioural therapy for anxiety and depression in primary care: Randomised controlled trial. *The British Journal of Psychiatry*, *185*(1), 46–54. doi:10.1192/bjp.185.1.46 PMID:15231555

Rojas, G., Fritsch, R., Solis, J., Jadresic, E., Castillo, C., González, M., ... Araya, R. (2007). Treatment of postnatal depression in low-income mothers in primary-care clinics in Santiago, Chile: A randomized controlled trial. *Lancet*, *370*(9599), 1629–1637. doi:10.1016/S0140-6736(07)61685-7 PMID:17993363

Ruaro, L. (2013). *The experience of mother who received therapy of PND. A qualitative study* [Professional Doctorate in Counselling Psychology].

Turner, K. M., Chew-Graham, C., Folkes, L., & Sharp, D. (2010). Women's experiences of health visitors delivered listening visits as a treatment for postnatal depression: A qualitative study. *Patient Education and Counseling*, *78*(2), 234–239. doi:10.1016/j.pec.2009.05.022 PMID:19574015

Wan', J., Hu, B., Moore, P., & Ashford, R. (2008). Intelligent mobile computing to assist in the treatment of depression. *Pervasive Computing and Application, IEEE, 2*, 650–655.

World Health Organisation. (2003). *Adherence to long-term therapies: evidence for action.*

Yonkers, K. A., Lin, H., Howell, H. B., Heath, A. C., & Cohen, L. S. (2008). Pharmacological Treatment of Postpartum Women with New Onset Major Depressive Disorder: A Randomized Controlled Trial with Paroxetine. *The Journal of Clinical Psychiatry, 69*(4), 659–665. doi:10.4088/JCP.v69n0420 PMID:18363420

This research was previously published in the International Journal of Public Health Management and Ethics (IJPHME), 2(1); edited by Qiang (Shawn) Cheng; pages 1-18, copyright year 2017 by IGI Publishing (an imprint of IGI Global).

APPENDIX

Questionnaire

1. What therapy did you use for postnatal depression? (*Please tick all that apply*)
   - Cognitive Behavioural Therapy
   - Monitoring and assistance (by a GP, Nurse or Therapist)
   - Medication
   - Psycho-education and information
   - Self-help from peer group
   - Interpersonal Therapy
   - Well-being Therapy
   - Problem-solving Therapy
   - No treatment
   - Other
2. Which ONE of these therapies did you find MOST effective for postnatal depression? (Please choose one)
3. How effective was the therapy you chose in question 2 in addressing the following?
   - It helped to reduce my isolation
   - It helped me talk to other people
   - It helped me prioritise demands on things I have to do
   - It helped my relationship with my children
   - It helped reduce my stress
   - It helped me to manage negative thoughts
   - It helped me to have faith in myself
4. How long did it feel you had to wait between when you were diagnosed with postnatal depression and when you started receiving therapy? (Please choose one)
5. When you had appointments to receive therapy, how convenient was the location of the facility for you?
6. How affordable was the cost of therapy to you? Costs include bus fare, travel costs, child care or time of work.
7. Thinking about the time you spent on each appointment, how acceptable did you find the length of time spent receiving treatment
8. How long did you have to use your most successful therapy for postnatal depression until recovery?
9. How often did you follow instructions specific to using your therapy when you had postnatal depression?

10. How frequently did you use your most successful therapy for postnatal depression?
11. How long did you have to use your most successful therapy for postnatal depression until recovery?
12. How often did you follow instructions specific to using your therapy when you had postnatal depression?

Chapter 15
Communicating "What's Not Said":
Mobile Apps for Psychological Wellbeing

Marguerite Barry
Trinity College Dublin, Ireland

Kevin Doherty
Trinity College Dublin, Ireland

Gavin Doherty
Trinity College Dublin, Ireland

ABSTRACT

Technologies designed to access our personal worlds have the potential to profoundly influence the way we live and to promote human flourishing. They also require an ethical approach to their design that takes human values into account. Mobile technologies for psychological wellbeing present particular challenges that require a sustainable approach to ethical reflection from early in the design process. This paper offers insights into ethical approaches to design, through projects that explore the potential for using mobile apps for reporting psychological wellbeing. It reports on feedback from a focus group with valuable insights for app design in particular contexts of use that help to inform discourse more generally around designing technologies for wellbeing. The discussion focuses on the practical and cultural issues that arise and explores how technologies can mediate self-knowledge and information in ways that might otherwise remain unsaid, but is crucial for successful outcomes both clinically and in design.

DOI: 10.4018/978-1-7998-2351-3.ch015

INTRODUCTION

Digital technologies for health and wellbeing are growing in use and sophistication, presenting both opportunities and challenges in their design. The increasing use of mobile apps in this context offers the potential to improve public health and a rich source of material for design research. However, their relatively recent arrival and short time frame of adoption means we are still at the early stages of understanding of how and why they work best (Walsh et al., 2016). In order to build a sustainable body of knowledge we need to understand how these apps differ from other digital technologies in terms of context and strategy of communication and examine the ethical implications for design.

Mental health is a major determinant of wellbeing and a concern for society (WHO, 2012). Mobile devices can help identify people who are struggling with depression, by delivering validated psychological health screening surveys, with the benefit of 'anytime, anywhere' usage. In addition, smartphones and tablets can support the implementation of data collection techniques, such as the on-going and remote monitoring of mood and other symptoms (Matthews & Doherty, 2011). A number of commercial smart phone applications have been developed in recent years to support psychological wellbeing among the general population, such as offering mindfulness techniques (Headspace), improving sleep and rest skills (DeepSleep), using CBT therapy (MoodGym) or specific tools to assess anxiety, PTSD and depression (CPT Coach, What's My M3). Some apps focus on physical and mental health during particular life events such as bereavement (Grief: Support for Young People), illness (CaringBridge) or pregnancy (Baby Bump, Mind The Bump). Others offer tools, planning and reporting facilities towards healthier lifestyles (e.g. Balanced, Life Charge). Menstruation tracking apps such as 'Clue' offer a combination of mood tracking, symptom analysis, fertility awareness and feedback for monitoring physical and psychological aspects of the cycle.

Mobile technologies for psychological wellbeing have also been developed for use in controlled clinical releases, involving individual users whose specifications go beyond standard (UX) research and design requirements for the general user. For example, apps focusing in particular on young people and teenagers have been designed to allow them to record and monitor symptoms of depression and anxiety which therapists can review (Matthews & Doherty, 2011), or for tracking mood and feelings to enhance personal autonomy for young people with chronic health problems in transition from paediatric to adult medicine (van der Velden & Machniak, 2016). Further studies have utilised automatic smartphone sensing to generate passive data for monitoring mood rhythms of individuals with bipolar disorder (Abdullah et al., 2016).

Such mHealth applications operate in a design space that needs to accommodate complex issues involving intimate interactivity with personal information, where offline communications frequently reflect poor communication, strategic or deliberate lack of engagement and mixed outcomes. Therefore, the design process needs to include collaboration with mental health professionals as well as deeper research on potential end-users at a very early stage with a particular focus on encouraging engagement (Doherty et al., 2010b). Where active input and interactivity is required, design also needs to support client-therapist relationships without placing excessive burdens or expectations on either (Doherty, Coyle & Matthews, 2010).

Psychological wellbeing during pregnancy is a particularly serious public health issue due to its impact on women's lives, birth outcomes and on children's development. Perinatal depression (PND) is one of the most common psychiatric disorders during pregnancy, affecting up to 15% of women during pregnancy or within one year of giving birth (Bauer et al., 2014, Yazici et al., 2015). However, its frequency is probably higher as it often goes undiagnosed (Ko et al., 2012). Human computer interaction researchers have been examining how technology can benefit pregnancy and motherhood, for example in studies that use social media to identify women at risk of PND (De Choudhury, Counts & Horvitz, 2013) and designing more context-sensitive post partum technologies (D'Ignazio et al., 2016). This paper offers insights from the early stages of design for a research project concerning the use of mobile apps to support psychological wellbeing in pregnancy. It reports on reflections from design feedback sessions and explores the design and structural decisions involved. Through examining the value-sensitive issues that arise, we offer these insights as inputs into a more sustainable ethical reflection process for design (Shilton & Anderson, 2016).

Through analysis of discourses around design in the very early stages, we identify some points in the process where important values relating to wellbeing can become embedded within system designs. We discuss how such projects benefit from interdisciplinary research with an emphasis on diversity and honest critical feedback – both personal and professional – with value for improving our understanding of how mobile technologies can help to promote wellbeing and human flourishing.

DESIGN FOR SELF-REPORTING

As users of digital technologies, we are increasingly voluntarily engaged in processes of self-reporting, through social media networks, technologies for behaviour tracking and intervention, apps for wellbeing and more. Such self-report data is a valuable component in psychological therapy and treatment and therefore in mobile health application design (Doherty et al., 2010). The challenge for HCI is to find ways to understand and design for this valuable self-report data both for the human but also other potential participants in the interactive loop, where feedback, social communication or other forms of automated response are included.

Design requirements for mobile apps are generated through well established HCI principles and frameworks including technical and functional task specifications, expert development of or feedback on content, field knowledge of participant roles and responsibilities, extensive user studies and so on. These approaches have been developed over decades in the refinement of user experience (UX) research broadly in HCI as well as in subfields focussing on specific contexts of use such as education or the commercial workplace. Studies on mobile healthcare applications have also adopted fieldwork and ethnographic approaches in order to reflect the specific requirements of complex healthcare contexts (Doherty et al., 2010a). However, while generating valuable information for specific applications, these approaches are often difficult to generalise and tend to produce a proliferation of choice where the conceptual framework used frequently shapes the requirements generated (ibid).

Meanwhile, our understanding of the role of interactivity in digital applications is improving and moving away from the instrumental view that sees it as a technical characteristic of technology towards a more nuanced understanding of its different modes and layers (Barry, 2014). Recent research has identified its capacity for empowering participants in interactive communications to differing extents through outcomes at an individual level but also at a wider level through its 'channelling' and community building effects (Barry & Doherty, 2016). This may be a vital ingredient in developing a sense of how values can become embedded in interactive design. This research aims to investigate how interactivity may 'empower' the target group for an app for psychological wellbeing, through analysis of insights from design feedback sessions.

Technologies allow us to create, interpret and narrate our experiences and facilitate the actions possible through their design. The field of human computer interaction (HCI) focuses on complex psychological phenomena involved in our responses to design, such as motivation, empathy, compassion, positive emotions and so on and is increasingly focused on research towards 'positive computing' (Calvo & Peters, 2014) as well as actively designing technology for 'good' (for example the ACM CHI conference 2016 theme "CHI4Good"[1]).

Our approach draws upon digital media and communications studies and philosophy of technology as well as HCI research and methodologies. Implementing this analysis in a ground-up approach to design and its cross-pollinating effects offers many potential outputs for these fields. It involves the kind of dialogue and collaboration considered essential for a consideration of 'virtue ethics' and how technologies can help in the pursuit of the 'good life' (Spiekermann, 2015; Ess, 2015).

EARLY DESIGN EVALUATION

User studies and participatory design are well established in HCI and digital media design, in order to identify and cater for user needs (Muller, 2010). Such design sessions are particularly important in a mental health context, given the motivations and personal nature of technology use for such applications. Feedback and evaluation studies are integral to the early stage of any design process and are essential in HCI, particularly in designing for specific groups and contexts of use. Early stage non-clinical evaluation design sessions involving experts, who can contribute feedback on context, practice and outcomes is particularly recommended for designing mobile technologies for mental health (Doherty et al., 2010).

Sharing responsibility and ideas during the process of design is considered to lead to more positive outcomes (Siegel & Beck, 2014). Including the participation of target users with health challenges in the design of their own interactive technologies can result in 'creative and important contributions to the design process' (van der Velden & Machiak, 2016). Thus, design feedback sessions form a key aspect of the design process for an app focused on psychological wellbeing in pregnancy and to the optimal support of the psychological needs of pregnant women.

We held a number of design sessions with a variety of expert groups including healthcare professionals, in different places of work including maternity services. Locating the design sessions in a real world context at an early stage, allowed for contributions anchored within the daily working routine. Mutual recognition of the everyday real world requirements of both researchers and participants is important for an informed design process. It allows for an approach that values 'ground up' knowledge or 'phronesis', based on everyday experiences and produces practical wisdom for particular applications (Ess, 2013; Eubanks, 2012). It also allows values to arise as local phenomena that are 'discovered' through design, as part of a continuing process of what it means to be value-sensitive in design (Le Dantec et al., 2009)

In total, 21 participants took part in five design sessions, both male and female and ranging in age from c.25 – 55, each with various levels of experience with pregnant women through practice and research. Each design session was recorded and transcribed and the data then anonymised and subjected to a thematic analysis. During the sessions, the researchers sought to elicit feedback on app design and functionality but also to facilitate informal conversation between the participants on general issues around psychological wellbeing in pregnancy, where insights might emerge. Participants assessed prototype screen designs offering feedback on potential content, functionality, design etc. but were asked no structured or leading questions. The following sections outline some preliminary insights on the feedback we received on app design, combined with observations and subsequent discussion from the research team. We do not present findings as such, but offer themes arising from discussion which we suggest are relevant to an ethical design approach, to be subjected to further analysis as the project continues.

ETHICAL AND CULTURAL ISSUES IN THE DESIGN DISCOURSE

A number of ethically relevant cultural issues were observed before and during the discussions that are pertinent to the interpretation, communication and understanding of feedback and discussion of the app design and content. These are of course relevant to technology design generally, yet may not always be acknowledged as such.

Gender

Considering the target user group for mental health in pregnancy and the particular context of experience, gender is highly relevant to design. The core researchers are male (including authors of this paper), while another project advisor (also author) is female with experience of pregnancy and childbirth. Participants in one feedback session were all female but other sessions with relevant clinicians involved male psychology and perinatal health researchers. We all bring different professional and life experiences as well as gendered perspectives and assumptions to the design process which must be acknowledged and addressed as early as possible.

Geography

The researchers are based in different geographic locations with different structures around delivery of mental health services. This may have somewhat political implications for expectations around the provision of physical and psychological perinatal services and how new technology might be adopted, used and received.

Ethnic Background

The design sessions involved participants from many different cultural backgrounds, which enrich the project enormously, and are particularly represented in feedback on concerns about specific cultural groups.

Interdisciplinary Interests

The researchers represent HCI, computer science, medical science, psychology and media and communications fields, each with different interests, foci, methodologies and theoretical frameworks as well as differing approaches to ethical and value considerations.

Values

HCI studies recognises that values have a deep impact on shaping technological design as well as its adoption and use (Shilton, 2012, Friedman & Nissenbaum, 1993). Studies are frequently concerned with whose values are guiding design and how these become embedded through design and development processes, prompting moves towards 'value sensitive design' approaches (Friedman, 1996, Shilton & Anderson, 2016). We take an ethical pluralism perspective (Ess, 2013), where the background of each researcher and participant and their individual values should be interpreted with regard to design. In addition, there is a commitment to noting that the target user group is highly heterogeneous i.e. all pregnant women are not the same. This follows the acknowledgement in HCI research that user studies are too often constructed as abstract ideal or 'intensional' users (Bardzell, 2009) rather than actual users whose responses to digital technologies and interactivity are individualised and inherently strategic (Barry & Doherty, 2016). Therefore each aspect of design is interrogated in the context of establishing the origin of value statements and the possibility of competing values.

Each of these attributes – and more that no doubt arise as such projects progress – represents the different circles of cultural influence from the personal to the institutional for participants and researchers, of which we must remain aware. Each has implications for a full consideration of ethical reflections in design and is included here for the purposes of disclosure as we focus on preliminary themes in feedback.

FEEDBACK

Language is only part of a detailed design process that involves every element of text, graphics, colour, imagery, sound and other multimedia content on screen, even before we arrive at how its interactivity might operate or the feedback from relevant participants. There are many opportunities to interrogate and reflect on decisions made and rationales given. The following outlines a brief selection of responses from the participants on general and specific aspects of design, to illustrate how such feedback provokes reflection. These are not findings per se, but selected contributions that illustrate issues for consideration in design.

Subjective and Objective Forms of Communication

P1: "I'd like to see it compared though…with…human contact... in exactly the same way, that would be really good…"
P2: "Well that's very subjective isn't it whereas this is more… objective…"

This exchange honestly reveals an aspect of the face-to-face form of conversation around mental wellbeing that occurs with any individual, where a 'subjective' judgment is formed on the part of the clinician. That an app might offer more 'objective' forms of information (in their words) opens up a discussion among the participants around how such an app could empower those experiencing mental health problems by allowing them more control over own self-knowledge and possibly offer alternative outcomes for judgment or what is done with such information. However, an individual may also form her own subjective judgment of her wellbeing based on her interaction with the app. Trust in our own subjectivity is of course directly relevant to our psychological wellbeing. This issue provoked an internal discussion for example around language within app design because depending on whether we use the first person or second person 'voice' in onscreen information, we shape how the someone communicates with and therefore internalises her relationship with the app and with herself.

"What's Not Said"

I'm going to be really honest with you, I really have a problem with the [points to app] interface rather than face to face when you're talking about…um…sensitive... um… subjects like mental health, because it's all about body language and what's not said?

We usually think of communication as an active thing, something that is done. In researching communications, we focus on the spoken, written, digital actions and interactions, what is done to send/receive messages, the meanings that are imparted and so on. We use technologies to actively, even interactively mediate these communications. But there is still much that is left out in communication. Can digital technology mediate and communicate that which is not said?

This participant has valid concerns that technology is a poor replacement for the multisensory signals picked up in an interview about emotional wellbeing, which often lead to a diagnosis. However, this provokes further questions around whether we can actively use technology to consider more deeply the kind of deliberate withholding of communications, often subconsciously or unconsciously done. In relation to psychological wellbeing, this can be manifested in the many subtle ways we learn to cope with presenting our 'front stage' face and disguise what is happening backstage (Goffman, 1963). For some more than others, this coping mechanism is a continuous daily effort and challenge, yet it is precisely the kind of information that clinicians and psychologists need in order to understand, to explore with individuals, to intervene if necessary and to help improve their psychological wellbeing.

Can digital technology somehow be used for our benefit in recording forms of non-communication? Despite the concerns expressed above, by providing a channel for a pregnant woman to talk to herself in private, such an app may be able to form part of the backstage 'cast' that helps to mediate what is or is not said. Other participants later acknowledge that this aspect may indeed appeal particularly to some younger women who they cannot engage with through existing mental health services communication channels.

Cultural Sensitivity

P1: You're going to get many of the same kind of women...motivated articulate intelligent interested in their own well being... and the ones that we really want to target...probably don't have... access to... and you think... of our Asian population...their mobile phones...actually their husbands have the phones

The participants expressed valid concerns about the demographics where assumptions might be made around ownership of smart phones, personal access to apps and purchasing power as well as privacy and autonomy over communications. It must be emphasised that the participant group themselves represented a variety of ethnic groups, including those under discussion, and so these comments could be seen to reflect both professional and personal community knowledge. This illustrates the value of eliciting feedback from those operating closely with a target community who can identify assumptions and vulnerabilities in design. While such an app may not immediately provide a solution for this issue, it might assist in driving discussion around the wider context of how we design technologies and how they might be accessible for more challenged communities in the context of healthcare delivery.

A Tool for Good

If it's a tool to elicit their true feelings, then that's only going to be good isn't it?

A major concern for healthcare professionals is getting people to admit to their 'true' feelings on emotional wellbeing, in whatever form they communicate. Clearly, an app such as this cannot assess 'truth' in communication (although arguably neither can a clinician in a face to face encounter). However, an app might facilitate communication where none was previously forthcoming. Mental health struggles are still highly stigmatised in the general community but even more so among pregnant women, who have real fears that by admitting to experiencing difficulties their child might be taken from them, a point made repeatedly by participants. An app could provide crucial access again particularly to younger people whose smartphones are an essential communication tool and to the many for whom admitting struggles with emotional wellbeing is still taboo. This illustrates how digital technologies can quite simply operate as a tool to mediate what is not said or what cannot be said to another human being in another context.

The Language of App Structures

There are striking elements to the language used in design discourse, influenced by the diverse cultural inputs along the lines outlined earlier. Apps for psychological wellbeing require care in the language and terminology used, a concern expressed also in non-digital communications[2]. Even app names can provoke detailed discussion. Ultimately however, app development is constricted by the names 'available' on app stores and as domain names for an accompanying web site. Although unique display names are not required, the technological superstructure – in this case Apple developer or Google Play developer stores – still somewhat dictates the language we use in their design. For example, app stores require the set up of a 'merchant' account so that publishers are instantly commercialised, even though these apps may ultimately be for the benefit of public health. Apps are produced in an international context for a potentially international audience, albeit with options for 'localisation', within guidelines produced by Apple and Google. Their language around design could be said to be culturally homogenising which may have an impact on our ability to build in an ethical and culturally sensitive approach to design from the beginning.

This raises questions for research about whether we can envisage a space where mobile digital applications are made available outside this industry-defined structure. Can we think outside the rounded-bevelled-cornered-logo-box that apps are presented in onscreen, and imagine different ways to engage with such apps that can promote wellbeing? Could we see a new kind of public 'app-casting' space that facilitates digital apps with a perceived inherent, even ethical 'good'? This may offer a way for technology to assist in the 'moral upskilling' of individuals (Vallor, 2014), or at least one way to more fully realise it.

CONCLUSION

This project looks at how everyday media technologies can have an effect on wellbeing by specifically targeting a group with health vulnerabilities. Vulnerability is one area where the difference between human and machine offers a space to design technology to positively intervene and assist. By focusing on known human vulnerabilities and conditions that impact on our ability to flourish offline, perhaps we can begin to envisage how technology can help, not by replacing other forms of communication or conversation but adding to the information gain, by providing for 'what is not said' online.

By facilitating different types of self-reporting via apps for psychological wellbeing over an extended period of time, and by offering access to reports and results individually and collectively, each person can have access to longitudinal information on their own wellbeing. On an individual level, this has empowering potential in relation to self-knowledge and personal autonomy with respect to this information being used in any subsequent intervention, diagnosis or treatment. On a wider social level however, the collective use of such apps could have empowering effects (building on previous studies) in providing a sense of community, which may have a role to play in de-stigmatising general and perinatal mental health issues.

If we are increasingly 'relational selves' (Ess, 2014; Broadbent et al., 2013) then we need to ask what aspects of this include our ability to hide or avoid certain types of relationality, or to cultivate one that recognises and respects what Goffman (1963) would call the gap between virtual social identity and actual social identity where he locates 'stigma'. Further research could examine if such digital technologies could be designed to help break social stigma, or at least to challenge the social and communication structures that allow them to persist. Aspects of human life are stigmatised by those who fear their impact on social cohesion and identity. However, digital interactivity may help produce a form of community around human vulnerabilities that strengthens efforts to de-stigmatise and support them.

We have reported some very preliminary insights from a design process involving a phronetic approach to show how we might go about designing technologies that provide a very internal but profound kind of empowerment that comes with self-knowledge. Vallor (2014) notes that 'self-knowledge' is one of the virtues that social network communications can provide, along with reciprocity, empathy and a shared life. However, in order to perform, never mind flourish in the social network, we must first flourish in our own internal network. In order to perform as a free and relational self, we must be empowered with knowledge of ourselves – which includes the ability to communicate 'what is not said' by ourselves, to ourselves and to others.

REFERENCES

Bardzell, J. (2009). Interaction Criticism and Aesthetics, *CHI Proceedings of the ACM* 2009

Barry, M. (2014). Please do touch: Discourses on aesthetic interactivity in the exhibition space. *Participations Journal of Audience & Reception Studies, 11*(1). Retrieved from http://www.participations.org/Volume 11/Issue 1/13.pdf

Barry, M., & Doherty, G. (2016). What we talk about when we talk about interactivity: Empowerment in public discourse. *New Media & Society*. doi:10.1177/1461444815625944

Bauer, A., Parsonage, M., Knapp, M., Iemmi, V., & Adelaja, B. (2014). *The cost of perinatal mental health problems*. London: Centre for Mental Health, London School of Economics.

Broadbent. (2014) *The Onlife Manifesto: Being Human in a Hyperconnected Era, European Commission*. Retrieved from https://ec.europa.eu/digital-single-market/en/onlife-manifesto

D'Ignazio, C., Hope, A., Michelson, B., Churchill, R., & Zuckerman, E. (2016). A Feminist HCI Approach to Designing Postpartum Technologies: "When I first saw a breast pump I was wondering if it was a joke. *Proceedings of CHI '16*. ACM 10.1145/2858036.2858460

De Choudhury, M., Counts, S., & Horvitz, E. (2013). Predicting Postpartum changes in emotion and behavior via social media. *Proceedings of CHI 2013*. ACM 10.1145/2470654.2466447

Doherty, G., Coyle, D., & Matthews, M. (2010). Design and evaluation guidelines for mental health technologies. *Interacting with Computers*, *22*(4), 243–252. doi:10.1016/j.intcom.2010.02.006

Doherty, G., McKnight, J., & Luz, S. (2010). Fieldwork for requirements: Frameworks for mobile healthcare applications. *International Journal of Human-Computer Studies*, *68*(10), 760–776. doi:10.1016/j.ijhcs.2010.06.005

Ess, C. (2013). *Digital Media Ethics* (2nd ed.). Cambridge: Polity.

Ess, C. (2015) The Good Life: Selfhood and virtue ethics in the digital age. In H. Wang (Ed.), *Communication and "The Good Life." Proceedings of the International Communication Association (ICA) Annual Conference Theme Book.* Peter Lang Publishing Group

Eubanks, V. (2012). Feminist Phronesis and Technologies of Citizenship. In B. Flyvbjerg, T. Landsman, & S. Schram (Eds.), *Real Social Science: Applied Phronesis.* New York: Cambridge University Press. doi:10.1017/CBO9780511719912.013

Friedman, B. (1996). Value Sensitive Design. *interactions,* December 1996

Friedman, B., & Nissenbaum, H. (1993) User autonomy: Who should control what and when? *Proceedings of CHI '96* (p. 433). ACM.

Goffman, E. (1981). *Forms of Talk.* Philadelphia: University of Pennsylvania Press.

Kahneman, D., Riis, J., (2005) Living, and thinking about it: Two perspectives on life. In *The science of well-being* (pp. 285-304).

Ko, J. Y., Farr, S. L., Dietz, P. M., & Robbins, C. L. (2012). Depression and Treatment Among U.S. Pregnant and Nonpregnant Women of Reproductive Age, 2005 – 2009. *Journal of Womens Health, 21*(8), 830–836. doi:10.1089/jwh.2011.3466 PMID:22691031

Le Dantec, C. A., Poole, E. S., & Wyche, S. P. (2009) Values as lived experience: evolving value sensitive design in support of value discovery. *Proceedings of CHI '09* (pp. 1141–1150). 10.1145/1518701.1518875

Muller, M. J. (2003). Participatory design: the third space in HCI. In *Human-computer interaction: Development process.*

Shilton, K. (2012). Values levers: Building ethics into design. *Science, Technology & Human Values, 38*(3), 374–397. doi:10.1177/0162243912436985

Shilton, K., & Anderson, S. (2016). Blended not Bossy: Ethics, roles, responsibilities and expertise in design. *Interacting with Computers, 2016.* doi:10.1093/iwc/iww002

Siegel, M. A., & Beck, J. (2014). Slow change interaction design. *Interaction, 21*(1), 28–35. doi:10.1145/2542649

Spiekermann, S. (2015). *Ethical IT innovation: A Value-Based System Design Approach.* Taylor & Francis. doi:10.1201/b19060

Vallor, S. (2014). Moral Deskilling and Upskilling in a New Machine Age: Reflections on the Ambiguous Future of Character. *Philosophy and Technology, 28*(1), 107–124. doi:10.100713347-014-0156-9

Van der Velden, M., & Machiak, M. (2016). Moodline and MoodMap: Designing a mood function for a mobile application with and for young patients. *Proceedings of eTELEMED 2016: Conference on eHealth, Telemedicine, and Social Medicine.*

Walsh, S., Golden, E., & Priebe, S. (2015). Systematic review of patients' participation in and experiences of technology-based monitoring of mental health symptoms in the community. *British Medical Journal.*

World Health Organization. (2011). mHealth: New horizons for health through mobile technologies, Geneva, Switzerland.

World Health Organization. (2013). Investing in Mental Health: Evidence for Action, Geneva, Switzerland.

ENDNOTES

1. http://chi2016.acm.org/wp/
2. See 'Terminology' at https://www.bestbeginnings.org.uk/helping-parents-with-mental-health-issues

This research was previously published in the International Journal of Sociotechnology and Knowledge Development (IJSKD), 8(3); edited by Lincoln Christopher Wood and Brian J. Galli; pages 46-55, copyright year 2016 by IGI Publishing (an imprint of IGI Global).

Chapter 16
User Experiences and Perceptions of Internet Interventions for Depression

Filip Drozd
National Network for Infant Mental Health, Norway

Silje Marie Haga
National Network of Infant Mental Health, Norway

Caroline Emilie Andersen
University of Oslo, Norway

Kari Slinning
National Network for Infant Mental Health, Norway

Cato Alexander Bjørkli
University of Oslo, Norway

ABSTRACT

The purpose of this chapter is to review qualitative research on user experiences with internet interventions for depression and present original results from in-depth interviews from a preventive unguided intervention for postpartum depression. The first part reviews the literature on qualitative studies of client experiences and perceptions of internet interventions for depression. The next part describes original data from a study investigating participants' experiences using semi-structured interviews, following the modified SWOT-format (i.e., strengths, weakness, opportunities, and threats). In total, 10 pregnant and postpartum women aged 28 to 41 were interviewed. Insights from the current review and study are used as a point of departure for discussing future directions in research on internet interventions for depression. This chapter should be valuable for clinicians, researchers, and other health professionals interested in the applicability of internet interventions for their clients, design of future studies, and development of internet interventions.

DOI: 10.4018/978-1-7998-2351-3.ch016

INTRODUCTION

Depression is one of the leading causes of years lost due to disability and shortened life expectancy, affecting about 350 million people worldwide every year (Marcus, Yasamy, van Ommeren, Chisholm, & Saxena, 2012; World Health Organization, 2009). The estimated lifetime prevalence rate is about 20% with about 10% affected by depression each year (Mykletun, Knudsen, & Mathiesen, 2009). However, less than half (in some countries, fewer than 10%) have access to or seek professional help (World Health Organization, 2010). Internet interventions are suggested as a supplement to primary and secondary care to help overcome barriers to help-seeking associated with depression such as stigma, reluctance for emotional disclosure, undertreatment, and lack of trained providers and resources (Dennis & Chung-Lee, 2006; Goodman, 2009; Overland, Glozier, Krokstad, & Mykletun, 2007). Systematic reviews show that both unguided and therapist-supported internet interventions can be of benefit for people with depression (Cuijpers et al., 2011; Cuijpers, Donker, van Straten, Li, & Andersson, 2010). Such findings have contributed to the inclusion of guided internet-based cognitive behavior therapy (iCBT) in several national guidelines for treatment of mild-to-moderate depression (e.g., Australian Psychological Society, 2011; Norwegian Directorate of Health, 2009; The National Board of Health and Wellfare, 2010).

Despite promising studies of efficacy and the inclusion of iCBT in national guidelines, few studies have asked end-users to reflect on their experiences of internet interventions. Such reflections can provide a deeper and richer understanding of the uptake and use of internet interventions, the therapeutic processes, and generate hypotheses for future research. They can provide us with complementary knowledge to the many randomized trials and inform us about (1) why some users adhere to internet interventions and others do not, (2) how users change by using internet interventions (i.e., the therapeutic process), and (3) help to determine what internet interventions may be appropriate for whom. In addition, it would not be safe to assume that user experiences in face-to-face psychotherapy can be generalized to automated or computer-mediated protocols delivered over the internet. Therefore, this chapter starts by reviewing the literature on qualitative studies on user experiences and perceptions that can either facilitate or impede adherence to internet interventions, how internet interventions can instigate important therapeutic processes, and which interventions may be appropriate for whom. Finally, we present findings from a qualitative study on women's experiences from an unguided intervention designed to prevent postpartum depression.

LITERATURE REVIEW

A recent meta-synthesis of user experiences of computer-based interventions identified two overarching themes (Knowles et al., 2014); (1) First, interventions need to be more personalized and sensitive to the individual users' needs, so that users can identify with the program and relate the program content to themselves and their daily lives (e.g., use of role models, examples, and homework assignments). Second, the level of support and guidance, either by a professional or lay person, is experienced as contradictory. For some, support may help identify different clinical needs and relate program content to the user's situation, and recognize and acknowledge personal emotional and motivational difficulties. For others, support may be experienced negatively (e.g., perceptions of high demands or expectations from the therapist). The authors also concluded that these findings may not generalize to other user groups (e.g., ethnic minorities, elderly or pregnant women) and approaches other than cognitive behavior therapy (CBT). In addition, this synthesis included mixed qualitative studies on anxiety and depression, and 7 out of 8 included studies were desktop-based CBT interventions. Thus, it is necessary to examine experiences among other user groups, include different therapeutic approaches, and examine user experiences that are specifically related to internet interventions for depression.

Adherence

Accessibility, convenience, flexibility, and anonymity and privacy, are some of the major advantages of internet interventions for depression (e.g., completing the program at home and around family obligations, and reducing stigma), and important for uptake and adherence (Beattie, Shaw, Kaur, & Kessler, 2009; O'Mahen et al., 2015; Pugh, Hadjistavropoulos, Hampton, Bowen, & Williams, 2015). Those who persist with interventions for depression report intrinsic motivation such as valuing task completion, a sense of empowerment and control, and recognize the need for external motivators to aid the development of habits for program use (Donkin & Glozier, 2012; Wilhelmsen et al., 2013). They are proactive users of the programs and are able to identify with and relate the program content to their daily lives (Bendelin et al., 2011; Gerhards et al., 2011). Highly motivated users also take more time and words to describe their problems in the program and, hence, are better able to utilize the program and may expect greater improvements (Van Der Zanden et al., 2014). They attribute personal benefits to the program and usually go on to complete treatment as planned (Donkin & Glozier, 2012; Svartvatten, Segerlund, Dennhag, Andersson, & Carlbring, 2015). However, finding program content personally relevant is key for users to learn and acquire new knowledge and skills, but not all users succeed in translating program contents and adaptations to real life (e.g., Lillevoll et al., 2013).

According to a review that examined adherence to guided iCBT and individual face-to-face CBT, adherence to iCBT and CBT may be equal (van Ballegooijen et al., 2014), although the researchers did not take into account that in-person CBT usually consists of more sessions than guided iCBT (12–28 vs. 5–9 sessions). Thus, therapist-support may help balancing the need for privacy, independence, and active engagement, and the need for assistance, dependence, and help to restructure the newly acquired knowledge to user's problems, thereby ensuring adherence (Wilhelmsen et al., 2013). In a study by Lillevoll and colleagues (2013), users emphasized the importance of dialogue with a professional to ask questions, discuss issues with someone, receive trustworthy feedback, be supported and acknowledged. A lack of support or "check-ins" with a therapist (or lay person) may lead users to consider that how they engage with the program is irrelevant and decrease their motivation to use the program as prescribed or completing it (e.g., using filler-words such as "blah, blah, blah …" instead of completing a written assignment in a meaningful way; Donkin & Glozier, 2012; Gerhards et al., 2011). It reduces any obligations to log on to the program, feelings of commitment, and sense of accountability. At the same time, users have reported being stressed by high expectations and demands from the therapist (Bendelin et al., 2011). In addition, guided self-help may also generate concerns such as loss of anonymity, feeling of being more exposed, and becoming a more passive recipient of treatment. Overall, internet interventions may solve issues with accessibility, reduce stigma, provide users with a sense of control for taking action and seeking help, but it also introduces new issues. On the one hand, the free nature of unguided self-help programs may attract users and make them engage in help-seeking behaviors, but also cause users to place less value on completing it (i.e., that it was without costs, time restrictions, therapist guidance, etc.). On the other hand, a sense of obligation to others, can make some users more reluctant to seek internet interventions, but be important for those who engage and who, for example, have doubts about internet interventions or experience delayed perceptions of their usefulness.

The Change Process

There are concerns about users withholding and not disclosing personal and relevant information that may be important for a therapist, and users have reported that the mode of communication has limited their ability to meaningfully convey their feelings or the therapists' ability to fully understand their problem (Beattie et al., 2009). However, most users establish a good therapeutic relationship with their therapist rather quickly, which enables them to commit and be honest, and perhaps even more so by the idea of "anonymity" online (Andersson et al., 2012; Beattie et al., 2009). Since online communication with the therapist is mostly text-based, it also enables users to see and review their responses on the screen, reflect and let things sink in, and gives them time and opportunity to formulate their thoughts. These reflective processes are likely to occur with unguided interventions as well. However, the most interesting in the absence of therapist-support, is that users may anthropomorphize the system such as describing a fully automated intervention as a social agent they “didn’t want to disappoint” (Farzanfar, Frishkopf, Friedman, & Ludena, 2007). Such findings are in line with the seminal work by Reeves and Nass (1996), Bickmore and Gruber (2010), and others who have demonstrated that it is possible to design systems that can build a sense of trust, rapport, and convey empathy, without therapist-support. However, fully automated responses and interventions may more easily come about as insensitive and be perceived more negatively (Gega, Smith, & Reynolds, 2013).

Case studies illustrate how therapists may work to instill hope, raise awareness, reinforce adherence, and build a therapeutic relationship, by offering support and an understanding of a user’s needs, thoughts, and feelings. For example, Pugh, Hadjistavropoulos, and Fuchs (2014) described a program module focused on activity planning and, although the user was successful in scheduling and carrying out activities, how the therapist was able to address her needs and worries unrelated to activity planning, but to so-called “first experiences” with a newborn baby (e.g., the baby having her first cough or cold). At the present, no fully automated systems can follow the ebbs and flows, and adapt to the user’s needs such as a human in this case. In another case study, Pugh, Hadjistavropoulos, Klein, and Austin (2014) demonstrated how a therapist assisted a depressed male, in reinforcing adherence and applying his newly acquired knowledge and skills. The user opened up regarding his difficulties with relaxation when feeling down. The therapist provided words of encouragement (e.g., “nice to hear that you tried the relaxation exercises despite feeling low”), normalized his feelings (e.g., “many find it difficult to practice relaxation techniques at first”), and assisted with considering an action plan for his down days (e.g., “It will be your go-to plan when you are feeling unmotivated. Do you have any ideas what this plan might look like?”).

As a result of internet interventions, users may also start to question the validity of their own thoughts, avoid categorical thinking, reality-check their depressive ideas, and engage in more flexible thinking (e.g., exploring alternative interpretations; Lillevoll et al., 2013). Such changes may, in turn, instigate behavioral changes and break cycles of inactivity (e.g., starting to play with kids or going to a dinner party). It is also interesting how language use may be an indicator or marker of treatment progress. In one study, researchers found that improvements in depression was predicted by use of more discrepancy words during treatment (e.g., “should”, “wish” or “hope”; Van Der Zanden et al., 2014). Discrepancy words may be a linguistic marker for future aspirations and not merely shortcomings in the past or present.

In another study, Svartvatten and colleagues (2015) identified how the content in e-mail exchanges between therapists and users can serve as an indication of treatment progress. More specifically, they found that user statements related to "observing positive consequences" (e.g., "When I went for a walk when feeling down, I noticed how it put me in a better mood") and "alliance" (e.g., "Thank you for your ideas. I think this exercise might prove be useful to me") were positively related to changes in depressive symptoms. Thus, there are issues that may be more specific to internet interventions such as worries about being misunderstood or avoidance of difficult therapeutic tasks in the absence of anyone to "check in" on the user (Gega et al., 2013). However, it appears that the ingredients in the therapeutic processes such as alliance, regardless of whether the intervention is designed with or without therapist-support, are similar to traditional psychotherapy.

Adverse Effects

Barak and colleagues (2009, p. 5) define the purpose of internet interventions as "*... to create a positive change and/or improve/enhance knowledge, awareness, and understanding via the provision of sound health-related material and use of interactive web-based components*". Most will agree with the purpose to create a positive change, but it is also important not to forget that there may be negative changes as a consequence of using internet interventions. However, only one study has explicitly examined the side-effects of internet interventions (Rozental, Boettcher, Andersson, Schmidt, & Carlbring, 2015). As with face-to-face therapy, the researchers found that increased awareness and insight into the user's own problems occasionally lead to, at least, a temporary deterioration. Learning about their condition may cause users to pay more attention to negative events, feeling vulnerable, anxious or regretful, noticing new problems, facing problems that were previously avoided, or increase subjective health complaints (e.g., headaches or muscle tensions). Another side-effect was the exhausting program schedule (Rozental et al., 2015). Given that most internet interventions follow a regular schedule, some felt pressured by tight time schedules and lack of flexibility, particularly by having to complete many tasks during a short time interval, and eventually falling behind schedule and becoming frustrated. Life events, positive or negative, may also interfere with users' experiences and ability to adhere to internet interventions. In a study by O'Mahen and colleagues (2015), postpartum women reported that the demands of motherhood directly interfered with their ability to complete the program. This, in turn, increased their feelings of hopelessness which is characteristic of depression. Some women also felt overwhelmed by the program and found the flexibility and minimal support difficult to manage. In such a case, it is important that the failure to use and benefit from an internet intervention, does not add to the burden of being depressed and nourish feelings of hopelessness.

For Whom

Most studies have been concerned with experiences related to adherence and the change process as reviewed above. Based on this, it is clear that internet interventions may be appropriate for intrinsically motivated users (e.g., desire to learn more about themselves) and users who have perceptions of benefit (e.g., their general physician recommending a program that may be helpful). However, only one study has looked directly into who benefits from internet interventions for depression. Bendelin and colleagues (2011) identified three types of users; (a) readers, (b) strivers, and (c) doers. Readers were typically characterized as not able or willing to put their new insight into practice and working sporadically through the materials. The autonomy of working through the guided intervention proved to be an obstacle for adherence, and they wished for more help and support. Strivers worked with the program in a practical way and succeeded to integrate some of the program contents into everyday life. However, they also expressed ambivalence towards working on their own, had doubts about treatment effects, and were not able to fully profit from treatment. They wished for more contact with their therapist to overcome barriers during treatment, but, at the same time, felt stressed by the demands from the therapist. Doers applied the program to their daily experiences and real-life events, in structured and methodic manner. This systematic and practice-oriented approach seemed to help overcome many barriers, and was often described as the most valuable lessons. They also appreciated working on their own and the responsibility that came with the program. More research is, however, needed to investigate who these readers, strivers, and doers are, and whether these represent different groups of users for whom internet interventions may be appropriate (or not) and that can be reliably identified, or whether experiences can vary within users (Knowles et al., 2014).

MAIN PURPOSE OF THIS STUDY

The literature review shows that unguided and guided internet and computer-based interventions are experienced and perceived both positively and negatively in terms of adherence, the change process, and for whom such interventions may be appropriate. It also shows that more qualitative research is needed for preventive interventions and interventions using therapeutic approaches other than CBT, as most of the qualitative studies have been conducted on CBT programs for users with sub-clinical depression (e.g., Pugh et al., 2015; Svartvatten et al., 2015; Van Der Zanden et al., 2014; Wilhelmsen et al., 2013). The main objective for this study was, therefore, to gain insight into users' experiences of an internet intervention for perinatal depression by acquiring knowledge and an understanding of how the program is perceived among pregnant and postpartum women. The study was set up investigate positive and negative factors that could affect adherence to the program, and identify opportunities for further development and risks that need to be addressed. More generally, this study can contribute to the strategic planning and development of the current and future interventions.

METHODS

Study Design and Participants

This study used semi-structured interviews by following the strengths, weaknesses, opportunities, and threats (SWOT) format and surveying participant characteristics. Participants were recruited through a randomized controlled trial (RCT), after being randomly assigned to receive the internet intervention. All participants were enrolled for the study, the intervention, and invited for an interview, consecutively. Inclusion criteria for being invited for interview were either: (a) completing the intervention or (b) no program activity during the last 4 weeks or (c) lagging 3 or more sessions behind prescribed intervention schedule. The criteria for participation in the study was being 18 years or older, and being pregnant between gestation week 21 and 25. There were 10 participants partaking in the study, all females, who were either pregnant or had given birth at the time of the interview.

Measures

Demographic information such as age, due date, number of children, education, occupation and relationship status, and native country, was collected at baseline. In addition, participants completed the following measures:

The *Edinburgh Postnatal Depression Scale* (EPDS; Cox, Holden, & Sagovsky, 1987) which is a 10-item self-report scale that is used to assess depressive symptoms in the past 7 days among mothers, during pregnancy and after childbirth (e.g., "*I have been so unhappy that I have had difficulty sleeping*"). Items are scored on a scale from 0 to 3 and yield a total score from 0 to 30 with higher scores indicating more depressive symptomatology. A score of 10 or greater indicates a possible depression.

The *Satisfaction with Life Scale* (SWLS; Diener, Emmons, Larsen, & Griffin, 1985) is a 5-item self-report scale designed to assess people's overall cognitive judgment of their life. Participants rate items such as "*My life is in many ways close to my ideal*", on a scale from 1 ("*completely disagree*") to 7 ("*completely agree*"). Total scores range from 5 to 25 with higher scores indicating greater life satisfaction.

The *Positive and Negative Affect Schedule* (PANAS; Watson, Clark, & Tellegen, 1988) consists of two 10-item self-report scales that measure positive (e.g., "*alert*" and "*enthusiastic*") and negative (e.g., "*anger*" and "*nervousness*") dimensions of affect. Participants indicated to what extent they had felt this way during the past 7 days on a scale from 1 ("*Not at all*") to 5 ("*Very much*").

Interviews

In the present study, semi-structured interviews were conducted based on the open-ended Strengths, Weaknesses, Opportunities, and Threats (SWOT) format. The open-ended format encourages participants' free reflections on the use of the intervention, with minimal interruptions from the interviewer. It does, however, provide a certain structure to participant's reflections without specifying a particular type of answers (Lone et al., 2013). Each of the participants were asked the following four questions:

Please tell me about what you perceive as the advantages of and that seems to work well with Mamma Mia; we refer to this as the strengths of the program.

Please tell me about what you perceive as the disadvantages of and that does not seem to work well with Mamma Mia; we refer to this as the weaknesses of the program.

Please tell me about what you consider to be the possibilities of improving the quality of Mamma Mia; we refer to this as the opportunities of the program.

Please tell me about what you consider to be the obstacles to Mamma Mia; we refer to this as the threats to the program.

The first part of the interview consisted mainly of allowing participant to speak freely about the different SWOTs (i.e., open-ended part). This ensures that the interviewer influences the participant's answers or drives the conversation in a certain direction, only to a minimal degree. This open-ended structure generally results in a wider range of information retrieved. In the second part (i.e., explorative part), the interviewer used probing questions to obtain additional information and richer descriptions of the SWOTs identified in the open-ended part of the interview such as "Could you please provide an example of [...]", "What do you mean by [...]?", or "Do I understand you correctly when you say that [...]". Based on the answers given in part one, the interviewer systematically worked through the various SWOTs, as identified by the participant, to clarify specific issues. Two interviewers conducted the interviews separately. Interviews were conducted during the period of March to September in 2014. Five of the interviews were carried out at the Regional Center for Child and Adolescent Mental Health (RBUP), Eastern and Southern Norway, two at home visits, and three by telephone. The length of the interviews ranged between 30 minutes to 77 minutes (*mean* = 53.0 minutes). All interviews were recorded and transcribed electronically.

Mamma Mia

In this study, Mamma Mia was deployed as an unguided, universal intervention designed to (1) prevent the onset and development of perinatal depression and (2) enhance subjective well-being, among pregnant and postpartum women. The intervention consists of 44 sessions over a period of 11 ½ months, starting in pregnancy between gestational week 17 to 24, and lasts into the postpartum period, 6 months after childbirth. Mamma Mia is available on both PC/Mac, tablets, and mobile phones. The woman receives an e-mail with a unique hyperlink for every new session that becomes available. By clicking the hyperlink, she is directed to the unique program contents for that particular session. The core organizing principles for the delivery of the program and its contents is the tunneled design. This means that each session, which is designed to take 10 to 15 minutes, must be completed before proceeding to the next session. In a similar way, the program content is presented in a predetermined sequence on a page-by-page basis. There are 5 main components in the Mamma Mia program; (1) monitoring and identification of depressive symptoms by means of the EPDS, (2) help and support for managing depressive symptoms (e.g., ask for partner support), (3) mother's mental health and well-being (e.g., adopting a relaxing mindset), (4) partner relationship (e.g., expressing more positive emotions toward partner), and (5) the child and her development (e.g., demonstrating the infant's socio-emotional competence). These protective and risk factors have previously been identified as important with regard to the development of emotional distress in mothers and children during pregnancy and postpartum. For a comprehensive and systematic description of Mamma Mia, please access the intervention protocol (Drozd, Haga, Brendryen, & Slinning, 2015).

Data Analysis

Descriptives and frequencies were used to describe the sample characteristics. Interviews were transcribed verbatim, anonymized, and unitized into small, but meaningful statements, prior to the main qualitative analysis. A statement was defined as the smallest, meaningful analysis unit that expressed a logic, consistent, and separate point of view, and that can be a part of a sentence, several sentences or other fractions of communication (Hoff, Straumsheim, Bjørkli, & Bjørklund, 2009; Neuendorf, 2002). Data were then analyzed by the use of an inductive thematic analysis (Braun & Clarke, 2006), to identify women's experiences and perceptions of

Mamma Mia. A thematic analysis is a flexible and inductive, data-driven approach, which is particularly compatible with the open-ended SWOT format. The analytic process was iterative, systematically going back to revise codes and themes in a non-linear fashion to improve analysis. In this regard, we employed participative inquiry, in which co-authors that did not take part of the thematic analysis, reviewed and commented on the coding along the way, ensuring reflection and refinement of the codes and coding process (Reason, 1994). Finally, residual statements that could not be coded onto any of the SWOTs were examined to determine whether these units contained any relevant information regarding women's experiences and perceptions of Mamma Mia.

RESULTS

Participants

All participating mothers were expecting one child and were aged from 28 to 41 with a mean age of 33.5 years. Seven women were first-time mothers, one had a child from before, and two women had two children prior to the current pregnancy. The women were highly educated, only one woman had a bachelor's degree, while three had a master's degree and six women had a degree requiring more than five years at a university or college. All of the participants were currently employed, either fulltime or part-time, or currently on maternity leave. Five of the women were married, while the remaining five women were living together with a partner. Seven women were native Norwegian and three were from Sweden, Denmark, and Iceland, respectively. By examining their depressive symptoms and subjective well-being, it was clear that these women had few symptoms of depression (*mean (M)* = 3.5; *standard deviation (SD)* = 2.7), were very much satisfied with their life (*M* = 22.9; *SD* = 1.6), and experienced more positive (*M* = 37.9; *SD* = 6.6) than negative emotions (*M* = 14.4; *SD* = 2.3).

SWOT Categories

Unitizing resulted in 790 statements with a mean of 79 (*SD* = 40) statements per participant. Three-hundred and forty (43.0%) statements were extracted from the open-ended part of the interview, 260 (32.9%) from exploration, and 190 (24.1%) statements were unrelated to women's experiences with Mamma Mia (e.g., reflections on their pregnancy, partner or experiences from perinatal care). Consequently, 600 (75.9%) statements were identified and deemed relevant for analysis. Of these, 531 (88.5%) were coded onto one of the SWOT categories; 208 (34.7%) were coded as strengths, 114 (19.0%) as weaknesses, 170 (28.3%) as opportunities, and 39 (6.5%) as threats, not taking into account that some SWOTs may be counted several times. It is noted that 69 (11.5%) statements were coded as residuals (i.e., statements not captured by the SWOT dimensions). However, there were no emerging themes in the residual category that could add to the women's experiences with Mamma Mia. Thus, data from the residuals are not reported herein.

Key Themes

There were two emerging superordinate themes across each of the SWOT dimensions and that are related to; (1) the design of the program and (2) transition to motherhood. All women consistently emphasized both themes, but the fact that the themes were superordinate and spanned across the SWOTs, suggested that the program design and the way Mamma Mia supports women in their transition to becoming a mother, was a mixture of both positive and negative experiences.

Program Design

Strengths

First of all, women emphasized the accessibility of the program and using the internet as a channel for disseminating information, as one of its' major strengths. Being able to perform the program at home and at their own convenience was considered positive. The program contents and some of the exercises were seen as pleasant and rather easy to carry out, and conveyed in a light tone-of-voice. Especially, the combination of accessibility and pleasant exercises was highlighted.

For most of the time, I've been at home when I've done the exercises. That worked for me. If not, I wouldn't have bothered doing them. They are pleasant exercises. They help you find some peace [...] – Respondent 118

Mamma Mia came across as containing brief, yet quality assured information. It was often compared to other typical online sources of information many women often use during pregnancy and after giving birth. The participants favored Mamma Mia over other such websites and described it as more structured and trustworthy.

We receive so much input from all over, so the more information gathered ... it feels easy to deal with than that other mess. – Respondent 242

It was described as professional and highly credible, without being clinical. The credibility to the program was partly attributable to the fact that some women were recruited to the study at the hospital.

... it's good to have a service that is research-based and scientifically grounded, because if you look online ... on antenatal and postnatal mental health, it is easy to wind up on blogs where there are a lot of expressions of opinion ... Those are not scientifically grounded, you get different answers, or you look for answers that you want, adapted to your situation. – Respondent 226

Weaknesses

The weaknesses related to the program design concerned the depth and relevance of information, and lack of flexibility. The content was, at times, perceived as obvious and lacking in depth, containing information easily retrieved from other sources such as magazines. The lack of depth was especially apparent among multiparous women, who emphasized that the program targeted young, first-time mothers, and was less suitable for multiparous women or women with pregnancy complications.

I feel like it appeals to first-time mothers who are in new relationships. And by young, I mean younger than twenty. I get a teenage-mom feeling, that they recently got together and wonder if they know each other. – Respondent 242

We had a different type of pregnancy than people generally have. There were no questions about that in the Mamma Mia program. Is the baby ill? Or do you know if you are getting a healthy baby? Our situation has been quiet different than those who get healthy babies. – Respondent 346

A lack of flexibility was reported, in general, as a weakness. Some women mentioned the lack of flexibility as not always finding an appropriate answer to the built-in EPDS in the program, or wanting to report the reason why they may, at times, have felt depressed, without being misunderstood or stigmatized.

[...] you had to answer for the last week if you felt overwhelmed. I thought to myself that I feel pretty tired, that's why things feel overwhelming, but in a manageable way. It's not like I'm about to slip into a depression kind of overwhelming. [...] I get why the questions were as generic as they were, but I miss the opportunity to say why I answered as I did. – Respondent 213

This lack of flexibility was also mentioned in relation to subjects that women wanted to learn more about. Some sessions were considered too brief and superficial, with no links or suggestions as to where users could retrieve more information on the subject. This was clearly formulated by one woman who was annoyed by the "one-to-one problem-solution" formula.

There are too many times where only one approach is presented as a solution for a problem, without any alternative options. No possibility to ask for advice or be guided further if you tried something and it didn't work. – Respondent 242

Opportunities

Participants listed a number of opportunities for improvement, most of which were intended to deal with the weaknesses of the program (see above). However, they often made suggestions for new subjects regarding more practical care such as health behavior (e.g., indoor environment for babies), labor rights and workplace facilitation during pregnancy, and necessary safety-equipment. Further, the participants expressed a desire to manage the course of the program themselves, including choosing to go deeper into one subject of interest, or skip one. According to the women, this could also be resolved by adding links to other websites on various subjects, or connecting to a web portal with more information.

Threats

Threats were mostly concerned with the (automated) program schedule in the postpartum period. Due to a peak in depressive symptoms 4 to 6 weeks after birth, the frequency increases to three sessions per week for a period of 6 weeks. At the same time, the demands of motherhood, especially for new mothers, made it difficult to follow the program on a weekly basis postpartum. It felt a bit overwhelming and resulted in lagging behind schedule, which, in turn, was identified as a risk of discontinuing the program.

It's mostly the risk of not following through that I consider to be the biggest threat. Even though I have been healthy and had excess energy during my pregnancy, I thought it was a bit difficult. All of a sudden there were two or three sessions piled up. For instance, if I would struggle mentally, become apathetic, or had become depressed, then I would not have been able to do it. – Respondent 167

Transition to Motherhood

Strengths

Regarding the transition to motherhood, the program seemed comforting and preparing, being something the women looked forward to, and feeling like she was being taken care of and in good hands. Participants reported that the program was normalizing and non-judgmental, and has helped them look at things more positively in their everyday life.

...mental health is being talked about in a very nice and natural manner. I think that is great, that you can be prepared, knowing that many women go into a postpartum depression ... – Respondent 167

It has also reminded me to be present, that's what the audio file [mindfulness exercise] highlights. So getting that reminder has helped me be more present when I walk to work, I notice the nice things around me, like birds and flowers. I am more attentive now. – Respondent 167

The psychoeducational information was also well received. They emphasized themes containing information about the baby as one of the strengths. The information createed awareness and self-reflection, and contained important reminders facilitating attachment and connecting with the baby.

I have a pretty hectic life, and when I sit down with the program, I fully focus on the pregnancy. This is pregnancy number three, so I barely remember what gestational week I'm in. It has just sort of run its course. So, that has been okay. I think it [the program] has made me pay more attention than I would normally. – Respondent 226

Weaknesses and Threats

Mamma Mia was perceived as not sufficiently taking into account the demands of motherhood (e.g., baby's irregular sleeping patterns, loss of energy, caretaking, etc.), which was both perceived as a weakness and a threat to the program. Women did not always have the time to complete the sessions as prescribed according to the program schedule, thus, falling behind and having more to do in the upcoming week. The relevance of information was thus affected by the tunneled design (i.e., having to complete one session before proceeding to the next). This resulted in perceiving the program as a nuisance or stressful. More importantly, by lagging behind, there was a risk of the information becoming irrelevant because it would no longer be aligned with, for example, gestational week during pregnancy or the baby's development after birth, eventually leading to discontinuation of the program.

Opportunities

Women suggested a parallel program dealing with problem-areas concerning difficulties relevant to multiparous women. Some participants also wished that the program facilitated more reflection, particularly self-reflection around subjects such as the partner relationship, transitioning into parenthood, and raising a child.

I think a well-designed program like this can lead to reflection or a conversation between partners. What do I really think, what do I really mean, how do I live my life? [...] Having these thoughts make me self-reflect. Or that my partner and me can clarify certain standpoints. I think a program like this should manage that. – Respondent 242

Including partner and significant others in what the mother is going through emotionally was also suggested, especially help to distinguish between postpartum blues and postpartum depression.

DISCUSSION

The purpose of this chapter was to review user experiences with internet and computer-based interventions for depression and add to this literature by presenting results from in-depth interviews of women's experiences from a preventive, unguided intervention for postpartum depression, and thereby identify factors that could potentially affect adherence and improve the quality of the program. There were two emerging, superordinate themes that spanned across the SWOTs; (1) program design and (2) transition to motherhood. Superordinate themes across SWOTs indicates that aspects of the program design and transition to motherhood were perceived both positively and negatively.

Women unanimously emphasized accessibility as a positive design characteristic. Designing accessible internet interventions addresses one of the important barriers for the prevention or treatment of perinatal depression, including lack of time and excess energy that many women experience during pregnancy (Goodman, 2009). The brief information in the program was valued, potentially contributing even further to the accessibility of Mamma Mia (i.e., being time-efficient). So far, the results from this study are aligned with the reviewed literature on user experiences with internet interventions for depression. However, despite that the content was considered trustworthy and generally likeable; several women emphasized its lack of depth as a weakness. This was particularly apparent among multiparous women, who claimed that parts of the content were irrelevant to their situation and contained things they already knew (e.g., from prior pregnancies), and that could possibly result in higher attrition among these women. Therapist-support could have been useful to help these women adapt program contents to their situation to some extent, but it is possible that multiparous women represent a different segment of the target population that are in need of different program content (e.g., sibling preparations or prior birth experiences).

The most consistent weakness of the program, however, was the intensity of the automated program schedule, in particular during the postpartum period. This was also considered a threat to adherence and relevance of the program, and unhelpful in the transition to motherhood. In the short term, this lead to irritation and stress, while in the longer term it contributed to a misalignment between the program content and the baby's actual age and development, thereby making the content personally irrelevant. Several women also explicitly and consistently expressed dissatisfaction with the tunneled sequence, which was characterized as inflexible. Tunneling, which does not allow skipping parts or going fast forward, could, in combination with the automated program schedule, contribute to sessions piling up and making it difficult use the program as prescribed.

Finally, Mamma Mia initiated cognitive processes such as increased awareness and reflection, and emotional processes such as comfort and normalization. They considered these processes to contribute to their well-being, attentiveness towards their pregnancy, and facilitating attachment to the baby. Furthermore, such cognitive and emotional processes could also prevent depressive symptoms and may potentially help women take early action when they start to feel more down (see e.g., Pugh, Hadjistavropoulos, Klein, et al., 2014).

SOLUTIONS AND RECOMMENDATIONS

The internet appears to be an important medium for the prevention of perinatal depression in terms of being accessible. The intention to use a program such as Mamma Mia, is dependent on its perceived unobtrusiveness and fit with users' daily lives (Drozd, Lehto, & Oinas-Kukkonen, 2012; O'Mahen et al., 2015). Once users start engaging with internet intervention, it should aim to instigate important cognitive and emotional processes that can promote maternal mental health and bonding with the baby by providing brief and concise contents. However, the brevity of information may lead to perceptions of program contents as lacking in depth or being superficial. There are several possible solutions to this problem; First, is to include links to more information for those who are interested. Second, add dynamic content that goes more in-depth on certain subjects at a web portal or program home page. Third, add tailoring to adapt the contents to the individual user's needs and to make it more relevant (e.g., parity or prematurity). It is also important that interventions establish credibility early on. Credibility is important both for the uptake of interventions and their continued use (Jimison et al., 2008). In Mamma Mia, this is partly done by initially mentioning who has financed and developed the program (assuming that these are credible sources). It is unlikely that women would request more information in Mamma Mia, if they did not experience the program as credible. This may explain why women suggested more information on health behaviors such as physical activity and nutrition, practical information on workplace adaptations for pregnant women, safety equipment, and help to handle a changing body image.

Mamma Mia is a narrative-based program designed to build a relationship with the user and follow a certain program structure and chronology. This is the reason a tunneled design is used and, although it is known to have a negative effect on user's perception of efficiency (i.e., easy search and access to information in a program), tunneling leads to higher adherence (i.e., more time spent on website and pages visited) and increased knowledge gains (Crutzen, Cyr, & de Vries, 2012). This may, however, have unintended negative side effects in Mamma Mia and unguided interventions in general, especially in combination with an automated program schedule and a lengthy program (e.g., failure to adhere to the program may lead to increased hopelessness). As such, a module-based program with more separable components and/or some degree of (optional) support would seem beneficial for pregnant and postpartum women. In Norwegian perinatal care, midwives and public health nurses at well-baby clinics, and general physicians, are in position to provide such support. The anonymity and freedom of using internet self-help also seems to be a two-edged sword according to previous research. For some, this may motivate and lower the barrier to help-seeking, empower users, and provide a sense of mastery and control (e.g., Gerhards et al., 2011). For others, this may lead to a lack of commitment and lead to the discontinuation of the program unless some support is provided. Thus, Mamma Mia should be offered as both a guided and unguided option, depending on the woman's needs.

FUTURE RESEARCH DIRECTIONS

This study has two main limitations that are important to bear in mind while interpreting the results and directing future research. First, participant characteristics suggested that the women interviewed for this study were typically well-educated, employed, and living with partners. They also scored low on depressive symptoms and high on subjective well-being. After all, Mamma Mia is a program that is intended to be offered to all pregnant women. It is necessary to reach as many women as possible for preventing postpartum depression, including those who are doing well, because maternal mental health may change during pregnancy and postpartum (Wisner et al., 2013). The homogeneity of women in this study, however, does limit the generalizability of the results. Thus, a more diverse sample should be included in future studies by including women with lower socioeconomic status, single mothers, and women with a history of depressive disorders or current mild-to-moderate symptoms of depression (e.g., EPDS score $\geq$ 10).

This study adds to the literature by examining women's experiences with a program, which is based on principles other than CBT. However, a second limitation is the eclectic approach of Mamma Mia (see, Drozd et al., 2015). Mamma Mia is not limited to any one approach and utilizes principles from CBT, positive psychology, attachment-based methods, and several others. This adds a degree of uncertainty to the generalizability of the results to other internet interventions, particularly those based on a singular approach, although the findings in this study are recognizable from findings in other studies on women's experiences with iCBT (O'Mahen et al., 2015; Pugh, Hadjistavropoulos, & Fuchs, 2014). Therefore, on the one hand, future research should continue to examine user experiences with singular approaches to internet interventions other than CBT. On the other hand, more eclectic and module- or component-based approaches should be investigated. A meta-analysis of parent training programs has demonstrated that not all program components are equal (Wyatt Kaminski, Valle, Filene, & Boyle, 2008). Some are consistently associated with larger effects (e.g., parent-child interaction) and others with smaller effects (e.g., problem-solving). Consequently, future research should identify and test core program components that are consistently associated with larger effects and that can be combined in an eclectic approach (i.e., delivering evidence-based kernels), and potentially give a greater effect than any singular approach.

CONCLUSION

This chapter has reviewed the literature on user experiences with internet and computer-based interventions, and presented results from women's experiences with a universal, unguided intervention for the prevention of perinatal depression. The review showed that highly motivated users adhere to these programs and experience positive changes. The change process shares similarities with face-to-face therapy, but it is not entirely clear who may benefit from using internet interventions. Some of the results in the present study are aligned with the existing literature such as accessibility, but have also added implications for the future development of the design of unguided interventions for pregnant and postpartum women. These should offer more flexibility and support, which is particularly important to avoid adverse effects of using Mamma Mia in a hectic period in life and better support women in their transition to motherhood. Nevertheless, women found the program to be accessible and requested more content that could be attributable to the credibility of the program. Mamma Mia also offered comfort, self-reflection, and maternal bonding with the baby, and seemed to provide a viable platform for the prevention of perinatal depression.

ACKNOWLEDGMENT

Mamma Mia was developed by Changetech in collaboration with the Regional Centre for Child and Adolescent Mental Health (RBUP) for the Norwegian Women's Public Health Association (N.K.S.). This research was funded by the Norwegian Women's Public Health Association (project no.: H3/2013) and the Research Council of Norway (project no.: 213737).

REFERENCES

Andersson, G., Paxling, B., Wiwe, M., Vernmark, K., Felix, C. B., Lundborg, L., ... Carlbring, P. (2012). Therapeutic alliance in guided internet-delivered cognitive behavioural treatment of depression, generalized anxiety disorder and social anxiety disorder. *Behaviour Research and Therapy*, *50*(9), 544–550. doi:10.1016/j.brat.2012.05.003 PMID:22728647

Australian Psychological Society. (2011). *Guidelines for providing psychological services and products using the internet and telecommunications technologies.* Melbourne, Australia: Australian Psychological Society.

Barak, A., Klein, B., & Proudfoot, J. G. (2009). Defining Internet-supported therapeutic interventions. *Annals of Behavioral Medicine*, *38*(1), 4–17. doi:10.100712160-009-9130-7 PMID:19787305

Beattie, A., Shaw, A., Kaur, S., & Kessler, D. (2009). Primary-care patients expectations and experiences of online cognitive behavioural therapy for depression: A qualitative study. *Health Expectations*, *12*(1), 45–59. doi:10.1111/j.1369-7625.2008.00531.x PMID:19250152

Bendelin, N., Hesser, H., Dahl, J., Carlbring, P., Nelson, K. Z., & Andersson, G. (2011). Experiences of guided Internet-based cognitive-behavioural treatment for depression: A qualitative study. *BMC Psychiatry*, *11*(1), 107. doi:10.1186/1471-244X-11-107 PMID:21718523

Bickmore, T. W., & Gruber, A. (2010). Relational agents in clinical psychiatry. *Harvard Review of Psychiatry*, *18*(2), 119–130. doi:10.3109/10673221003707538 PMID:20235777

Braun, V., & Clarke, V. (2006). Using thematic analysis in psychology. *Qualitative Research in Psychology*, *3*(2), 77–101. doi:10.1191/1478088706qp063oa

Cox, J. L., Holden, J. M., & Sagovsky, R. (1987). Detection of postnatal depression. Development of the 10-item Edinburgh Postnatal Depression Scale. *The British Journal of Psychiatry*, *150*(6), 782–786. doi:10.1192/bjp.150.6.782 PMID:3651732

Crutzen, R., Cyr, D., & de Vries, N. K. (2012). The role of user control in adherence to and knowledge gained from a website: Randomized comparison between a tunneled version and a freedom-of-choice version. *Journal of Medical Internet Research*, *14*(2), e45. doi:10.2196/jmir.1922 PMID:22532074

Cuijpers, P., Donker, T., Johansson, R., Mohr, D. C., van Straten, A., & Andersson, G. (2011). Self-guided psychological treatment for depressive symptoms: A meta-analysis. *PLoS ONE*, *6*(6), e21274. doi:10.1371/journal.pone.0021274 PMID:21712998

Cuijpers, P., Donker, T., van Straten, A., Li, J., & Andersson, G. (2010). Is guided self-help as effective as face-to-face psychotherapy for depression and anxiety disorders? A systematic review and meta-analysis of comparative outcome studies. *Psychological Medicine*, *40*(12), 1943–1957. doi:10.1017/S0033291710000772 PMID:20406528

Dennis, C. L., & Chung-Lee, L. (2006). Postpartum depression help-seeking barriers and maternal treatment preferences: A qualitative systematic review. *Birth*, *33*(4), 323–331. doi:10.1111/j.1523-536X.2006.00130.x PMID:17150072

Diener, E., Emmons, R. A., Larsen, R. J., & Griffin, S. (1985). The satisfaction with life scale. *Journal of Personality Assessment, 49*(1), 71–75. doi:10.120715327752jpa4901_13 PMID:16367493

Donkin, L., & Glozier, N. (2012). Motivators and motivations to persist with online psychological interventions: A qualitative study of treatment completers. *Journal of Medical Internet Research, 14*(3), e91. doi:10.2196/jmir.2100 PMID:22743581

Drozd, F., Haga, S. M., Brendryen, H., & Slinning, K. (2015). An Internet-based intervention (Mamma Mia) for postpartum depression: Mapping the development from theory to practice. *JMIR Research Protocols, 4*(4), e120. doi:10.2196/resprot.4858 PMID:26476481

Drozd, F., Lehto, T., & Oinas-Kukkonen, H. (2012). Exploring perceived persuasiveness of a behavior change support system: A structural model. In M. Bång & E. Ragnmalm (Eds.), *The 7th Conference on Persuasive Technology* (pp. 157–168). Linköping, Sweden: Springer-Verlag. 10.1007/978-3-642-31037-9_14

Farzanfar, R., Frishkopf, S., Friedman, R., & Ludena, K. (2007). Evaluating an automated mental health care system: Making meaning of human-computer interaction. *Computers in Human Behavior, 23*(3), 1167–1182. doi:10.1016/j.chb.2004.11.015

Gega, L., Smith, J., & Reynolds, S. (2013). Cognitive behaviour therapy (CBT) for depression by computer vs. therapist: Patient experiences and therapeutic processes. *Psychotherapy Research, 23*(2), 218–231. doi:10.1080/10503307.2013.766941 PMID:23390994

Gerhards, S. A. H., Abma, T. A., Arntz, A., de Graaf, L. E., Evers, S. M. A. A., Huibers, M. J. H., & Widdershoven, G. A. M. (2011). Improving adherence and effectiveness of computerised cognitive behavioural therapy without support for depression: A qualitative study on patient experiences. *Journal of Affective Disorders, 129*(1-3), 117–125. doi:10.1016/j.jad.2010.09.012 PMID:20889214

Goodman, J. H. (2009). Womens attitudes, preferences, and perceived barriers to treatment for perinatal depression. *Birth, 36*(March), 60–69. doi:10.1111/j.1523-536X.2008.00296.x PMID:19278385

Hoff, T., Straumsheim, P., Bjørkli, C. A., & Bjørklund, R. A. (2009). An external validation of two psychosocial work environment surveys - A SWOT approach. *Scandinavian Journal of Organization Psychology, 1*(1), 12–19.

Jimison, H. B., Gorman, P., Woods, S., Nygren, P., Walker, M., Norris, S., & Hersh, W. (2008). *Barriers and drivers of health information technology use for the elderly, chronically ill, and underserved*. Rockville, MD: Agency for Healthcare Research and Quality.

Knowles, S. E., Toms, G., Sanders, C., Bee, P., Lovell, K., Rennick-Egglestone, S., ... Bower, P. (2014). Qualitative meta-synthesis of user experience of computerised therapy for depression and anxiety. *PLoS ONE*, *9*(1), e84323. doi:10.1371/journal.pone.0084323 PMID:24465404

Lillevoll, K. R., Wilhelmsen, M., Kolstrup, N., Høifødt, R. S., Waterloo, K., Eisemann, M., & Risør, M. B. (2013). Patients experiences of helpfulness in guided internet-based treatment for depression: Qualitative study of integrated therapeutic dimensions. *Journal of Medical Internet Research*, *15*(6), e126. doi:10.2196/jmir.2531 PMID:23786763

Lone, J. A., Bjørklund, R. A., Østerud, K. B., Anderssen, L. A., Hoff, T., & Bjørkli, C. A. (2014). Assessing knowledge-intensive work environment: General versus situation-specific instruments. *European Journal of Work and Organizational Psychology*, *23*(3), 469–482. doi:10.1080/1359432X.2012.750449

Marcus, M., Yasamy, M. T., van Ommeren, M., Chisholm, D., & Saxena, S. (2012). *Depression: A global public health concern*. Geneva, Switzerland: World Health Organization.

Mykletun, A., Knudsen, A. K., & Mathiesen, K. S. (2009). *Psykiske lidelser i Norge: Et folkehelseperspektiv* [Mental disorders in Norway: A public health perspective]. Oslo, Norway: Norwegian Institute of Public Health.

Neuendorf, K. A. (2002). *The content analysis guidebook*. Thousand Oaks, CA: Sage Publications Inc.

Norwegian Directorate of Health. (2009). *Nasjonale retningslinjer for diagnostisering og behandling av voksne med depresjon i primær- og spesialisthelsetjenesten* [National guidelines for diagnosis and treatment of adults with depression in primary and secondary care]. Oslo, Norway: Norwegian Directorate of Health.

O'Mahen, H. A., Grieve, H., Jones, J., McGinley, J., Woodford, J., & Wilkinson, E. L. (2015). Womens experiences of factors affecting treatment engagement and adherence in internet delivered behavioural activation for postnatal depression. *Internet Interventions*, *2*(1), 84–90. doi:10.1016/j.invent.2014.11.003

Overland, S., Glozier, N., Krokstad, S., & Mykletun, A. (2007). Undertreatment before the award of a disability pension for mental illness: The HUNT Study. *Psychiatric Services*, *58*(11), 1479–1482. doi:10.1176/ps.2007.58.11.1479 PMID:17978260

Pugh, N. E., Hadjistavropoulos, H. D., & Fuchs, C. M. (2014). Internet therapy for postpartum depression: A case illustration of emailed therapeutic assistance. *Archives of Women's Mental Health*, *17*(4), 327–337. doi:10.100700737-014-0439-2 PMID:24965602

Pugh, N. E., Hadjistavropoulos, H. D., Hampton, A. J. D., Bowen, A., & Williams, J. (2015). Client experiences of guided internet cognitive behavior therapy for postpartum depression: A qualitative study. *Archives of Women's Mental Health*, *18*(2), 209–219. doi:10.100700737-014-0449-0 PMID:25109484

Pugh, N. E., Hadjistavropoulos, H. D., Klein, B., & Austin, D. W. (2014). A case study illustrating therapist-assisted internet cognitive behavior therapy for depression. *Cognitive and Behavioral Practice*, *21*(1), 64–77. doi:10.1016/j.cbpra.2013.08.002

Reason, P. (1994). Co-operative inquiry, participatory action research, and action inquiry: Three approaches to participative inquiry. In N. K. Denzin & Y. S. Lincoln (Eds.), *Handbook of qualitative research* (pp. 324–339). Thousand Oaks, CA: Sage.

Reeves, B., & Nass, C. (1996). *The media equation: How people treat computers, television and new media like real people and places*. Stanford, CA: Cambridge University Press.

Rozental, A., Boettcher, J., Andersson, G., Schmidt, B., & Carlbring, P. (2015). Negative effects of internet interventions: A qualitative content analysis of patients experiences with treatments delivered online. *Cognitive Behaviour Therapy*, *44*(3), 223–236. doi:10.1080/16506073.2015.1008033 PMID:25705924

Svartvatten, N., Segerlund, M., Dennhag, I., Andersson, G., & Carlbring, P. (2015). A content analysis of client e-mails in guided internet-based cognitive behavior therapy for depression. *Internet Interventions*, *2*(2), 121–127. doi:10.1016/j.invent.2015.02.004

The National Board of Health and Wellfare. (2010). *Nationella riktlinjer för vård vid depression och ångestsyndrom 2010 - stöd för styrning och ledning* [National guidelines for care in cases of depression and anxiety disorders]. Stockholm, Sweden: The National Board of Health and Wellfare.

van Ballegooijen, W., Cuijpers, P., Van Straten, A., Karyotaki, E., Andersson, G., Smit, J. H., & Riper, H. (2014). Adherence to internet-based and face-to-face cognitive behavioural therapy for depression: A meta-analysis. *PLoS ONE*, *9*(7), e100674. doi:10.1371/journal.pone.0100674 PMID:25029507

Van Der Zanden, R., Curie, K., Van Londen, M., Kramer, J., Steen, G., & Cuijpers, P. (2014). Web-based depression treatment: Associations of clients word use with adherence and outcome. *Journal of Affective Disorders*, *160*, 10–13. doi:10.1016/j.jad.2014.01.005 PMID:24709016

Watson, D., Clark, L. A., & Tellegen, A. (1988). Development and validation of brief measures of positive and negative affect: The PANAS Scales. *Journal of Personality and Social Psychology*, *54*(6), 1063–1070. doi:10.1037/0022-3514.54.6.1063 PMID:3397865

Wilhelmsen, M., Lillevoll, K. R., Risør, M. B., Høifødt, R. S., Johansen, M.-L., Waterloo, K., ... Kolstrup, N. (2013). Motivation to persist with internet-based cognitive behavioural treatment using blended care: A qualitative study. *BMC Psychiatry*, *13*(1), 296. doi:10.1186/1471-244X-13-296 PMID:24199672

Wisner, K. L., Sit, D. K. Y., Mcshea, M. C., Rizzo, D. M., Zoretich, R. A., Hughes, C. L., ... Hanusa, B. H. (2013). Onset timing, thoughts of self-harm, and diagnoses in postpartum women with screen-positive depression findings. *Journal of American Medical Association Psychiatry*, *70*(5), 490–498. doi:10.1001/jamapsychiatry.2013.87.Onset

World Health Organization. (2009). *Global health risks: Mortality and burden of disease attributable to selected major risks*. Geneva, Switzerland: World Health Organization; doi:10.2471/BLT.09.070565

World Health Organization. (2010). Depression. Retrieved February 19, 2016, from http://www.who.int/mental_health/management/depression/en/

Wyatt Kaminski, J., Valle, L. A., Filene, J. H., & Boyle, C. L. (2008). A meta-analytic review of components associated with parent training program effectiveness. *Journal of Abnormal Child Psychology*, *36*(4), 567–589. doi:10.100710802-007-9201-9 PMID:18205039

KEY TERMS AND DEFINITIONS

Internet-Based Cognitive Behavioral Therapy (iCBT): The most commonly used psychotherapeutic approach for treating mental health problems on the internet based on the same principles as in-person cognitive behavior therapy.

Mamma Mia: An unguided internet intervention designed to prevent pre- and postnatal depression and promote subjective well-being among pregnant and postpartum women.

Perinatal Depression: Onset or elevated symptoms of depression during pregnancy and the first 6 months following childbirth.

Strengths, Weaknesses, Opportunities, and Threats (SWOT): A systematic method and tool for assessment of internal and external environments to support strategic planning and decision-making, and development of products, organizations, and services.

Subjective Well-Being: Refers to people's experience of the quality of their lives and encompasses cognitive evaluations of life and emotional reactions.

Tunneled Design: A directive information architecture that guides users step-by-step through a predetermined sequence of web pages and/or sessions in order to improve the chances of achieving a goal.

Unguided Intervention: A fully automated and self-guided internet intervention without any therapist-support or human involvement.

This research was previously published in Web-Based Behavioral Therapies for Mental Disorders edited by Sitwat Usman Langrial; pages 27-52, copyright year 2018 by Medical Information Science Reference (an imprint of IGI Global).

Chapter 17
Complexity of Breastfeeding on Child/Maternal Health and Counseling Intervention

Ogunlade Joseph Olurotimi
College of Education Ikere Ekiti, Ekiti State, Nigeria

ABSTRACT

This chapter is a critical review of the complexities of breastfeeding and its attending effects on the health of the Mother and Child. The researcher employs a historical research approach to gather both theoretical and empirical facts on this issue. It was discovered that in spite of the pragmatic and frantic efforts by different individuals, organizations, governments and non-governmental bodies in establishing a universal, healthy and safest method of breastfeeding through research, publications, workshops and so on, based on the unavoidable and uncompromising importance and benefits to maternal and child health, it is on record that the maternal behaviour is still obviously at variance to the acceptability of full breastfeeding as promulgated and declared by World Health Organization (WHO). A serious, dedicated, pragmatic and coordinated counseling approach is therefore recommended to be adopted to revive and strengthening a positive behaviour in women to foster positive attitude towards breastfeeding to guarantee 100% morbidity and mortality rate in Maternal and Child health.

ORGANIZATION BACKGROUND

Human beings belong to a group of animals referred to as mammals while mammals are the class of animals that give birth to babies and feed their young ones on milk from the breast through the mammary gland. Female human beings belong to the group of mammals with well-developed breasts

DOI: 10.4018/978-1-7998-2351-3.ch017

UNICEF (2002) explained that breast milk is an excellent source of nutrition for the first four to six months of a child's life and can continue to be an important part of a child's diet for many months and thereafter. Breast milk is an appropriate source of nutrients; it contains proteins, fats, carbohydrates, vitamins and minerals in correct proportions needed by the child.

Breastfeeding is the act of feeding the baby from the breast. According to WHO (2002) Breastfeeding confers substantial health benefits on both mother and child. For the infant, the principal advantages of breast milk are nutritional and immunological. For the mother, breastfeeding encourages the involution of the uterus and thus the rapid return of uterine tomb which helps the mother to regain her natural shape. It promotes an affectionate bond between mother and child. It is economical and it is convenient. Also, through the proclatin – elevating effect of nipple stimulation, breastfeeding delays the return of normal ovarian function and thereby lengthens the interval between births (McNeily 1999, Orubuloye 1979, Ogunlade 2010).

Without controversy, nature itself has natural provision that has been put in place in a young woman long before she prepares to procreate. At conception, the women body is naturally active to receive and feed an infant that is yet about eight months to come, thus the first physical sign in a young lady who is newly pregnant of a baby is the enlargement (engorgement) of the mammary gland, preparation to lactation at birth so as to feed the expected baby and nurse it to life when it finally arrives. This engorgement sign becomes noticeable around the sixth week of pregnancy or two weeks after amenorrhea (loss of menstruation). This is due to the growth and enlargement of the milk duct and the alveoli in the breast. This enlargement is due to the influence of estrogens and performance for preparation of the breast for all the important nursing care of the mother. Shortly before delivery the levels of estrogens and progesterone fall in order to stimulate the pituitary gland produce lactogenic hormone which act on the acini's cell in the breast to start the production of milk.

Ogunmodimu (2004) submitted that the sucking action of the baby on the breast stimulates the posterior pituitary gland to release an oxytocic or pressor factor. The oxytocic or pressor factor causes the plain muscles of the breast to contract thereby propelling the milk from alveolar along the lactatiferous duct into the ampullae's. The acini's cells are stimulated to produce more milk, as the breasts are empty. It should be noted that the oxytocic released during breast – feeding also causes uterine contractions; hence 'after pain' is felt more during feeding times. This how breastfeeding and involution of the uterus work.

According to WHO (2012) Breastfeeding confers substantial health benefits on both mother and child. For the infant, the principal advantages of breast milk are nutritional and immunological. For the mother, breastfeeding encourages the involution of the uterus and thus the rapid return of uterine tomb which helps the mother to regain her natural shape. It promotes an affectionate bond between mother and child. It is economical and it is convenient. Also, through the proclatin – elevating effect of nipple stimulation, breastfeeding delays the return of normal ovarian function and thereby lengthens the interval between births (McNeily 1999, Orubuloye 1979, Hatcher 2004).

Literature on Complexity in Breastfeeding

In spite of the importance of breastfeeding there is a notable reduction in breastfeeding duration. Several complexities have been identified as playing various significant roles in influencing breastfeeding behaviour of nursing mothers. Odu and Ogunlade (2011) opined that factors which have negative influence on breastfeeding are pressures on nursing mothers to return to the labour force, lack of family support in urban areas. This, in combination with the reality that many women cannot afford to take extended maternity leaves for either financial or career reasons, can make breastfeeding a complex assignment (Flower, 2008). Heinig (2009) Explain that as the roles of women in modern societies change, there is tension between motherhood and the various other roles that women play. Increasingly, both men and women work outside of the home and parenting of children is becoming more of a shared responsibility both between a woman and her partner as well as with extended family. Increasingly, having two incomes is a necessity for many families and thus a reason for complexity in breastfeeding.

Bailey (2007) posited that a major complexity to breastfeeding at the community level is the discomfort and embarrassment many women feel about breastfeeding in public, including at work or at school. Young people in particular express a lot of disapproval about breastfeeding in public. Many young women decide not to breastfeed or stop breastfeeding sooner than they intend to because of the sense of isolation that results from this reluctance to breastfeed in public places. A number of women talk about how returning to work and/or school is a major reason why they stop breastfeeding or decide not to start. Developing workplace and school policies and practices that actively support breastfeeding, as well as peer support initiatives can positively contribute to breastfeeding rates

Some notable researchers added that in addition to painful breasts or nipples, physical feeding issues that are widely described by women as part of complexities that warrant stopping breastfeeding early on are: the baby rejecting the breast or not sucking (Redshaw & Henderson, 2012); and perceived insufficient milk supply (Gatti, 2008; Twamley et al, 2011). Gatti's (2008) review of the literature concluded that many women discontinue breastfeeding during the first few weeks because of perceived insufficient milk supply. Approximately 35% of women who wean early report this as the primary reason for stopping. Gatti's review also notes that women primarily use infant satisfaction cues as their main indication of sufficient milk supply. They will discontinue breastfeeding if they perceive their infant is still hungry and/or not satisfied without any professional concurrent evaluation of their actual breast milk supply (Gatti, 2008). In response to an open-ended question asked in an Australian survey, the reason most commonly given for stopping breastfeeding in the second week (i.e., once breastfeeding was proceeding well) was that breastfeeding took too long or was too tiring (Redshaw & Henderson, 2012).

Some other complexities observed by the researcher as likely factors responsible for the declining rate in breastfeeding duration and child spacing practices are urbanization, industrialization, infant food industry marketing pressures, biases towards bottle feeding and confusing instruction from the medical professional, eradication of traditional values and modes of living such as decline in extended family system thought to have supported breastfeeding and the employment of women in faraway places of abode which makes it difficult for women to breastfeed on demand.

Another complexity is the strength of the mother's desire for a healthy infant combined with her knowledge about the benefits of breastfeeding. If she believes breastfeeding benefits the child as she strongly desires a healthy child, she will be more likely to breastfeed. A second issue is a mother's understanding about the relationship between breastfeeding to her own health and fertility. It is believed that every woman possesses the ability to breastfeed her baby as asserted by the United Nations Children Fund (2012) (UNICEF) in their explanation they opined that the experience may be strange, tingling and exciting but in a matter of days, mother and baby will surely find a comfortable and enjoyable routine mutually beneficial to both.

Mooney (2005) emphasized that psychological and cultural changes related to modernization are known complexities that associated with decline in breastfeeding, such as perception of female breast as symbols of sexual attraction, women having the feeling that breastfeeding may make their breasts to sag or having a sense of modesty about breastfeeding, feeling shy to breastfeed in the public while some nursing mothers complain of insufficient milk. Concerned about breast size and shape seems to be one of the common bodily worries of women. Nigeria culture has created the exaggerated impression that large breasts are sexy and desirable, females now see their breasts as sex organ, women often perceive breasts as a source of sexual arousal and many women find that simulation of their breast especially the nipple is sexually arousing. Many women now prefer to present the breast as sexual organ than to breastfeed even though the breast is not a sex organ.

From news and reports, women in the south west are observed to appear deeply involved in acts or behaviour that negates breastfeeding such as inability to commence breastfeeding few hours after delivery due to perceive complexities as observed aboved, some appear not breastfeeding on demand as postulated by WHO (2001) that nursing mothers should breastfeed on cues i.e. exclusive for the first six months of life of the baby. It is even felt that complexity of bottle feeding appears to be a fashion among women. Recently, the method of child spacing through hormonal effect of lactation seems not to be appreciated. The importance of breastfeeding as a mechanism in controlling fertility and enhancing postpartum manipulation in southwest seems to be low. It is regarded as a good contraceptive, especially in a natural fertility situation by acting as an agent of child spacing

SUMMARY AND CONCLUSION

Giving credence to the question addressed through this literature review: What are the perceptions of women to the initiation and duration of breastfeeding on their health and their children? The main theme that emerged in response to this question is reflected in the title of this report: *"The Complexities of Breastfeeding on Child/ Maternal Health"*.

Many women intend to breastfeed, and the majority of women in Nigeria and Sub-Sahara countries do initiate breastfeeding. Some women struggle early on with the physical challenges associated with breastfeeding such as latching issues that result in painful nipples and bad feeding experiences. Other women may overcome these physical issues but continue to struggle trying to integrate breastfeeding into modern life, with a major complexity here being the discomfort many women experience with breastfeeding in public places. The result is that far fewer women are breastfeeding exclusively at six months than who successfully initiated breastfeeding.

The majority of women do understand the benefits of breastfeeding, but knowledge of the health benefits of breastfeeding alone is clearly not enough to enable women to breastfeed. One key complexity is the mixed messages that women get. Many women describe receiving conflicting advice early in the postnatal period about mastering the technical nuances of breastfeeding. A number of societal-level mixed messages seem to be even more problematic with respect to their influence on women who are trying to integrate breastfeeding into their lives. Some of the mixed messages we identified through this review of the literature are summarized below.

Breastfeeding is natural, something every woman can easily do, but it does require a lot of persistence, commitment, practice and technical support.

1. Breastfeed because it is best for your baby, but do not do so in public because it makes people uncomfortable.
2. Your breasts are made to feed babies, but in many of our modern societies breasts are predominantly viewed and 'advertised' as sexual objects.

3. Fathers should be playing a bigger role in their children's lives and it is important that they bond with and share in the care of their baby, but the mother should breastfeed.
4. To be a modern woman it is important to take your career seriously, but if you are a good mother you will breastfeed your baby - but not at work.
5. If you are a young mom we really want you to stay in school, but breastfeeding is not part of the teen culture so you might not want to breastfeed at school.

To conclude, although breastfeeding may be a health issue it is also very much a societal one. Health professionals who work directly with women and their partners to support them in their infant feeding decisions, and public health professionals working on initiatives to increase breastfeeding rates should be mindful about viewing breastfeeding within this broader context. Like many health issues, infant feeding choices are not made by individuals based solely on research evidence about what is best for the baby's and the mother's short and long term health. Rather, these are decisions embedded in real lives that are informed and influenced by many factors, including societal structures, norms, values, attitudes and beliefs. The health sector has an important role to play in contributing to the development of a society that truly supports women to breastfeed their babies. This includes the development of healthcare cultures that support health professionals to practice patient- and family-centred care, but goes far beyond this to contributing to an opening up of public discourse into how breastfeeding fits in the real world.

REFERENCES

Bailey, J. (2007). Modern parents' perspectives on breastfeeding: A small study. *British Journal of Midwifery*, *15*(3), 148–152. doi:10.12968/bjom.2007.15.3.23034

Becerra, L. E. (2009). Sources and acceptance of infant-feeding advice among low-income women. *Journal of Human Lactation*, *25*(2), 163–172. doi:10.1177/0890334408329438 PMID:19136396

Gatti, L. (2008). Maternal perceptions of insufficient milk supply in breastfeeding. *Journal of Nursing Scholarship*, *40*(4), 355–363. doi:10.1111/j.1547-5069.2008.00234.x PMID:19094151

Heinig, M. J., Ishii, K. D., Banuelos, J. L., Campbell, E., & O'Loughlin, C. (2008). Understanding breastfeeding initiation and continuation in rural communities: A combined qualitative/quantitative approach. *Maternal and Child Health Journal*, *12*(3), 402–414. doi:10.100710995-007-0248-6 PMID:17636458

Ogunlade, J. O. (2010). *Breastfeeding and child spacing among women in Nigeria* [Unpublished Ph.D Thesis]. Ekiti State University. Ado-Ekiti, Nigeria.

Ogunmodimu, E. F. (2006). The effects breastfeeding on the rate of conception. *Proceeding of the International Population Conference,* London (Vol. 2, pp. 129-136).

Odu, B. K., & Ogunlade, J. O. (2011). Breastfeeding behavior among women in Nigeria. *Conference Proceeding Canada International Conference on Education.* Retrieved from www.Ciceducation.org

Orubuloye, I. O. (1979). The significance of breastfeeding on fertility and mortality. *Journal of Tropical Pediatrics and Environmental Child Health.*

Mcneilly, A. S. (1999). Relationship of feeding patterns, proclaction and resumption of ovulation postpartum. In G. I. Zatuchini, M. H. Labbok, & J. Sciarra (Eds.), *Research frontiers in fertility regulation.* New York.

Redshaw, M., & Henderson, J. (2012). Learning the hard way: Expectations and experiences of infant feeding support. *Birth (Berkeley, Calif.)*, *39*(1), 21–29. doi:10.1111/j.1523-536X.2011.00509.x PMID:22369602

Lactational Amenorrhea Method (LAM). (2012). UNICEF. Georgia University, Institute for Reproductive Health.

The State of the World children. (2004). *UNICEF.* London: Oxford University Press.

Interactions of nutrition and infections. (2002). *World Health Organization.*

Does maternal smoking have a negative effect on breastfeeding? (2012World Health Organization.

The World Health Report: Make Every Mother and Child Count. (2002). *WHO.*

Breastfeeding counselling: A training course. (2001World Health Organization. Geneva.

KEY TERMS AND DEFINITIONS

Breastfeeding: It is simply the act of feeding the baby directly from the breast of the mother.

Complexity: This is used in this study as barriers/challenges to breastfeeding.

Counseling: In this work is a process of helping breastfeeding mother to appreciate the benefits of breastfeeding to their health and that of their baby so as to encourage them to breastfeed appropriately.

Maternal Health: It is the complete physical, mental and social well-being of the mother.

This research was previously published in the Handbook of Research on Chaos and Complexity Theory in the Social Sciences edited by Şefika Şule Erçetin and Hüseyin Bağcı; pages 382-387, copyright year 2016 by Information Science Reference (an imprint of IGI Global).

Chapter 18
Breastfeeding, Authority, and Genre:
Women's Ethos in Wikipedia and Blogs

Alison A. Lukowski
Christian Brothers University, USA

Erika M. Sparby
Northern Illinois University, USA

ABSTRACT

This chapter is concerned with women's mis- or underrepresentation in knowledge creation, particularly when it comes to their bodies. In this chapter, the authors examine how Wikipedia's generic regulations determine that women's often experiential ethos is unwelcome on the site. Thus, women are often unable to construct knowledge on the "Breastfeeding" entry; their epistemological methods are ignored or banned by other contributors. This chapter also examines six breastfeeding-focused mommyblogs, proposing blogs as an alternative genre that welcomes women's ethos. However, the authors also recognize that such blogs are not a perfect epistemological paradigm. The chapter closes with an examination of the implications of this work for academic collaboration across fields and for women's agency.

INTRODUCTION

Women often struggle to find a place online to express themselves and to create credible knowledge. Whether women write about issues as mundane as wedding dresses or as important as health issues, they are often harassed and silenced by a

DOI: 10.4018/978-1-7998-2351-3.ch018

variety of strategies as overt as trolling and as opaque as editing. Previous research about breastfeeding rhetoric (Koerber, 2013; Koerber et al, 2012; Koerber, 2006) demonstrated that breastfeeding is situated in disciplinary and discursive contexts that control women's bodies, such as science, medicine, and education. One way discursive power manifests online is through controlling sources of knowledge. This chapter offers case studies of the Wikipedia "Breastfeeding" entry and six blogs written by nursing mothers, mommyblogs, to show how feminist standpoint theory (Haraway, 1988) and apparent feminism (Frost, 2015) reveal that some spaces use a guise of balance, impartiality, and free speech to hinder women's processes of knowledge creation, while other spaces welcome experiential ethos. This study of knowledge production and ethos, which is grounded in the authority and credibility to create and evaluate that knowledge, reveals a reciprocal relationship between the knower and the known. The authors find that women prefer alternative *ethea* and are excluded because of cultural norms and hierarchies rather than truth or reality. Based on feminist standpoint theory and apparent feminism, this article rhetorically analyzes Wikipedia's "Breastfeeding" entry and its Talk page and six mommyblogs.

Collaborative writing has the potential to provide multiple viewpoints, but Wikipedia contributors—nearly 90% of whom are male (Simonite, 2013)—dismiss the credibility of women, even on issues of women's health. This work suggests that the design of Wikipedia's site and the culture it supports enforce a "neutral point of view" (NPOV) that excludes women's experiences because they are underrepresented in normative discourses of medicine, science, and philosophy. Wikipedia's generic conventions necessitate that contributors engage in debates about epistemology, truth, verifiability, and validity (McIntyre, 2010; Kennedy, 2009; Garfinkel, 2008). These conventions lead editors to question, challenge, or dismiss women's ethos when discussing an epistemology of their own bodies, thus silencing many female contributors. As a result of this persistent exclusion, women often avoid collaboratively curated sites like Wikipedia altogether (Hargittai & Shaw, 2015; Eckert & Steiner, 2013; Reagle & Rhue, 2011; Reagle, 2009). The consequences of these rhetorical moves have implications beyond digital spaces and contribute to society's persistent negative view of breastfeeding as something that must always happen in the margins.

In contrast, blogs provide a refreshing look at breastfeeding and women's digital ethos, giving women a forum in which to speak. However, the personal and individual nature of blogs prevents women from contributing to official narratives about their own bodies on a more public level: while their knowledge is marginalized, they continue to be ostracized for and banned from public breastfeeding despite the efforts blogs make to reverse such restrictions. The authors selected six mommyblogs—*The Breastfeeding Mother* (*TBM*), *Chronicles of a Nursing Mom* (*CoaNM*), *Paa. la, Unlatched, Dispelling Breastfeeding Myths* (*DPM*), and *Breast for the Weary* (*BftW*)—because they appeared in a list of top breastfeeding blogs and/or were top results in a Summer 2015 Google search for the keywords "breastfeeding" and "blog." The bloggers at *TBM*, *Unlatched*, and *BftW* no longer update their pages, but the information they provide therein remains relevant and sought after; *CoaNM*, *Paa.la*, and *DPM* continue to post updates. A brief note on data presentation is in order here because the authors will reference multiple posts from each blog, the date of the post will appear next to its quote or summary, but no direct links will appear in the text or references.

This chapter will examine Wikipedia and mommyblogs post-publication to determine how each site uses generic design and cultural expectations to signal to their users what kinds of ethos is welcomed. Rhetorical analysis will reveal that the epistemologies behind these culturally saturated sites mirror how our society values different forms of knowledge. Rhetorical analysis is a suitable method for this study because of the nature of this inquiry. As Koerber (2013) suggested, "[R]hetorical analysis can enrich our understanding of the manner in which expert knowledge is produced and the channels through which individuals in the public sphere receive and relate to such information" (p. 7). Likewise, Selzer (2004) explained rhetorical analysis as "studying carefully some kind of symbolic action, often after the fact of its delivery and irrespective of whether it was actually directed to you or not, so that you might understand it better and appreciate its tactics" (p. 281). This chapter also answers Novotny's (2015) call to "build and take up feminist methodologies that intervene in the designs of policies and projects that regulate female health" (p. 62). The authors examine the tensions between Wikipedia and mommy blogs to determine how women can find digital voices and create their own epistemologies. Rhetorical analysis enables the authors to recognize that because the values behind mommy blog epistemologies risk excluding others—including women of color, working-class women, and women for whom breastfeeding may not be an option—they are not a perfect paradigm. Nonetheless, opening Wikipedia and blogs to various standpoints creates more accurate and verifiable claims about breastfeeding while building a digital ethos of women writers.

BACKGROUND

This project is indebted to a long-standing tradition of work in credibility scholarship. The early 2000s saw an upswing in the debate about credibility online as more and more people adopted digital modes of publishing. The ways authors developed and used ethos becomes a central concern for digital rhetoric scholarship. The following scholars directly influenced this essay. Several scholars address credibility in the digital age: Johnson & Kaye (2004, 2010, 2011) showed how a user's demographic features and political affiliations influence his/her perceptions of credibility, and

Flanagin and Metzger (2008) and Metzger (2007) illustrated that each user's perceptions of credibility depend on how the source content meets his/her unique needs and expectations. Scholars have also addressed the credibility of Wikipedia since its inception in 2001 (Chawner & Lewis, 2004; Giles, 2005; Chesney, 2006; Fallis, 2008; Garfinkel, 2008; Brooke, 2009; Brown, 2015). Gruwell (2015) argued that a critical feminist approach to Wikipedia is necessary to understand and remedy the lack of women contributors. Blogs also receive attention from credibility scholars (Johnson & Kaye, 2004; Armstrong & McAdams, 2009; Johnson & Kaye, 2010; Johnson & Kaye, 2011). Winter and Krämer (2014) concluded that female writers are more credible on topics relating to issues with which they would be expected to establish a deeper connection and thus about which they would know more, such as violence in the media (p. 450).

Credibility and epistemology have been an essential facet of feminist research for decades because all knowledge is situated within a larger cultural context (Hartsock, 1983; Rose, 1983; Haraway, 1988; Harding, 1993). Like credibility scholarship, feminist scholarship addresses the role of digital media in the early to late 2000s. Two particular strands of feminist criticism, standpoint theory and apparent feminism, shape the approach of this work. In Harding's (1993, 2003) standpoint theory, strong objectivity is reached when oppressed and marginalized perspectives are shared. Johnston, Friedman, and Peach (2011) claimed that new media technologies play a role in how women participate in knowledge generation in political blogs. Scott and White (2013) explained that standpoint theory's strength is its recognition "that we construct our knowledge by interacting with each other from our respective and situated social positions" (pp. 61-2). Apparent feminism (Frost, 2013; 2014a; 2014b; 2015) is a methodology that fights the post-feminist notion that society has moved beyond the need for feminism and shows places where women and other marginalized identities continue to face resistance and/or oppression, particularly in spaces that support a guise of neutrality or democracy. Its three goals are key to this approach: "[1] making more apparent the need for feminist interventions, [2] hailing nonfeminists as allies, and [3] demystifying the relationship between feminism and efficiency" (Frost, 2015, p. 9). Novotny (2015) employed apparent feminism by "advocating for the incorporation of diverse stakeholders" (p. 68) to engage in knowledge production.

This chapter draws on a long tradition of digital credibility, epistemology, and feminist scholarship. In doing so, the authors demonstrate an ongoing need to analyze and understand how digital genres shape knowledge about women's bodies.

DESIGN AND KNOWLEDGE/KNOWLEDGE AND DESIGN

Design and culture and the origins of knowledge are key aspects of epistemological creation on Wikipedia and blogs. The design and culture of the sites influence what kinds of actions users take and what they access, while each site has rules governing from where knowledge must come. Although this chapter isolates each aspect to discuss it separately, it is worth noting that such a construction is artificial. In reality, the design and culture and the rules that govern origins of knowledge work recursively to reinforce and construct each other. Wikipedia's encyclopedic genre dictates specific rules for the origins of knowledge (design dictates origins of knowledge), but a blog's freedom from the need for typical scholarly sources enables users to include hyperlinks to outside articles or uploads of personal photos as evidence (origins of knowledge dictate design). Thus, the reader should be aware that although this chapter addresses each phenomenon separately, each is always influenced by the other.

Design and Culture

Analyzing design is useful for discussing epistemology in Wikipedia and blogs because each space follows specific generic guidelines that govern how users can participate in the act of knowledge construction. Design choices can also reveal authorial values: the images used, page hierarchies, and font choices demonstrate how the contributors think users will engage with their content. Furthermore, the design of a site also reveals the culture it supports. For instance, Wikipedia's design privileges a polished entry page and hides the creation of that knowledge in small links to "Talk" and "History" pages; this results in an exclusive culture available only to a small percentage of page visitors. Conversely, blogs expose collaborative processes of knowledge creation by placing the entry and comments on the same page level, which results in a culture of collaboration and relevance. Rhetorical analysis of design and culture uncovers the complex relationship between knowledge and the presentation of that knowledge.

Despite its innovative use of open source and collaborative knowledge creation, Wikipedia recapitulates traditional print methods of knowledge creation because it relies on outside and verifiable sources for validation. The reliability and accessibility of its information makes Wikipedia one of the top ten sites in terms of web traffic (Brooke, 2009; Fallis, 2011; Simonite, 2013). Wikipedia differs from other reference materials such as *Encyclopedia Britannica* and *Webster's Dictionary* because its content is generated and verified by a community of volunteers rather than professional writers and researchers (Loveland & Reagle, 2013). Wikipedia's design creates a space for people to collaborate and debate the value of knowledge. As an exercise in mass-collaboration and groupthink, Wikipedia has potential to provide a voice to the marginalized. Gruwell (2015) agreed that the space could disrupt notions of single authority generated knowledges: "Wiki technology presents the potential to create a constantly evolving space that privileges collaborative writing (and meaning-making), undermining the notion that a single, unified identity is the preferred authorial position" (p. 119). Unfortunately, as Gruwell also noted, this has not been the case. Instead, Wikipedia often reflects the knowledge of the normalized majority and reenacts cultural values that minimize the contributions of women and minorities.

Furthermore, the design of Wikipedia affirms hierarchies by presenting the entry first and displaying tabs for "Talk" and "View History" secondarily; these tabs reveal how the page is constructed and who contributes to it, but they are almost invisible in the larger context of the article. As Brooke (2009) suggested, "Each entry on Wikipedia is, in fact, the tip of a much larger iceberg of activity … If a user visits Wikipedia and simply samples an entry, she or he may be missing out on a great deal of the information the site can provide" (p. 191). For instance, on the Breastfeeding "Talk" page contributors discussed whether to include a section sex and breastfeeding, during which one contributor noted that, "this article's presentation of the facts about breastfeeding does not feel encyclopedic, and most definitely does not feel comprehensive" (Breastfeeding: Talk, 2015a). In other words, readers who do not read "Talk" pages may think the entry is an objective and encyclopedic representation of breastfeeding rather than the contributions of individuals who debate the relevance and salience of each section. While every version of a page is saved and the construction of knowledge can be traced, few users actually contribute to entries or access the "Talk" and "View History" pages where the debates about truth and verifiability occur. In a single month, Wikipedia has over 370 million views worldwide and over 60 million views in North America (Wikimedia Report, 2015), yet only 70,000 users actively contribute to Wikipedia and share in creating this knowledge (Wikipedia, 2015b). While users can participate in knowledge generation, many of them do not, perhaps because the murky nature of these tabs covertly (or overtly) excludes them.

The Wikipedia interface and "Talk" and "History" pages also follow a set of editing conventions that discourage new contributors. Wikipedia acknowledges this failing: "Editors who fail to comply with Wikipedia cultural rituals, such as signing talk pages, may implicitly signal that they are Wikipedia outsiders, increasing the odds that Wikipedia insiders may target or discount their contributions" (Wikipedia, 2015b). Wikipedia even has an entry titled "Please Do Not Bite the Newcomers" that outlines a series of tools and reminders for regular editors to encourage and gently correct inexperienced contributors. Wrapped in the flag of NPOV, long-standing contributors can flag and delete edits or entries they deem unverifiable or irrelevant, which often deters newcomers from the editorial process. One editor on the Breastfeeding Talk page qualifies her meaningful contributions by pleading ignorance and using humility instead of stating that she has as much right to make changes as other contributors: "I am not a regular editor here, and I honestly don't have time to learn things like which sources are valid and how to avoid original research … I'm just someone who fixes bad spelling or syntax or throws in an episode list for a TV show I like" (Wikipedia, 2015a). Although this editor has valuable information to add to the page, she preempts an attack from the regular editors who may recognize her as an outsider. Moreover, this issue is compounded for the few women who contribute to Wikipedia because the site reflects broader cultural problems that exclude women from computing, software development, and technology in general. Gruwell (2015) suggested that women may be underrepresented on Wikipedia because the interface itself requires familiarization with basic computer coding to fully participate in the community (p. 125); historically, women have had limited access to these skills, so they may feel discouraged from participating.

In fact, we may never fully know how many women contribute to Wikipedia because the design enables users to make changes anonymously. In 2004 and 2007, Wikipedia's self-studies found that "over 80% of edits by unregistered users" are meaningful contributions. If we accept Virginia Woolf's notion that Anonymous was "often a woman," then the number of contributions women make in Wikipedia may never be quantified. And yet, if women contributors remain anonymous, we should interrogate why women choose not to identify their gender. Gruwell (2015) suggested women editors fear accusations of bias simply because they are women: one of her study participants, Sylvia, "feared that because she was a 'female writing about women,' other editors would dismiss her writing as simply the work of someone 'writing about women because they're hot.' Sylvia worried that the community would not recognize her expertise because of her embodied identity position" (p. 127). Since Wikipedia's default NPOV is heterosexual, white, and male, contributions centering on women are often trivialized. Women may not feel comfortable entering a rhetorical situation in which they are marked as outsiders; they tend to migrate to knowledge-constructing sites that contrast Wikipedia's culture of exclusion, such as blogs.

In general, blogs are designed to fit within a few generic guidelines. They operate via posts from the blog's owner, or blogger, and appear in reverse chronological order. In general, all of the different styles of blog can be boiled down to three subgenres: 1) link-driven, which compiles hyperlinks; 2) diaristic, which offers personal reflections; and 3) a hybrid that does both (Blood, 2000). The blogs examined in this chapter are largely the latter, discussing relevant breastfeeding media items and offering individual narratives to develop individual digital ethos. In particular, the benefits of this kind of knowledge include the bloggers sifting "through the mass of information packaged daily for our consumption and pick[ing] out the interesting, the important, the overlooked, and the unexpected" (Blood, 2000). Then, the blogger "may provide additional information to that which corporate media provides, expose the fallacy of an argument, perhaps reveal an inaccurate detail" (Blood, 2000). Thus, readers are able to quickly understand the issue at hand while also engaging with one or more additional perspectives.

This design creates a culture of *kairos*, or timeliness and relevance. *TBM*, *CoaNM*, *Paa.la*, *Unlatched*, *DPM*, and *BftW* offer unique opportunities for knowledge creation because each blogger responds directly to issues that are relevant to her and her readers. For example, Rachelle (*Unlatched*) and Paala (*Paa.la*) both closely follow Facebook's restrictions against posting breastfeeding photos to social media sites. Rachelle (Aug 20, 2013; Aug 27, 2013; Aug 29, 2013) and Paala (Jun 10, 2014; Jun 21, 2015; Jul 14, 2015) not only post links to external articles and websites that deal with this issue, but they also share screencaps and stories from readers and their own experiences while, most importantly, explaining why it is so important to fight back against Facebook's policies. These posts are *kairotic*; they would not have had as great an effect (or potentially any effect) had they been written months later or even preemptively months earlier. However, because they respond to the events as they are unfolding, updating the blogs' readers in real-time, they are relevant.

Another key design feature of blogs leads to a culture of collaboration: the comments section. Here, bloggers can elaborate on or defend their posts while conversing with their readers. Wikipedia editors can do so to an extent as well, but the genre necessitates that these interactions take place on a separate page. Notoriously reluctant to make extra effort, Wikipedia users must find the right link and click through to find the debates about truth and knowledge. Conversely, on blogs, the comments section is connected directly to the original blog post. Comments do not appear on the blog homepage, but each post has a unique URL that links to a separate page where the comments will appear just below it. Such placement suggests a continuity between the blogger's post and her readers' comments or her own clarifications. Because they are openly displayed with the blog post, they are held in nearly as high esteem as the main post and thus promote an interactive knowledge creation among bloggers and readers that values each other as equals.

The six breastfeeding blogs at hand display interactive knowledge creation regularly. Jenny (*CoaNM*), Paala, Teglene (*TBM*), Rachelle, and Shannon (*BftW*) all support comments from readers that provide additional information. In particular, Anne's (*DPM*) post on tongue tie (Feb 2013)—a condition resulting from a short frenulum that attaches the tongue to the lower floor of the jaw—shows her readers contributing to the information she provides in her posts. Anne explains that many doctors and other medical professionals often tell mothers whose babies have tongue tie that it either doesn't exist or doesn't affect breastfeeding; she goes on to cite advice from International Board Certified Lactation Consultants (IBCLCs) that say otherwise and points to the need for more research. Her post has received over two-dozen supportive comments, many from IBCLCs who verified that tongue-tie is often misunderstood or misdiagnosed. Several hyperlink other sources on the same topic. Taken together, the post and comments work collaboratively to provide credible knowledge about what tongue tie is and how to spot and fix it. Notably, Wikipedia's entry on "Ankyloglossia" (the medical term for tongue-tie) only includes two brief paragraphs on the condition's impact on infant feeding, and the "Breastfeeding" entry only has two sentences on it, little of it useful for a breastfeeding mother seeking information.

Although all six blogs this chapter studies enabled their comments sections, not every blog is required to do so. Such restrictions limit this valuable knowledge creation from happening on their site and, frankly, limit the authority of the blog because readers cannot offer insight that may contradict or correct the information in the posts. Sometimes bloggers may moderate their comments to restrict who leaves feedback, although it is generally considered bad blogging ethics to do so (Blood, 2000). In an interview, Rachelle admits that she moderates the comments on her blog: "I moderate my comments, so I have control over what does get published, but I don't really censor people and approve almost all comments, even if they are negative" (personal communication, June 2014). Rachelle would seem to be in the majority of mommybloggers. Typically, bloggers allow readers to comment freely on their page, in a large part because that's what many consider to be the point of a blog: to spread information collaboratively through posts and comments.

The explicit design of blogs keeps knowledge creation at the forefront. The hybridity of the link-driven and diaristic styles of blogs creates a culture that values relevance and collaboration. This is distinct from Wikipedia's two-pronged problem: women's voices *and* women's issues are often excluded. On breastfeeding blogs, women use their individual digital *ethea* to collaboratively create knowledge; however, on Wikipedia, men edit entries that should appeal to women, such as "Breastfeeding," which may misrepresent the experience and concerns of breastfeeding. Whether uninitiated Wikipedia visitors are not aware that epistemological discussions are happening just a click away or whether they do not feel welcome to join the conversation, Wikipedia's collaborative, free-access, and free-content encyclopedic genre discourages the participation of all but a select few, particularly women. However, the transparency of blogs' epistemologies provides space for women and other minorities to exercise authority in ways that Wikipedia prohibits them from doing so.

Origins of Knowledge

A second factor that influences knowledge construction on Wikipedia and blogs is how they craft their credibility and ethos. As an encyclopedic genre, Wikipedia is concerned with credibility, or the outward appearance of authority through neutrality and verifiability. As such, it maintains a NPOV and requires secondary sources to verify all knowledge claims. However, women's knowledge is often grounded in testimony and folk wisdom, which Wikipedia's generic constraints disallow; thus Wikipedia tends to silence their epistemological contributions. On the other hand, blogs are predicated on individual ethos, or identity factors—such as firsthand experience or acquired credentials—that lead to authority. Because blogs are open to multiple viewpoints and experiences, they give women and other marginalized identities a place from which to speak.

Wikipedia's "Talk" page provides a space for contributors to shape the debate about what knowledge is relevant to the entry. Wikipedia depends on the collaborative writing process for fact checking and neutrality; its entries rely on verifiable sources with citations so "that anyone using the encyclopedia can check that the information comes from a reliable source" (Wikipedia, 2015c). Many of the individuals who contribute to Wikipedia are volunteers and do not have professional or educational expertise in the pages they edit; they often have little individual ethos on most topics. For instance, one of the top editors of the breastfeeding entry is Gandydancer who also wrote significant portions of the "Gandy Dancer" and "Yodeling" entries. The "Talk" page could be a space for women to control knowledge about their bodies, but instead the generic requirements for neutrality and verifiability often silence them. On the "Breastfeeding" "Talk" page, user Fabiola Grojan requested the addition of a section entitled "breastfeeding fashion" so that mothers can "avoid the unwanted attention when breastfeeding in public without using their scarf to cover up." However, another user, SummerPhD, responded that Fabiola needs to provide "reliable sources discussing 'breastfeeding fashion' to add it to the article." The difference between the opinion of the contributor and a reliable resource seems moot here; Fabiola could easily find support from a credible source, such as an article from *The Guardian* or perhaps *Parenting*. While McIntyre (2010) argued that Wikipedia's collaborative process, verifiability, and NPOV make it verifiable and not a source of objective truth, the authors find this distinction disingenuous. Even as Wikipedia encourages contributors to cite verifiable sources such as scholarly articles and textbooks, they privilege some forms of knowledge over others, thus making them appear as objective truth. In other words, some types of sources are considered more "true" (verifiable) than others; peer-reviewed articles are more "true" than personal blogs, and any source is more "true" than personal experience or individual ethos.

But perhaps more troubling are instances when the user has direct knowledge and experience, but, by championing neutrality, Wikipedia ignores these testimonial forms of evidence. Technology futurist Jaron Lanier (2006) tried to delete parts of his own entry that called him a filmmaker because he made "one experimental short film about a decade and a half ago." However, he found himself in a battle with other Wikipedians who "corrected" the changes Lanier made. Lanier's own life experience was less important than the verifiability of his sources. For women, this bias can have devastating effects. Historically, women have been excluded from creating scholarly and verifiable research, and, in some cases, the only way to encounter the perspective of non-academic women is through experiential accounts. Cassel (2011) explained, "despite Wikipedia's stated principle of the need to maintain a neutral point of view, the reality is that it is not enough to 'know something' about friendship bracelets or 'Sex and the City.'" In her study of several regular women contributors, Gruwell (2015) shared a similar experience to Fabiola's. One study participant, Janet, explained, "'Sometimes you just can't [find citations]. Sometimes particularly for stuff you know' … 'Where do you find a source that tells you there isn't a high school in a particular suburb? I mean, I know that. I've lived there for twenty-something years'" (p. 126). While Janet's knowledge may be useful and interesting to other users, the generic requirements for citation of verifiable sources preclude any appeals to direct experience. Fabiola's and Janet's voices are silenced by a generic need for NPOV and verifiability that in turn excludes their *ethea*. Similarly, the Breastfeeding "Talk" page demonstrates how personal experience is unwelcome in Wikipedia: Gandydancer, a prolific editor, noted that her experiential ethos is not a legitimate source, but she feels the need to share it nevertheless: "From a personal POV, which I suppose I should not mention but will anyway, thinking back to my own experience, loss of interest in sex was more of my experience than feeling 'sexy' while I nursed." Regardless of her experience, Gandydancer must provide verifiable sources to justify the editorial direction of the entry.

Because they are predicated on personal ethos, blogs offer a counter-authority to Wikipedia's encyclopedic genre. For instance, Paala frequently praises pop culture figures who support breastfeeding (Jun 14, 2014) and addresses Facebook's anti-nipple policy that prohibits users from posting breastfeeding photos (Jun 10, 2014). Teglene (*TBM*) also discusses her personal experiences in relation to larger cultural norms. In one post (Sep 6, 2014), she examines the common myth that busy women should be excused from breastfeeding because it is inconvenient. She uses her own experience to claim how a mother can work breastfeeding into any schedule, particularly if she recruits help from her family. Here, Paala and Teglene both provide personal ethos to contextualize breastfeeding issues and give advice to their readers. And their readers respond positively, despite their lack of "reliable sources." Wikipedia would not allow such material because these posts and others like them express both opinions and experiences and often do not draw upon outside verifiable sources.

The value of this experiential digital ethos is that the bloggers can explain how they came to their knowledge. They can describe what happened to them and how they handled it; readers have insight into the logic that goes into the bloggers' decisions, which can help them reach their own conclusions on related issues. To illustrate, Jenny (*CoaNM*, Mar 11, 2014) advises pregnant women how to prepare for breastfeeding. She uses her experiential ethos to help women determine what is best for them. Likewise, Shannon (*BftW*, May 11, 2011) writes a lengthy post on law and justice in regard to an incident in which she was illegally ejected from a store for breastfeeding in public. She hyperlinks several outside resources, each of which pertains to the event at the store and the ensuing aftermath, including media coverage and out-of-court settlements. Although she does not cite any scholarly sources, Shannon documents her journey through this event and advises other women in similar situations on how to exercise their agency and receive restitution. In both instances, Jenny and Shannon not only share knowledge, but they also contextualize where it comes from.

Notably, this study's mommybloggers use their own credentials and outside research to boost their digital *ethea*, although the blog genre does not require them to do so. First, they are mothers who breastfeed their children, so they offer firsthand experience to substantiate their claims. In addition, several of these bloggers train in lactation and breastfeeding. Jenny has L.A.T.C.H. (Lactation, Attachment, Training, Counseling, Help) training, Anne (*DPM*) has experience as a peer supporter with her local Healthcare Trust and as a birth and postnatal doula, and Rachelle (*Unlatched*) works as a breastfeeding counselor and advocate while studying to become an IBCLC. These three women have background experience beyond their own to supplement their *ethea*. On their blogs, this *ethea* lends authority and adequately legitimizes the knowledge they produce. On Wikipedia, other contributors would reject this firsthand knowledge.

Despite the genre's freedom from the need for secondary sources, the breastfeeding bloggers still tend to draw from external materials, most frequently from sources such as *KellyMom* and *La Leche League International*, two well-reputed websites on breastfeeding and parenting. Many posts include a list of references at the end: Anne (Jul 10, 2010) hyperlinked six sources in a post about drinking alcohol while nursing (on Aug 19, 2010, her post includes a 17-item reference list), and Teglene (Dec 14, 2010) includes both hyperlinks and an APA-formatted list of references in a post about low milk production. Notably, these lists include scholarly articles and books written by healthcare professionals and breastfeeding experts with strong reputations. In the instances when the mommybloggers cite secondary sources, they demonstrate that they are well-informed readers on breastfeeding topics. All six blogs utilize some level of research, although how much and how often varies entirely by the blog post and the blogger's preferences.

Blogs show that people can have similar experiences and still learn from each other. For example, if a mother is having a hard time breastfeeding (maybe the baby isn't latching or often becomes colicky after feeding), she is certainly not the only woman who has encountered these problems. Thus, blogs lend authority to bloggers who exercise their digital *ethea*. However, because Wikipedia relies on the credibility of verifiable sources to establish authority, the "Breastfeeding" page reflects a clinical concern with how breastfeeding works. By reading on breastfeeding blogs about other women's experiences, a mother might find solutions to her problems quickly and easily without needing to spend time and money on a doctor's visit. Even though blogs are renowned for focusing on the individuals writing them, these six women have shown how the genre can balance both researched facts and personal experience in a meaningful way, something Wikipedia denies its users.

Blogs and Privileged Epistemologies

The traditional view of blogs is that they level the playing field for those who wish to write; all a person needs to do is sign up, log in, and go. Arguably, since blogs do not restrict who writes or comments, they provide marginalized voices a place from which to finally speak (Coleman, 2005). At the very least, blogs connect people all over the globe and alert each other to culturally distinct viewpoints on similar topics. At first, these six mommyblogs seem to fit with this utopian view of blogs as empowering and globally diverse: Jenny (*CoaNM*) is from the Philippines, Shannon (*BftW*) is from Canada, Anne (*DPM*) is from the United Kingdom, and Rachelle (*Unlatched*) and Paala are American; Teglene (*TBM*) does not disclose her geographical location. However, as Ratliff (2007) quoting Fraser (1992, p. 120) pointed out, "The blogosphere, like any other rhetorical situation, is 'situated in a larger societal context that is pervaded by structural relations of dominance and subordination.'" Thus, because blogs can reflect the same social strife and discrimination that exist offline, they are not always a perfect paradigm of digital credibility equality.

Gaining access to the blogosphere and having your voice heard is based on privilege, and, in our society, certain genders, races, and socioeconomic statuses still carry privilege over others. Friedman's (2010) analysis of mommyblogs revealed that women of color, queer mothers, women with disabilities, and other non-normative identities are often underrepresented on mommyblogs, in part because of marginalized identities' link to socioeconomic status. Friedman concludes that, while blogs provide opportunities for diverse experiences, "white, married, middle- or upper-class women are… perceived as not simply common, but normal" (p. 203). Indeed, not only are most of the six mommybloggers at hand racially white and apparently heterosexual-identifying, they are also all predominantly influenced by Anglo-American ideologies and narratives about breastfeeding. Although these bloggers come from diverse backgrounds, they are not representative of all breastfeeding mothers worldwide. They are not even representative of many non-normative mothers in their own countries. Their digital ethos, although valuable, has limits. And these limits have the potential to be dangerously exclusive.

Friedman (2010) examined how the "good mother" narrative in mommyblogs influences and reflects cultural norms, and the authors have noticed a similar trend in the six breastfeeding blogs. One theme ties them together: the "breast is best," or at least the "breast*milk* is best" philosophy. A quick look at some recent posts from all six bloggers reveals a bias against bottlefeeding:

- On October 18, 2014, Jenny posts a "Quick Guide to Breastfeeding Challenges," which asserts that "medical and physical reasons" should not limit a woman's ability to breastfeed.
- On September 6, 2012, Teglene tells her readers that being busy is not a valid excuse for mothers to choose not to breastfeed.
- On July 4, 2015, Paala posts photos of fellow mothers in her community breastfeeding their children. She also frequently shares breastfeeding selfies ("brelfies," as she calls them).
- On December 16, 2012, Anne asserts "birth and breastfeeding—they are connected."
- On December 12, 2012, Rachelle defends milksharing (which is when a nursing mother donates her milk to another mother so her baby can receive breastmilk).
- On April 8, 2011, Shannon tells a story about how she explained to her children (who, she makes a point to mention, were all breastfed) why they went to a nurse-in.

All of these instances may not seem significant, but together and compounded with the multifarious other times these bloggers make similar implicit and explicit assertions, they speak to a larger cultural assumption that good mothers supply their children with breastmilk. These women establish digital credibility by drawing on their credibility as "good" mothers who breastfeed.

The authors of this chapter do not intend to disparage the value of breastfeeding. Too many studies to cite here have shown that breastmilk, preferably the mother's, is healthier for babies and that formula-feeding may be risky. But because many mommyblogs refuse to consider any other viewpoints, the implication behind these "good mother" narratives is that bottlefeeding mothers are the opposite—bad mothers—and that their digital ethos is less valuable, thus depriving them of digital authority. Jenny's and Teglene's posts explicitly state that mothers do not have an excuse for not breastfeeding. Some bloggers suggest alternative options: Rachelle's post cited above offers milksharing as a substitute for breastfeeding, while Jenny (May 7, 2012) and Anne (Feb 25, 2013) propose breastpumps as another method for mothers to feed breastmilk to their children. However, these posts do not acknowledge that not all mothers have access to donor milk nor can all mothers afford expensive breastpumps. Only Anne and Paala concede that breastfeeding is not available to some mothers. Paala (Oct 23, 2015) openly addresses her breastfeeding bias while offering advice to bottlefeeding mothers. Anne (Mar 30, 2015) admits that sometimes women just cannot breastfeed even though they may want to; she emphasizes that they do not deserve scorn because of it. However, posts like Paala's and Anne's are rare. The collective ethos of the mommblogging community is reflected in posts like Jenny's and Teglene's assertions that all mothers should breastfeed or Rachelle's, Jenny's, and Anne's alternative suggestions. Such comments reveal that alternative *ethea* about breast- and bottlefeeding is not always valued in normative narratives of the "good mother." Blogs are more inclusive than Wikipedia when deciding what sources of knowledge they consider authoritative, but, as this case study of breastfeeding blogs shows, they are also culturally saturated spaces that can reinscribe cultural privilege through both implicit and explicit narratives of what it means to be a "good mother."

FUTURE RESEARCH DIRECTIONS

This chapter has provided case studies of Wikipedia and blogs to support an argument that while Wikipedia's generic constraints silence women's digital credibility and authority, blogs' generic affordances provide a space from which women use their authority to create knowledge about such important topics as health and childcare. The authors find three potential avenues for further research:

1. Digital social media may provide a different way of reaching collaborative knowledge,
2. Digital social media may still marginalize women, and
3. Wikipedia and digital social media may marginalize other identities.

Although the authors originally determined blogs to be a digital genre in which women are more likely to share information and experiences, these case studies reveal that women also use various digital social media sites (SMS) to perform these tasks. Many of the breastfeeding blogs this article examines have links to Facebook pages, Google+ accounts, and other SMS, and often the bloggers appear to use these sites more regularly than their blogs. Rachelle has not updated *Unlatched* in nearly a year, but she updates her blog's Facebook page daily (Rachelle, 2015); likewise, Anne updates *DPM* every few months, but her blog's Facebook page almost weekly (Anne, 2015b). In an interview, Rachelle explained why she uses social media more often than her blog to connect with her readers: "I use [Facebook] usually on a daily basis, whereas my blog is reserved for topics that I feel are under-covered by others. I feel that being active on social media is extremely important as a breastfeeding professional because… We need to meet moms where they are at. Facebook has given me the opportunity to connect with and help so many mothers" (personal communication, June 2014). Further research on the digital authority of women's health pages on sites like Facebook could examine if and why social media is better suited to spreading this knowledge to a larger audience.

Facebook is one of the most popular websites in the world and can certainly reach a wide audience, but what is interesting is how it limits women's expression in a way similar to Wikipedia. Paala and Rachelle both document on their blogs how Facebook deletes photos or suspends and bans accounts that violate the strict rules against showing breastfeeding photos. As a corporate entity, Facebook can control the media added by its users. Facebook (2015a) plainly states that the users own and control any content they publish to the site, but it also has equally clear Community Standards (2015b) that dictate what content is allowed to be posted and what content will be removed if published. Similarly Wikipedia (2015b) states, "Contributions remain the property of their creators," but as the "Talk" and "About" pages illustrate, content should only be published if there is communal consensus about it. These rules limit what users can publish on these corporate sites in ways that blogs typically do not. Stories that show the censorship of women on sites like Facebook and Wikipedia are troubling, and more research is needed into how the corporatization of digital social media influences how women and other marginalized identities are able to exercise digital credibility and authority in those spaces.

Finally, the authors suspect that women are not alone in their encyclopedic silencing and that race, class, and sexuality also have an impact on how knowledge is created on Wikipedia. A search for articles on these identities and Wikipedia reveals that virtually no research has been done to examine how Wikipedia excludes or empowers people of color and non-white ethnicities. Wikipedia also appears to exclude impoverished people, many of whom, as Balit (2007) found, access the Internet by mobile device only. Noam Cohen (2014) noted that less than one percent of the edits made to Wikipedia come from mobile devices, thus suggesting an implicit discrimination against people of lower socioeconomic status. Finally, only one article (Raval, 2014) touched on sexuality and Wikipedia. This may be because, although Wikipedia measures the gender, age, and nationality of its contributors (Wikipedia, 2015d), it does not measure their racial identities, socioeconomic standing, or sexuality. More research is certainly needed to explore how these factors affect editing practices on Wikipedia.

CONCLUSION

The case studies in this chapter have implications for collaborative writing in academia. There are many benefits to collaborative work (Lunsford & Ede, 2012). First, when the processes of knowledge creation are open and obvious, writers and readers on the margins can learn the rules and join the conversation. As Brooke (2009) mentioned, the final product of a Wikipedia entry is only a small representation of the epistemological activity that happens on the site. When users look at the "Talk" pages and see the debates between collaborators, they gain a better understanding of what all sides are saying about an issue and which side wins. Second, when collaboration is open and respectful to all perspectives, many standpoints may be represented, which may in turn prevent the tyranny of normativity. In particular, such valuing of multiple perspectives opens up the opportunity for alternative *ethea* when discussing knowledge.

However, there is a darker side to collaboration. Although it has the potential to open knowledge creation to multiple *ethea*, this chapter shows it does not always do so. This remains particularly true in academia, where collaboration is increasingly becoming a respected mode of authorship, not just in rhetoric and composition studies, but in many other fields. The sciences have long supported co-authored works, and fields as disparate as literature and medicine are also realizing the benefits of co-written scholarship (Kutner et al, 2006). However, a bias against experiential ethos in many fields undermines the potential value of collaboration. For instance, in 2015, evolutionary science academics Fiona Ingleby and Megan Head received a review from a peer editor who explained that their work on "gender differences in the PhD to postdoc transition" (Bernstein, 2015) was unfit for publication on the basis of the gender of the writers. The anonymous reviewer explained, "It would probably… be beneficial to find one or two male biologists to work with (or at least obtain internal peer review from, but better yet as active co-authors), to serve as a possible check against interpretations that may sometimes be drifting too far away from empirical evidence into ideologically biased assumptions" (Ingleby, 2015). This example shows that while academia has become more accepting of collaboratively written scholarship, it still does not hold alternative *ethea* equal to a normative, empirical ethos. This exclusion leads to the continued silence of women and other minority identities whose *ethea* are based in alternative epistemologies that may include experiential authority. Collaborative composition needs policing; we need more users who do not represent normative ideologies to participate in knowledge creation, lest we risk silencing valid *ethea*.

The case studies presented in this chapter also have implications for how women exercise agency over their own bodies. For instance, in 2012, Todd Akin, in a stunning display of ignorance about female anatomy, declared, "If it's a legitimate rape, the female body has ways to try to shut that whole thing down" (Eligon and Schwirtz, 2012). The authors believe that such obliviousness reveals two troubling issues. First, it speaks to the long history of physicians' and researchers' lack of consideration for women's health issues. Fausto-Sterling (2012) pointed out that research into female genetic development is decades behind research into male genetic development because of our society's implicit belief that femaleness is often defined simply as a lack of maleness. Furthermore, Fausto-Sterling explained that this gendered research disparity is slowly being rectified, but it still has a long way to go. More importantly, Fausto-Sterling's research helps explain why Akin knew so little about how female bodies work. They are deemed as less important to learn about. Society believes women's health is women's problem.

Second, Akin's comment showcases how legislators and policy makers devalue women's ethos. When women are unable to make knowledge about their own bodies, they are stripped of agency for how their bodies are controlled in public. For instance, many of the breastfeeding bloggers are also self-proclaimed lactivists who actively fight for women's rights to breastfeed in public, and they are often met with vehement resistance. Lunceford (2012) pointed to this resistance as indicative of "a strong desire to discipline and control female bodies" that arises from the internalized "belief that the breast is solely there as a sexual object" and not as a functional one (p. 51). He also explains, "[T]he cultural construction of the female breast as a sexual object… stands in the way of widespread acceptance of public breastfeeding" (Lunceford, 2012, p. 37). If women's *ethea* is accepted on a global and societal level—not just on niche blogs—their experiential knowledge could put an end to unnecessary sexualization and ignorance by informing more people about their bodies from their own perspective, which would in turn facilitate more agency when it comes to public policy and perception about issues like breastfeeding.

Above all, this case study reveals the pressing need to empower women and people of color to contribute to collaborative environments, particularly mainstream digital spaces like Wikipedia. One way to do this is to host and contribute to Wikipedia edit-a-thons and write-ins. These events are aimed at filling gaps in women's history on Wikipedia by editing, expanding, and/or creating entries. The Wikimedia Foundation often sponsors edit-a-thons in which experienced and novice editors can revise pages or create new ones. In 2012, Wikimedia Foundation community fellow Sarah Stierch "Missvain" organized an edit-a-thon at the Smithsonian to build entries about women scientists in their archives (Shen, 2012). While this is a step in the right direction, the focus on scientists implies that women are only valuable when they conform to normative discourses. However, the most famous write-in event, the Global Women Wikipedia Write-In (GWWI), does not focus solely on scientists; the GWWI solicits suggestions from the community on what needs to added or edited. Its goals are "to encourage new people to become Wikipedia editors, to provide support for new editors, and to develop best practices for rewriting Wikipedia" (Koh and Risam, 2014). Events like these empower women to exercise agency over their knowledge creation in mainstream spaces. This study also points to the need to change the rules and informal practices of collaborative environments to encourage contributors to think twice before automatically deleting entries and/or edits (a common practice on Wikipedia). Finally, the authors suggest that knowledge creators need to trust the process of open collaboration rather than thinking of themselves as gatekeepers of knowledge and truth. Only then will multiple *ethea* be considered credible and valuable, both online and off.

REFERENCES

Anne. (2015a). *Dispelling breastfeeding myths* [Blog]. Retrieved from http://mythnomore.blogspot.com/

Anne. (2015b). *Dispelling breastfeeding myths* [Facebook page]. Retrieved from https://www.facebook.com/DispellingBfMyths/

Armstrong, C. L., & McAdams, M. J. (2009). Blogs of information: How gender cues and individual motivations influence perceptions of credibility. *Journal of Computer-Mediated Communication*, *14*(3), 435–456. doi:10.1111/j.1083-6101.2009.01448.x

Balit, S. (2007). Communication for isolated and marginalized groups. In *Communication and sustainable development: Selected papers from the 9th UN roundtable on communication for development* (pp. 101-122). New York: FAO UN Press.

Bernstein, R. (2015, May 1). PLOS ONE outs review, editor after sexist peer-review storm. *Science Insider*. Retrieved from http://news.sciencemag.org/scientific-community/2015/04/sexist-peer-review-elicits-furious-twitter-response

Blood, R. (2000). Weblogs: A history and perspective [Blog]. *Rebecca's Pocket*. Retrieved from http://www.rebeccablood.net/essays/weblog_history.html

Brooke, C. G. (2009). *Lingua fracta: Towards a rhetoric of new media*. Cresskill, NJ: Hampton Press.

Brown, J. (2015). *Ethical programs: Hospitality and the rhetorics of software*. Ann Arbor, MI: University of Michigan Press. doi:10.3998/dh.13474172.0001.001

Cassel, J. (2011, Feb 4). A culture of editing wars. *New York Times Online*. Retrieved from http://www.nytimes.com/roomfordebate/2011/02/02/where-are-the-women-in-wikipedia/a-culture-of-editing-wars

Chawner, B., & Lewis, P. H. (2004, October). *WikiWikiWebs: New ways of interacting in a web environment*. Paper presented at the ALA (American Library Association) LITA National Forum.

Chesney, T. (2006). An empirical examination of Wikipedia's credibility. *First Monday*, *11*(11). doi:10.5210/fm.v11i11.1413

Cohen, N. (2014, February 4). Wikipedia vs. the small screen. *New York Times Online*. Retrieved from http://www.nytimes.com/2014/02/10/technology/wikipedia-vs-the-small-screen.html?_r=0

Coleman, S. (2005). Blogs and the new politics of listening. *The Political Quarterly*, 273–280.

Eckert, S., & Steiner, L. (2013). Wikipedia's gender gap. In C. L. Armstrong (Ed.), *Media disparity: A gender battleground* (pp. 87–98). New York: Lexington Books.

Eligon, J., & Schwirtz, M. (Aug 19, 2012). Senate candidate provokes ire with "legitimate rape" comment. *The New York Times Online*. Retrieved from http://www.nytimes.com/2012/08/20/us/politics/todd-akin-provokes-ire-with-legitimate-rape-comment.html

Facebook. (2015a). *Terms*. Retrieved from https://www.facebook.com/terms.php

Facebook. (2015b). *Community Standards*. Retrieved from https://www.facebook.com/communitystandards?ref=br_tf

Fallis, D. (2011). Wikipistemology. In A. Goldman & D. Whitcomb (Eds.), *Social epistemology: Essential readings* (pp. 297–313). New York: Oxford University Press.

Fausto-Sterling, A. (2012). *Sex/Gender: Biology in a social world*. New York: Routledge.

Flanagin, A. J., & Metzger, M. J. (2008). Digital media and youth: Unparalleled opportunity and unprecedented responsibility. In M. Metzger & A. Flanagin (Eds.), *Digital media, youth, and credibility* (pp. 5–27). Cambridge, MA: MacArthur Foundation Series on Digital Media and Learning.

Fraser, N. (1992). Rethinking the public sphere: A contribution to the critique of actually existing democracy. In C. Calhoun (Ed.), *Habermas and the public sphere* (pp. 109–142). Cambridge, MA: MIT Press.

Friedman, M. (2010). On mommyblogging: Notes to a future feminist historian. *Journal of Women's History*, *22*(4), 197–208.

Frost, E. A. (2013). *Theorizing an apparent feminism in technical communication.* (Doctoral dissertation). Retrieved from ProQuest. (Order No. 3574642).

Frost, E. A. (2014a). Apparent feminist pedagogies: Interrogating technical rhetorics at Illinois State University. *Programmatic Perspectives*, *6*(1), 110–131.

Frost, E. A. (2014b). An apparent feminist approach to transnational technical rhetorics: The ongoing work of Nujood Ali. *Peitho*, *16*(2), 183–199.

Frost, E A. (2015). Apparent feminism as a methodology for technical communication and rhetoric. *Journal of Business and Technical Communication*, 1-26.

Garfinkel, S. L. (2008). Wikipedia and the meaning of truth. *Technology Review*, *111*(6), 84–86.

Giles, J. (2005). Special report internet encyclopedias go head to head. *Nature*, *439*(12), 900–901. doi:10.1038/438900a PMID:16355180

Gruwell, L. (2015). Wikipedia's politics of exclusion: Gender, epistemology, and feminist rhetorical (in)action. *Computers and Composition*, *37*, 117–131. doi:10.1016/j.compcom.2015.06.009

Haraway, D. (1988). Situated knowledges: The science question in feminism and the privilege of partial perspective. *Feminist Studies*, *14*(3), 575–599. doi:10.2307/3178066

Harding, S. (1993). Rethinking standpoint epistemology: What is "strong objectivity?". In L. Alcoff & E. Potter (Eds.), *Feminist Epistemologies* (pp. 49–82). New York: Routledge.

Harding, S. (Ed.). (2003). *The feminist standpoint theory reader: Intellectual and political controversies*. New York: Routledge.

Hargittai, E., & Shaw, A. (2015). Mind the skills gap: The role of Internet know-how and gender in differentiated contributions to Wikipedia. *Information Communication and Society*, *18*(4), 424–442. doi:10.1080/1369118X.2014.957711

Hartsock, N. C. M. (1983). The feminist standpoint: Developing the ground for a specifically feminist historical materialism. In S. G. Harding & M. B. Hintikka (Eds.), *Discovering reality: Feminist perspectives on epistemology, metaphysics, methodology, and philosophy of science* (pp. 283–310). Boston: D. Reidel.

Ingleby, F. (2015, April 29). *and this is a bit hypocritical given the reviewer's own ideological biases throughout the review, for example: (3/4)* [Tweet]. Retrieved from https://twitter.com/FionaIngleby/status/593408350001471489

Jenny. (2015). *Chronicles of a Nursing Mom* [Blog]. Retrieved from http://www.chroniclesofanursingmom.com/

Johnson, T.J., & Kaye, B.K. (2004). Wag the blog: How reliance on traditional media and the internet influence credibility perceptions of weblogs among blog users. *Journalism & Mass Communication Quarterly September*, *81*(3), 622-642.

Johnson, T. J., & Kaye, B. K. (2010). Believing the blog of war: How blog users compare on credibility and characteristics in 2003 and 2007. *Media, War, and Conflict*, *3*(3), 315–333. doi:10.1177/1750635210376591

Johnson, T. J., & Kaye, B. K. (2011). Hot diggity blog: A cluster analysis examining motivations and other factors for why people judge different types of blogs as credible. *Mass Communication & Society*, *14*(2), 236–263. doi:10.1080/15205431003687280

Johnston, A., Friedman, B., & Peach, S. (2011). Standpoint in political blogs: Voice, authority, and issues. *Women's Studies*, *40*(3), 269–298. doi:10.1080/00497878.2010.548427

Kellymom. (2015). *KellyMom* [Website]. Retrieved from http://kellymom.com/

Kennedy, K. (2009). Textual machinery: Authorial agency and bot-written texts in Wikipedia. In M. Smith & B. Warnick (Eds.), *The responsibilities of rhetoric: Proceedings of the 2008 Rhetoric Society of America Conference*. Retrieved from http://surface.syr.edu/wp/1/

Koerber, A. (2006). Rhetorical agency, resistance, and the disciplinary rhetorics of breastfeeding. *Technical Communication Quarterly*, *15*(1), 87–101. doi:10.120715427625tcq1501_7

Koerber, A. (2013). *Breast or bottle? Contemporary controversies in infant-feeding policy and practice*. Columbia, SC: University of South Carolina Press.

Koerber, A., Brice, L., & Tombs, E. (2012, February). Breastfeeding and problematic integration: Results of a focus-group study. *Health Communication*, *27*(2), 124–144. doi:10.1080/10410236.2011.571754 PMID:21834716

Koh, A., & Risam, R. (2014). The global women Wikipedia write-in #GWWI. *Postcolonial digital humanities*. Retrieved from http://dhpoco.org/rewriting-wikipedia/the-global-women-wikipedia-write-in/

Kutner, J. S., Westfall, J. M., Morrison, E. H., Beach, M. C., Jacobs, E. A., & Rosenblatt, R. A. (2006). Facilitating collaboration among academic generalist disciplines: A call to action. *Annals of Family Medicine*, *4*(2), 172–176. doi:10.1370/afm.392 PMID:16569722

La Leche League International. (2015). *La Leche League International* [Website]. Retrieved from http://www.llli.org/

Lanier, J. (2006). Digital Maoism. *The Edge*. Retrieved from http://edge.org/conversation/digital-maoism-the-hazards-of-the-new-online-collectivism

Loveland, J., & Reagle, J. (2013). Wikipedia and encyclopedic production. *New Media & Society*, *15*(8), 1294–1311. doi:10.1177/1461444812470428

Lunceford, B. (2012). *Naked politics: Nudity, political action, and the rhetoric of the body*. Lanham, MD: Lexington Books.

Lunsford, A., & Ede, L. (2012). *Writing together: Collaboration in theory and practice, a critical sourcebook*. St. Martins.

McIntyre, A. M. C. (2010). The 'truthiness' of Wikipedia: An examination of the open content encyclopedia as a valuable vehicle in developing critical thinking in the classroom. *Access to Knowledge*, *2*(1), 2–8.

Metzger, M. J. (2007). Making sense of credibility on the Web: Models for evaluating online information and recommendations for future research. *Journal of the American Society for Information Science and Technology*, *58*(13), 2078–2091. doi:10.1002/asi.20672

Novotny, M. (2015). reVITALize gynecology: Reimagining apparent feminism's methodology in participatory health intervention projects. *Communication Design Quarterly*, *3*(4), 61–74. doi:10.1145/2826972.2826978

Paala. (2015). *Paa.la* [Blog]. Retrieved from http://paa.la/

Rachelle. (2014). *Unlatched* [Blog]. Retrieved from https://unlatched.wordpress.com/

Rachelle. (2015). *Unlatched* [Facebook page]. Retrieved from https://www.facebook.com/unlatched/

Ratliff, C. (2007). Attracting readers: Sex and audience in the blogosphere. *The Scholar and Feminist Online, 5*(2). Retrieved from http://sfonline.barnard.edu/blogs/ratliff_03.htm

Raval, N. (2014). The encyclopedia must fail! – Notes on queering Wikipedia. *ADA: A Journal of Gender, New Media, and Technology, 5*. Retrieved from http://adanewmedia.org/2014/07/issue5-raval/

Reagle, J. (2009). *Gender bias in Wikipedia coverage? Open communities, media, source, and standards*. Retrieved from http://reagle.org/joseph/blog/social/wikipedia/wp-eb-gender-bias-coverage

Reagle, J., & Rhue, L. (2011). Gender bias in Wikipedia and Britannica. *International Journal of Communication*, *5*, 1138–1158.

Rose, H. (1983). Hand, brain and heart: A feminist epistemology for the natural sciences. *Signs (Chicago, Ill.)*, *9*(1), 73–90. doi:10.1086/494025

Scott, K. A., & White, M. A. (2013). COMPUGIRLS' Standpoint: Culturally Responsive Computer and Its Effects on Girls of Color. *Urban Education*, *48*(5), 657–681.

Selzer, J. (2004). Rhetorical analysis: Understanding how texts persuade readers. In C. Bazerman & P. Prior (Eds.), *What writing does and how it does it* (pp. 279–308). Mahwah, NJ: Lawrence Erlbaum.

Shannon. (2011). *Breast for the Weary* [Blog]. Retrieved from http://breastfortheweary.com/

Shen, A. (Apr 4, 2012). How many women does it take to change Wikipedia? *Smithsonian Magazine.com*. Retrieved from http://www.smithsonianmag.com/smithsonian-institution/how-many-women-does-it-take-to-change-wikipedia-171400755/?no-ist

Simonite, T. (2013). The decline of Wikipedia. *The MIT Technology Review*. Retrieved from http://www.technologyreview.com/featuredstory/520446/the-decline-of-wikipedia/

Teglene. (2014). *The Breastfeeding Mother* [Blog]. Retrieved from http://thebreastfeedingmother.blogspot.com/

Wikimedia Report Card. (2015, August). Retrieved from http://reportcard.wmflabs.org/

Wikipedia. (2015a). *Breastfeeding:Talk*. Retrieved from https://en.wikipedia.org/wiki/Talk:Breastfeeding

Wikipedia. (2015b). *Wikipedia:About*. Retrieved from https://en.wikipedia.org/wiki/Wikipedia:About

Wikipedia. (2015c). *Wikipedia:Verifiability*. Retrieved from https://en.wikipedia.org/wiki/Wikipedia:Verifiability

Wikipedia. (2015d). *Wikipedia:Wikipedians*. Retrieved from https://en.wikipedia.org/wiki/Wikipedia:Wikipedians

Winter, S., & Krämer, N. C. (2014). A question of credibility – Effects of source cues and recommendations on information selection on news sites and blogs. *Communications*, *39*(4), 435–546. doi:10.1515/commun-2014-0020

KEY TERMS AND DEFINITIONS

Agency: The power a person has to act in a given situation.

Apparent Feminism: A methodology designed by Frost (2013, 2014a, 2014b, 2015) whose goal is to make apparent instances of gendered marginalization.

Collaborative Writing: A process of writing in which multiple authors, editors, and/or collaborators draft and revise a text.

Feminist Standpoint Theory: A method of knowledge creation first defined by Harding (1993, 2003) that presupposes complete objectivity can never be reached because all knowledge is culturally situated. Instead, researchers can achieve "strong objectivity" that acknowledges and includes many perspectives.

Kairos/Kairotic: The ancient Greek rhetorical concept that describes a timely response or rhetorical opportunity in a rhetorical situation that is both realist and constructivist.

Lactivism: A movement fueled by the belief that mothers should breastfeed their children. Many lactivists also believe mothers should be allowed to breastfeed in public.

Mommyblog: A genre of blog whose themes and topics pertain almost exclusively to motherhood.

This research was previously published in Establishing and Evaluating Digital Ethos and Online Credibility edited by Moe Folk and Shawn Apostel; pages 329-347, copyright year 2017 by Information Science Reference (an imprint of IGI Global).

Related Readings

To continue IGI Global's long-standing tradition of advancing innovation through emerging research, please find below a compiled list of recommended IGI Global book chapters and journal articles in the areas of pregnancy, childbirth, and reproductive health. These related readings will provide additional information and guidance to further enrich your knowledge and assist you with your own research.

Abelha, A., Pereira, E., Brandão, A., Portela, F., Santos, M. F., Machado, J., & Braga, J. (2015). Improving Quality of Services in Maternity Care Triage System. *International Journal of E-Health and Medical Communications*, *6*(2), 10–26. doi:10.4018/IJEHMC.2015040102

Adcock, A., Cram, F., & Lawton, B. (2019). E Hine: Young Māori Women's Journeys Through Pregnancy, Birth, and Motherhood. In D. Akella (Ed.), *Socio-Cultural Influences on Teenage Pregnancy and Contemporary Prevention Measures* (pp. 250–272). Hershey, PA: IGI Global. doi:10.4018/978-1-5225-6108-8.ch014

Akella, D. (2019). Bringing Culture Back In: Deconstructing Teenage Pregnancy. In D. Akella (Ed.), *Socio-Cultural Influences on Teenage Pregnancy and Contemporary Prevention Measures* (pp. 273–292). Hershey, PA: IGI Global. doi:10.4018/978-1-5225-6108-8.ch015

Akella, D. (2019). Situating Foucault in Teenage Pregnancy Prevention Measures. In D. Akella (Ed.), *Socio-Cultural Influences on Teenage Pregnancy and Contemporary Prevention Measures* (pp. 234–248). Hershey, PA: IGI Global. doi:10.4018/978-1-5225-6108-8.ch013

Akella, N. R. (2019). At the Mercy of Facebook: A Meta-Analysis on Impact of Social Networking Sites, Teen Brain on Teenage Pregnancies. In D. Akella (Ed.), *Socio-Cultural Influences on Teenage Pregnancy and Contemporary Prevention Measures* (pp. 129–149). Hershey, PA: IGI Global. doi:10.4018/978-1-5225-6108-8.ch008

Bata, H. (2019). Technology and Teenage Pregnancy: The Role of Technology as Double-Edged Sword. In D. Akella (Ed.), *Socio-Cultural Influences on Teenage Pregnancy and Contemporary Prevention Measures* (pp. 150–164). Hershey, PA: IGI Global. doi:10.4018/978-1-5225-6108-8.ch009

Boursier, V., Manna, V., Gioia, F., Coppola, F., & Venosa, N. (2018). Cyber-Moms Facing Motherhood: Holding Functions and Regressive Movements in Parenting Websites. In S. Sekalala & B. Niezgoda (Eds.), *Global Perspectives on Health Communication in the Age of Social Media* (pp. 29–58). Hershey, PA: IGI Global. doi:10.4018/978-1-5225-3716-8.ch002

Brandão, A., & Portela, F. (2016). Step towards Improving the Voluntary Interruption of Pregnancy by Means of Business Intelligence. In J. Machado & A. Abelha (Eds.), *Applying Business Intelligence to Clinical and Healthcare Organizations* (pp. 43–63). Hershey, PA: IGI Global. doi:10.4018/978-1-4666-9882-6.ch003

Carissoli, C., Villani, D., & Riva, G. (2016). An Emerging Model of Pregnancy Care: The Introduction of New Technologies in Maternal Wellbeing. In D. Villani, P. Cipresso, A. Gaggioli, & G. Riva (Eds.), *Integrating Technology in Positive Psychology Practice* (pp. 162–192). Hershey, PA: IGI Global. doi:10.4018/978-1-4666-9986-1.ch007

Drozd, F., Haga, S. M., & Slinning, K. (2018). From Science to Practice: Implementation and Clinical Guidelines for an Internet Intervention for Postpartum Depression. In S. Langrial (Ed.), *Web-Based Behavioral Therapies for Mental Disorders* (pp. 79–110). Hershey, PA: IGI Global. doi:10.4018/978-1-5225-3241-5.ch004

Eshiet, I. (2019). Sustainable Development Goal 3 and Maternal Health in Nigeria: Any Hope of Meeting the Target by 2030? In A. Eneanya (Ed.), *Human Rights, Public Values, and Leadership in Healthcare Policy* (pp. 247–271). Hershey, PA: IGI Global. doi:10.4018/978-1-5225-6133-0.ch012

Ferraz, M., Almeida, A. M., & Matias, A. (2016). The Decision-Making Processes of Pregnant Women at High Risk. In M. Cruz-Cunha, I. Miranda, R. Martinho, & R. Rijo (Eds.), *Encyclopedia of E-Health and Telemedicine* (pp. 901–909). Hershey, PA: IGI Global. doi:10.4018/978-1-4666-9978-6.ch069

Fields, M. D. (2019). Women in American Labour Movement: Overcoming Exclusion and Sex-Based Discrimination. *International Journal of Public and Private Perspectives on Healthcare, Culture, and the Environment*, *3*(2), 59–66. doi:10.4018/IJPPPHCE.2019070104

George, R. (2016). Developing SMS Health Messages for Pregnant Indigenous Australians Using Persuasive Technology. In J. Moon & M. Galea (Eds.), *Improving Health Management through Clinical Decision Support Systems* (pp. 81–107). Hershey, PA: IGI Global. doi:10.4018/978-1-4666-9432-3.ch004

Gnanabai, R. (2018). Health Information Systems and Their Usefulness Among the Women Folk of Kanyakumari District, India. In J. Jeyasekar & P. Saravanan (Eds.), *Innovations in Measuring and Evaluating Scientific Information* (pp. 36–49). Hershey, PA: IGI Global. doi:10.4018/978-1-5225-3457-0.ch003

Golman, M., Ricks, N., Gallegos, I. D., & Weaver, J. (2019). Utilizing the Socio-Ecologic Model as a Framework for the Prevention of Teen Pregnancy. In D. Akella (Ed.), *Socio-Cultural Influences on Teenage Pregnancy and Contemporary Prevention Measures* (pp. 208–233). Hershey, PA: IGI Global. doi:10.4018/978-1-5225-6108-8.ch012

Handwerk, S. E., & Handwerk, K. (2019). Teenage Pregnancy: From Research and Theory to Practice. In D. Akella (Ed.), *Socio-Cultural Influences on Teenage Pregnancy and Contemporary Prevention Measures* (pp. 1–32). Hershey, PA: IGI Global. doi:10.4018/978-1-5225-6108-8.ch001

Harris, K. R., & Hopper, M. T. (2019). Preventing Teen Pregnancy at Pre-Adolescence. In D. Akella (Ed.), *Socio-Cultural Influences on Teenage Pregnancy and Contemporary Prevention Measures* (pp. 166–188). Hershey, PA: IGI Global. doi:10.4018/978-1-5225-6108-8.ch010

Holloway, A. (2017). Teaching Childbirth Support Techniques Using the Prepared Partner and Digital Birth: The Design and Development of Games for Dads-To-Be. In B. Dubbels (Ed.), *Transforming Gaming and Computer Simulation Technologies across Industries* (pp. 154–182). Hershey, PA: IGI Global. doi:10.4018/978-1-5225-1817-4.ch009

Huidu, A. (2019). The Ethics of Embrionic Stem Cells Research: The Human Being in the Early Stages of Development – A "Medicine" or an End in Itself? In A. Sandu, A. Frunza, & E. Unguru (Eds.), *Ethics in Research Practice and Innovation* (pp. 244–263). Hershey, PA: IGI Global. doi:10.4018/978-1-5225-6310-5.ch013

Idowu, P. A., Balogun, J. A., & Alaba, O. B. (2017). Data Mining Approach for Predicting the Likelihood of Infertility in Nigerian Women. In N. Wickramasinghe (Ed.), *Handbook of Research on Healthcare Administration and Management* (pp. 76–102). Hershey, PA: IGI Global. doi:10.4018/978-1-5225-0920-2.ch006

Jordan, M. (2019). A Methodological Consideration and Methodological Design Suitable to Examine Teenage Pregnancy. In D. Akella (Ed.), *Socio-Cultural Influences on Teenage Pregnancy and Contemporary Prevention Measures* (pp. 33–42). Hershey, PA: IGI Global. doi:10.4018/978-1-5225-6108-8.ch002

Khalil, M. A., Jan, S., Ali, W., & Khan, A. (2019). MotherCare App for Expectant Mothers in Interior Parts of Pakistan. In S. Umair & M. Shah (Eds.), *Mobile Devices and Smart Gadgets in Human Rights* (pp. 132–152). Hershey, PA: IGI Global. doi:10.4018/978-1-5225-6939-8.ch006

Luk, C. Y. (2019). A Human Rights-Based Approach to Teenage Pregnancy Prevention in China. In D. Akella (Ed.), *Socio-Cultural Influences on Teenage Pregnancy and Contemporary Prevention Measures* (pp. 95–116). Hershey, PA: IGI Global. doi:10.4018/978-1-5225-6108-8.ch006

Monyai, R. B., & Metsing, K. M. (2019). Understanding Teenage Pregnancy in the South African Context. In D. Akella (Ed.), *Socio-Cultural Influences on Teenage Pregnancy and Contemporary Prevention Measures* (pp. 117–128). Hershey, PA: IGI Global. doi:10.4018/978-1-5225-6108-8.ch007

Nagarathna, R., & Chaku, R. (2018). Research-Based Applied Psychophysiology: Yoga for Women's Health. In S. Telles & N. Singh (Eds.), *Research-Based Perspectives on the Psychophysiology of Yoga* (pp. 121–150). Hershey, PA: IGI Global. doi:10.4018/978-1-5225-2788-6.ch008

Nanda, S. (2019). Sexual and Reproductive Health. In *Psycho-Socio-Physical Dimensions of Adolescent Health Management: Emerging Research and Opportunities* (pp. 101–117). Hershey, PA: IGI Global. doi:10.4018/978-1-5225-7384-5.ch004

Olukolu, Y. R. (2017). Harmful Traditional Practices, Laws, and Reproductive Rights of Women in Nigeria: A Therapeutic Jurisprudence Approach. In D. Halder & K. Jaishankar (Eds.), *Therapeutic Jurisprudence and Overcoming Violence Against Women* (pp. 1–14). Hershey, PA: IGI Global. doi:10.4018/978-1-5225-2472-4.ch001

Omisade, O., Good, A., Fitch, T., & Briggs, J. (2017). An Analysis of Factors Affecting Postnatal Depression Intervention Adherence. *International Journal of Public Health Management and Ethics*, *2*(1), 1–18. doi:10.4018/IJPHME.2017010101

Palza, E., Sanchez, J., Mamani, G., Pacora, P., Abran, A., & Moon, J. (2016). A Predictive Analytic Model for Maternal Morbidity. In J. Moon & M. Galea (Eds.), *Improving Health Management through Clinical Decision Support Systems* (pp. 108–126). Hershey, PA: IGI Global. doi:10.4018/978-1-4666-9432-3.ch005

Paraskou, A., & George, B. P. (2018). *Legal and Economic Considerations Surrounding Reproductive Tourism: Emerging Research and Opportunities*. Hershey, PA: IGI Global. doi:10.4018/978-1-5225-2694-0

Pereira, E., Brandão, A., Salazar, M., Portela, C. F., Santos, M. F., Machado, J., ... Braga, J. (2015). Pre-Triage Decision Support Improvement in Maternity Care by Means of Data Mining. In A. Azevedo & M. Santos (Eds.), *Integration of Data Mining in Business Intelligence Systems* (pp. 175–192). Hershey, PA: IGI Global. doi:10.4018/978-1-4666-6477-7.ch009

Pereira, E., Portela, F., & Abelha, A. (2016). A Clinical Recommendation System to Maternity Care. In J. Machado & A. Abelha (Eds.), *Applying Business Intelligence to Clinical and Healthcare Organizations* (pp. 64–83). Hershey, PA: IGI Global. doi:10.4018/978-1-4666-9882-6.ch004

Prabhu, D. F., & Larson, R. C. (2019). Scaling the Maternal and Newborn Survival Initiative (MANSI): Rural India. *International Journal of System Dynamics Applications*, *8*(1), 94–111. doi:10.4018/IJSDA.2019010106

Ramakrishnan, S., & Jayaraman, A. (2019). Pesticide Contaminated Drinking Water and Health Effects on Pregnant Women and Children. In K. Wani, & Mamta (Eds.), Handbook of Research on the Adverse Effects of Pesticide Pollution in Aquatic Ecosystems (pp. 123-136). Hershey, PA: IGI Global. doi:10.4018/978-1-5225-6111-8.ch007

Ramulumo, M. R. (2019). Causes and Factors Responsible for Teenage Pregnancy. In D. Akella (Ed.), *Socio-Cultural Influences on Teenage Pregnancy and Contemporary Prevention Measures* (pp. 44–63). Hershey, PA: IGI Global. doi:10.4018/978-1-5225-6108-8.ch003

Rausch, M. A., & Wikoff, H. D. (2020). Case Study for Counseling Same Sex Couples Through the Fertility Process: Jane and Kelsey. In B. King & T. Stewart (Eds.), *Cases on Cross-Cultural Counseling Strategies* (pp. 66–88). Hershey, PA: IGI Global. doi:10.4018/978-1-7998-0022-4.ch004

Rouhani, S., & Maryam MirSharif. (2018). Data Mining Approach for the Early Risk Assessment of Gestational Diabetes Mellitus. *International Journal of Knowledge Discovery in Bioinformatics*, *8*(1), 1–11. doi:10.4018/IJKDB.2018010101

Saeed, N., Khan, S. K., Raheed, H. M., & Hussain, M. Z. (2018). Empirical Analysis of Socio-economic Factors Effecting Nutritional Status of Children (1-5) of Age. *International Journal of Civic Engagement and Social Change*, *5*(4), 1–18. doi:10.4018/IJCESC.2018100101

Shema, C. R. (2019). Psychosocial and Cultural Contributing Factors of Teen Pregnancy in North America. In D. Akella (Ed.), *Socio-Cultural Influences on Teenage Pregnancy and Contemporary Prevention Measures* (pp. 64–76). Hershey, PA: IGI Global. doi:10.4018/978-1-5225-6108-8.ch004

Takahashi, M. (2018). Policy Narratives in Formation of Comprehensive Support System for Parenting and Child Care in Japan. *International Journal of Public and Private Perspectives on Healthcare, Culture, and the Environment*, *2*(1), 22–32. doi:10.4018/IJPPPHCE.2018010102

Tu, W. (2018). County Socioeconomic Deprivation and Preterm Birth Risk Between White and Black Mothers in Georgia, USA. *International Journal of Applied Geospatial Research*, *9*(3), 18–30. doi:10.4018/IJAGR.2018070102

Vidourek, R. A., & King, K. A. (2019). Preventing Teen Pregnancy Among Minority Populations: Risk and Protective Factors. In D. Akella (Ed.), *Socio-Cultural Influences on Teenage Pregnancy and Contemporary Prevention Measures* (pp. 189–207). Hershey, PA: IGI Global. doi:10.4018/978-1-5225-6108-8.ch011

Yildirim, F., Abukan, B., & Oztas, D. (2019). From Early Marriage to Adolescent Pregnancy in Turkey: A Review Study in Socio-Cultural Context. In D. Akella (Ed.), *Socio-Cultural Influences on Teenage Pregnancy and Contemporary Prevention Measures* (pp. 77–94). Hershey, PA: IGI Global. doi:10.4018/978-1-5225-6108-8.ch005

Youssouf, M., Kalia, A., Nabi, Z., & Malik, Z. A. (2019). Health Effects of Pesticides on Pregnant Women and Children. In K. Wani, & Mamta (Eds.), Handbook of Research on the Adverse Effects of Pesticide Pollution in Aquatic Ecosystems (pp. 105-122). Hershey, PA: IGI Global. doi:10.4018/978-1 5225-6111-8.ch006

Index

E

F

G

H

I

K

L

M

N

O

P

Q

R

S

T

U

W

www.ingramcontent.com/pod-product-compliance
Lightning Source LLC
LaVergne TN
LVHW080610300926
849162LV00005B/1105